T0289884

Pathology Research in the 21st Century

Pathology Research in the 21st Century

Edited by Cecilia Bryant

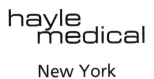

New York

Hayle Medical,
750 Third Avenue, 9th Floor,
New York, NY 10017, USA

Visit us on the World Wide Web at:
www.haylemedical.com

ISBN: 978-1-64647-514-8

Cataloging-in-Publication Data

Pathology research in the 21st century / edited by Cecilia Bryant.
    p. cm.
Includes bibliographical references and index.
ISBN 978-1-64647-514-8
1. Diagnosis, Laboratory. 2. Diagnosis. 3. Pathology. I. Bryant, Cecilia.
RB37 .C55 2023
616.075--dc23

Table of Contents

Preface

This book has been a concerted effort by a group of academicians, researchers and scientists, who have contributed their research works for the realization of the book. This book has materialized in the wake of emerging advancements and innovations in this field. Therefore, the need of the hour was to compile all the required researches and disseminate the knowledge to a broad spectrum of people comprising of students, researchers and specialists of the field.

Pathology studies the causes and effects of diseases. It addresses various components of a disease, like pathogenesis, morphologic changes and clinical manifestations. In general medical practice, it is focused on analyzing clinical abnormalities which are precursors and markers for infectious and non-infectious diseases. Pathology can be categorized into anatomical pathology and clinical pathology. Anatomical pathology diagnoses the diseases on the basis of molecular, gross, immunologic, microscopic and chemical examination of tissues, organs or whole bodies. Various subfields of anatomical pathology include forensic pathology, surgical pathology and cytopathology. Clinical pathology is involved in the diagnosis of diseases on the basis of laboratory analysis of tissues and body fluids like urine and blood, with the help of tools of molecular pathology, chemistry, hematology and clinical microbiology. Pathology work like blood tests, biopsy and resection are necessary for diagnosing various kinds of cancers. Similarly, blood and tissue analysis is important for the investigation of infectious diseases. This book explores all the important aspects of pathology in the present day scenario. It will help the readers in keeping pace with the rapid changes in this field.

At the end of the preface, I would like to thank the authors for their brilliant chapters and the publisher for guiding us all-through the making of the book till its final stage. Also, I would like to thank my family for providing the support and encouragement throughout my academic career and research projects.

Editor

Dedifferentiated Central Chondrosarcoma: A Clinical, Histopathological and Immunohistochemical Analysis of 57 Cases

Li-Hua Gong [1]*, Yong-Bin Su [2], Wen Zhang [1], Wei-Feng Liu [3], Rong-Fang Dong [1], Xiao-Qi Sun [1], Ming Zhang [1] and Yi Ding [1]*

[1] Department of Pathology, Beijing Jishuitan Hospital, The Fourth Medical College of Peking University, Beijing, China,
[2] Department of Radiology, Beijing Jishuitan Hospital, The Fourth Medical College of Peking University, Beijing, China,
[3] Department of Orthopedic Oncology Surgery, Beijing Jishuitan Hospital, Fourth Medical College of Peking University, Beijing, China

*Correspondence:
Li-Hua Gong
lhgong2005@126.com
Yi Ding
jst_blk@126.com

Dedifferentiated central chondrosarcoma (DCCS) is a rare cartilage tumor with invasive biological behavior and a poor prognosis. To better understand the morphological characteristics of this type of tumor and its internal mechanism of dedifferentiation, we retrospectively analyzed 57 cases of DCCS. A total of 29 female and 28 male patients were included, ranging in age from 20 to 76 years, with a median age of 54 years. Fifty-seven cases of DCCS occurred in the pelvis ($n = 29$), femur ($n = 17$), scapula ($n = 4$), tibia ($n = 2$), humerus ($n = 2$), metatarsals ($n = 1$), fibula ($n = 1$), and radius ($n = 1$). Radiologically, DCCS had two different appearances on imaging, with an area showing calcifications of the cartilage forming the tumor juxtaposed to a lytic area with a highly aggressive, non-cartilaginous component. Histopathologically, the distinctive morphological features consisted of two kinds of defined components: a well-differentiated cartilaginous tumor and non-cartilaginous sarcoma. The cartilaginous components included grade 1 ($n = 38$; 66.7%) and grade 2 ($n = 19$; 33.3%) cartilage. The sarcoma components included those of osteosarcoma ($n = 29$; 50.9%), undifferentiated pleomorphic sarcoma ($n = 20$; 35.1%), rhabdomyosarcoma ($n = 3$; 5.2%), fibrosarcoma ($n = 2$; 3.5%), spindle cell sarcoma ($n = 2$; 3.5%) and angiosarcoma ($n = 1$; 1.8%). Immunohistochemistry showed that the expression of p53 and RB in the sarcoma components was significantly higher than that in the cartilaginous components, suggesting that these factors play roles in the dedifferentiation process of chondrosarcoma. DCCS is a highly malignant tumor with a poor prognosis. Except for the patients who were lost to follow-up, most of our patients died.

Keywords: dedifferentiated, chondrosarcoma, central, imaging, immunohistochemistry

INTRODUCTION

Dedifferentiated chondrosarcoma (DCS) is a high-grade chondrosarcoma with the bimorphic histological appearance of a conventional chondrosarcoma with abrupt transition to non-cartilaginous sarcoma (1). In the literature, the reported incidence of DCS in chondrosarcoma cases is 10–15% (2). This type of tumor usually occurs between the ages of 50 and 60 years and occurs more frequently in males (3). It is most often located in the pelvis and long bones such as the proximal femur or humerus, the distal femur and the tibia. Dedifferentiation usually originates from either an enchondroma or a low-grade chondrosarcoma (dedifferentiated central chondrosarcoma, DCCS), but it can also originate from a low-grade peripheral chondrosarcoma secondary to a pre-existing osteochondrosarcoma or a solitary osteochondroma (dedifferentiated peripheral chondrosarcoma) (4). Histopathologically, the distinctive morphological features include two kinds of defined components, a well-differentiated cartilage tumor juxtaposed to a high-grade non-cartilaginous sarcoma, and the transition between the two is abrupt. The dedifferentiated components may be conventional osteosarcoma, telangiectatic osteosarcoma (5), undifferentiated pleomorphic sarcoma (UPS), or fibrosarcoma (6). Other rare histological subtypes of the differentiated components may include leiomyosarcoma (7), rhabdomyosarcoma (8), giant cell tumor-like (9–12), gastrointestinal stromal tumor (GIST)-like (13), or epithelial differentiation (14). To better understand the characteristics and dedifferentiation transformation mechanism underlying DCCS, we conducted a retrospective study to analyze the clinicopathological features of 57 patients with DCCS. Additionally, we carried out immunohistochemistry to explore the intrinsic mechanism involved in the process of dedifferentiation in these tumors.

METHODS
Patients and Surgical Specimens

With approval from the institutional ethics committee and following the research protocol, 57 DCCS cases were retrieved from surgical pathological records between January 2009 and December 2020 at the Department of Pathology, Beijing Jishuitan Hospital. All tissues were fixed in neutral buffered formalin and processed routinely *via* paraffin embedding, and then the sections were prepared and stained with hematoxylin and eosin (HE). Histopathological assessment was carried out according to the WHO Classification of Tumors of Soft Tissue and Bone and reviewed by three pathologists, while clinical and imaging information was obtained from online medical records and surgeons. All cases were treated by surgery, and 28 cases were treated with chemotherapy after surgery.

Imaging

Pre-operative imaging studies included plain radiographs, computed tomography (CT) and magnetic resonance imaging (MRI). As a routine examination protocol in our hospital, patients with bone tumors are assessed by contrast-enhanced

TABLE 1 | Antibodies used for immunohistochemical staining.

Antigen	Antibody	Source	Type	Dilution
Desmin	ZC18	Zymed	Monoclonal antibody	Prediluted
Myogenin	F5D	DAKO	Monoclonal antibody	1:200
RB	1FB	Zhongshan	Monoclonal antibody	Prediluted
CDK4	EP180	Zhongshan	Polyclonal antibody	Prediluted
Cyclin D1	SP4	Roch	Polyclonal antibody	Prediluted
p53	D0-7	Leica	Monoclonal antibody	1:100
p16	G175-405	Zymed	Monoclonal antibody	Prediluted
S-100	None	Leica	Polyclonal antibody	1:400
H3k27me3	None	Zhongshan	Polyclonal antibody	Prediluted
Ki-67	MM1	Leica	Monoclonal antibody	Prediluted

CT or contrast-enhanced MRI. Fifty-one patients underwent plain radiographs with at least two positions; 45 patients were evaluated with CT scans, and 38 patients were assessed by MRI. The images were reviewed on our PACS (Picture Archiving and Communication Systems) by two experienced radiologists (YS, WL).

Tissue Samples and Immunohistochemistry

Formalin-fixed, paraffin-embedded specimens of DCCS were available for immunohistochemical analysis. Immunohistochemical staining was performed with an automated immunostainer (Autostainer 720, Labvision, San Diego, CA) according to standard heat-induced epitope retrieval and the avidin-biotin-peroxidase complex method. The following cytophenotypic markers were detected: desmin, S-100, p16, RB, p53, Cyclin D1, CDK4, H3k27me3, and Ki-67 (**Table 1**). Simultaneously, appropriate positive and negative control sections were used. Positive immunostaining was characterized by brown nuclear or cytoplasmic staining under a microscope. Cytoplasmic staining was considered positive for desmin, and nuclear staining was considered positive for S-100, p16, RB, p53, Cyclin D1, CDK4, H3k27me3, and Ki-67. All slides were evaluated independently by two pathologists who were not provided clinical information. The grade of immunoreactivity was defined as follows: negative (−); focal positive (+): fewer than 75% of tumor cells were positive; and diffuse positive (++): more than 75% of tumor cells were positive. The Ki67 proliferation index was defined 25% as the threshold value. Agreement was reached by careful discussion when the opinions of the two pathologists (LG, YD) were different.

RESULTS
Clinical Characteristics

The patients included 29 females and 28 males, ranging in age from 20 to 76 years, with a median age of 54 years. Fifty-seven cases of DCCS occurred in the pelvis ($n = 29$), femur ($n = 17$), scapula ($n = 4$), tibia ($n = 2$), humerus ($n = 2$), metatarsals ($n = 1$), fibula ($n = 1$), and radius ($n = 1$). In our study, 12 cases (21.1%) were secondary DCCS occurring after central low-grade

TABLE 2 | Clinical summary of DCCS.

Age	n (%)
≥50 years	34 (59.7)
<50 years	23 (40.3)
Sex	
Female	29 (50.9)
Male	28 (49.1)
Location	
Pelvis	29 (50.8)
Femur	17 (29.8)
Scapule	4 (7.0)
Tibia	2 (3.5)
Humerus	2 (3.5)
Fibula	1 (1.8)
Radius	1 (1.8)
Metatarsals	1 (1.8)
Classification	
Primary	45 (78.9)
Secondary	12 (21.1)
Grade of chondrogenic component	
G1	38 (66.7)
G2	19 (33.3)
Type of dedifferentiation	
Osteosarcoma	29 (50.9)
UPS	20 (35.1)
Rhabdomyosarcoma	3 (5.2)
Fibrosarcoma	2 (3.5)
Spindle cell sarcoma	2 (3.5)
Angiosarcoma	1 (1.8)
Prognosis	
Disease-free survival	27 (47.4)
Dead	23 (40.3)
Missed follow-up	7 (12.3)

G1, grade 1; G2, grade 2; UPS, undifferentiated pleomorphic sarcoma.

chondrosarcoma recurrence. The other cases involved primary dedifferentiation (**Table 2**).

Imaging Characteristics

Most of the tumors were located in the pelvis and femur. Lesions often exhibit ill-defined intramedullary destruction with calcific foci and associated cortical permeation and soft tissue masses and with heterogeneous contrast enhancement on imaging. The most characteristic features of images consist of two different appearances on imaging, with an area showing calcifications or hyperintense chondral component of the cartilage-forming tumor juxtaposed to a lytic area involving a highly aggressive, non-cartilaginous component with a soft tissue mass, which frequently reflects the presence of undifferentiated pleomorphic sarcoma or osteosarcoma (**Figures 1, 2**). A total of 21.6% (11/51), 75.6% (34/45), and 50% (19/38) of lesions showed this biphasic pattern on plain radiograph, CT and MRI, respectively. This bimorphic pattern was characteristic and was appreciated more clearly on CT images than on radiography.

Gross Pathological Features

Grossly, the tumor was located in the medullary cavity. The cartilaginous and DCS components are distinct. The cartilaginous component was blue-gray, translucent and fragile, whereas the dedifferentiated components were fresh, pale, soft, tough or hard (**Figure 3A**). The sarcoma components could invade the cortex of bone, forming a soft tissue mass (**Figure 3B**).

Histopathological Features

Microscopically, the DCCS cases showed a typical chondrosarcoma structure and non-chondrogenic sarcoma structure. The types of chondrosarcoma include chondrosarcoma grade I and chondrosarcoma grade II. Grade I cartilage may mimic normal hyaline cartilage. In 38/57 cases, the cartilaginous component consisted of chondrosarcoma grade I, which is weakly to moderately cellular and hyperchromatic, with no mitoses (**Figure 4A**). Nineteen cases of chondrosarcoma grade II were found. Chondrosarcoma grade II is more cellular, with a greater degree of nuclear atypia, and mitoses can be found (**Figure 4B**). The perilobular and interlobular cells of chondrosarcoma grade II are rich and pleomorphic. Myxoid changes were found in 22 cases, primarily in chondrosarcoma grade II components.

The dedifferentiated components usually transition abruptly to distinct cartilaginous components. We observed an obvious line of demarcation as described in the WHO classification. Fiber bundles were present in some cases and absent in others (**Figure 4C**). Additionally, in some cases, sarcoma could be the major component, and the focal cartilaginous component was located in it, forming an island structure (**Figure 4D**). The dedifferentiated components showed multiple features, including those of high-grade sarcomas, namely, osteosarcoma ($n = 29$), UPS ($n = 20$), rhabdomyosarcoma ($n = 3$), fibrosarcoma ($n = 2$, the diagnostic criteria refer to adult fibrosarcoma in the WHO classification) and angiosarcoma ($n = 1$). Additionally, there were low-grade components, such as grade I or II spindle cell sarcoma ($n = 2$) (**Table 1**).

In the UPS, sarcoma showed high-grade cell pleomorphism and atypia, some zones with bizarre multinuclear tumorous giant cells (**Figure 5A**), and some zones with epithelioid morphology. The high-grade myxoid zone also existed, forming high-grade myxoid fibrosarcoma features. In two cases, pleomorphic rhabdomyosarcoma differentiation occurred. The cells were large, round or polygonal with abundant pink cytoplasm and unusual nuclei, similar to rhabdomyosarcoma (**Figure 5B**). In one case, the tumor invaded the lymph node. Only dedifferentiated components could be found in the lymph node without cartilaginous components.

In the osteosarcoma component, the cells were highly anaplastic and pleomorphic with enlarged and darkly stained nuclei (**Figure 5C**). A focal hemangiopericytoma-like pattern was also found (**Figure 5D**). The important and necessary characteristics for the diagnosis of osteosarcoma are the production of osteoids by malignant tumor cells. Osteoids

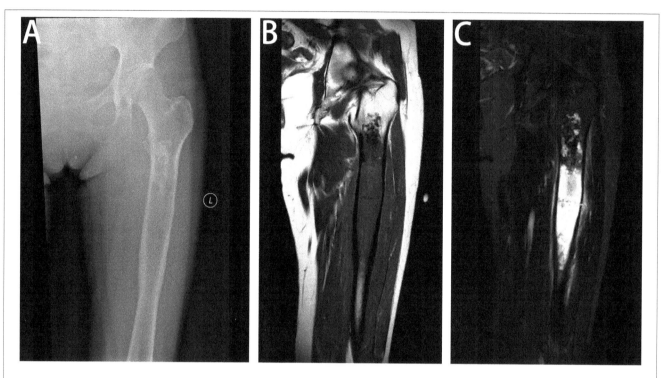

FIGURE 1 | Radiologic features of DCCS. **(A)** Anteroposterior view of the left femur. Radiographs show a large lytic lesion of the femur, with cortical remodeling and a poorly defined margin of the distal part. The proximal part of the lesion has popcorn-like matrix calcifications. **(B)** Coronal T1-weighted MR image of the left femur. MR imaging shows a large destruction in the medullary cavity of the femur, with low signal on the T1-weighted image. **(C)** Coronal fat-suppressed T2-weighted MR image of the left femur. On fat-saturated T2-weighted images, the existence of the two components is recognized. The proximal third of the lesion has areas of low signal representing matrix mineralization and areas of high signal representing the high water content of the cartilage matrix, but the distal two-thirds has a heterogeneous predominantly high signal and peritumoral edema, showing bimorphism of the lesion.

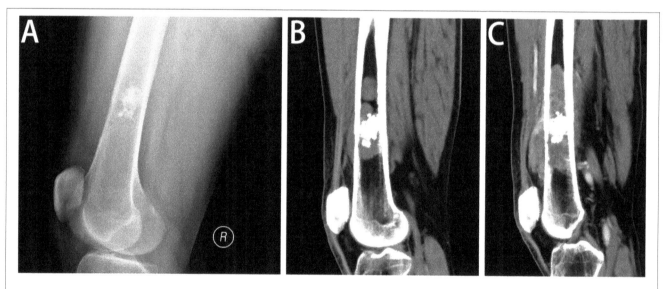

FIGURE 2 | Radiologic features of DCCS. **(A)** Lateral view of the left femur. Radiography of the distal femur shows a lesion in the medullary cavity with calcifications, with subtle destruction of the anterior cortex and anterior soft tissue mass. **(B)** Sagittal CT scan of the left femur in the soft tissue window. The sagittal CT images demonstrate that the lesion is multifocal, with penetration of the cortex and considerable soft tissue components. In addition to the calcific foci, the lesion contains more areas of lytic destructive changes. **(C)** Sagittal post-contrast CT scan of the left femur in the soft tissue window. One and a half months later, the sagittal post-contrast CT image in the soft tissue window shows the lesion expanding into a large area of bone destruction, with heterogeneous enhancement.

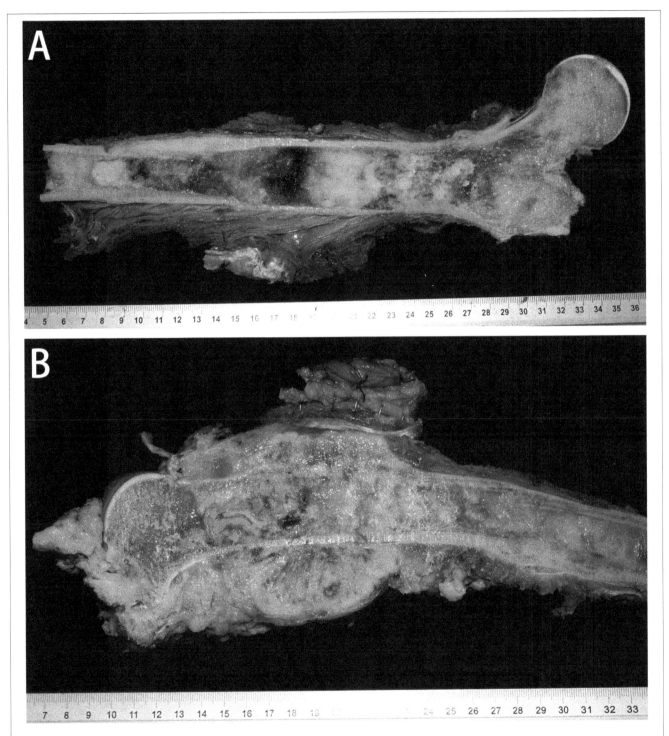

FIGURE 3 | Gross specimens of DCCS. **(A)** The tumor was located in the medullary cavity and was composed of porcelain white cartilage and red fish-like tissue. **(B)** The tumor in the marrow cavity was cartilage-like with invasion of the surrounding soft tissues, forming an osteosarcoma structure.

were dense, pink, and amorphous intercellular material with or without calcification. Osteosarcoma has a broad morphological spectrum. Small cell osteosarcoma had uniform small cells with scant cytoplasm, with little pink osteoid production. The nuclei were round to oval, and the chromatin was fine. The

osteoclast-type giant cells scattered in the tumor cells formed the giant cell-enriched variant of osteosarcoma in one case. Additionally, in this case, blood vessel invasion could be found (**Figure 5E**). Two cases showed focal telangiectatic osteosarcoma features. The tumor was composed of cystic spaces simulating

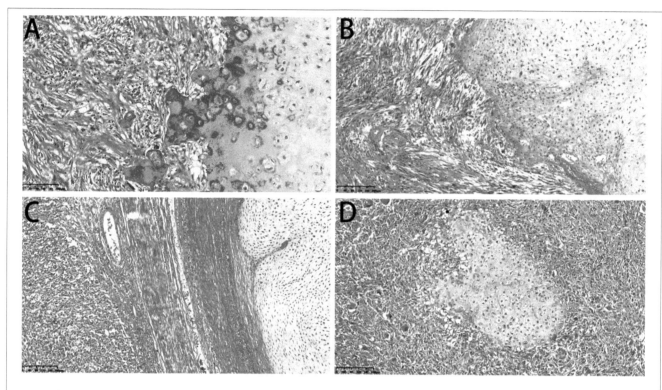

FIGURE 4 | Microscopical features of DCCS. **(A)** The cartilage component shows a grade I cartilage structure, and the sarcoma component shows a low-grade sarcoma morphology (HE, 200×). **(B)** The cartilage component shows a grade II cartilage structure, and the sarcoma component shows the morphology of myxofibrosarcoma (HE, 200×). **(C)** Thick fibrous separation was located between the cartilage component and the sarcoma component (HE, 100×). **(D)** Well-differentiated cartilage nodules surrounded by sarcoma components (HE, 100×).

an aneurysmal bone cyst, but pleomorphic tumor cells with focal osteoid formation were scattered in the septa-like structures.

One case showed epithelioid angiosarcoma features (**Figure 5F**). The fibrosarcoma was composed of relatively monomorphic spindle cells with a "herringbone" growth pattern and sometimes also formed a synovial sarcoma-like structure (**Figure 6A**). In some areas, the tumor cells were round and epithelioid with interstitial fiber formation, similar to sclerosing epithelioid fibrosarcoma features (**Figure 6B**). Two cases showed low-grade spindle cell sarcoma, with mild-moderate atypia, and some areas had storiform patterns, forming a benign fibrohistiocytoma structure (**Figure 6C**); some areas had a distinctive inflammatory infiltrate with aggregates of plasma cells and lymphocytes mimicking the inflammatory myofibroblastic tumor (**Figure 6D**).

Immunohistochemical Features

Immunohistochemical staining showed strong positivity for desmin in the rhabdomyosarcoma differentiation components in two cases (**Figure 7A**). The Ki-67 index revealed active cell proliferation in the sarcoma components; 79.3% cases showed a Ki-67 value >25%, with only individual cells in the cartilage portion showing proliferative activity, and the Ki-67 value was <25% in all cartilage portions (**Figure 7B**). Staining for p16 was negative in sarcoma and original cartilaginous lesions in most cases; only in some cases were both components positive,

and the sarcoma component showed stronger and more diffuse staining than the cartilaginous components (**Figure 7C**). Staining for p53 was diffusely positive in the nuclei of tumor cells in the dedifferentiated components of 54.4% cases (**Figure 7D**) but almost undetectable in the chondrosarcoma component, except for one case with grade II cartilage. The expression pattern of Cyclin D1 was similar to that of p16. In 29.9% of cases, the sarcoma was focal positive, while in only 5.3% of cases, the cartilage was positive. The expression intensity of the sarcoma portion was much higher than that of the cartilage portion (**Figure 7E**). In some cases, although CDK4 was positive in both the cartilage and sarcoma portions, the cartilage portion showed focal positive expression, while the sarcoma portions showed mainly diffuse expression (**Figure 7F**). RB was not expressed in the cartilage portion of all cases, but it showed positivity (73.7%) in the sarcoma portion (**Figure 7G**). H3k27me3 was diffuse positive in the cartilage in all cases, and the sarcoma components were diffuse positive in 89.5% of cases; in only six cases, H3k27me3 showed focal expression (**Figure 7H**). The results of immunohistochemical staining are depicted in **Table 3**.

PROGNOSIS

The patients were followed up from 2 to 127 months. The median follow-up time was 59 months. Seven patients were lost to follow-up. Twenty-three patients died of DCCS. The remaining

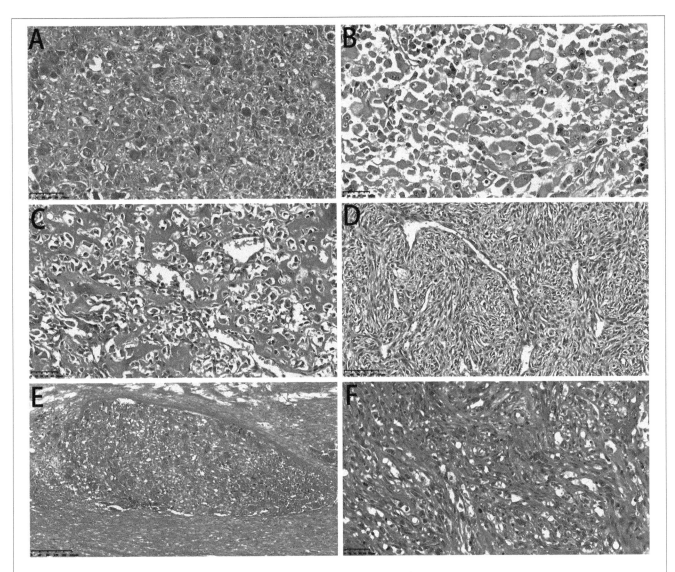

FIGURE 5 | Microscopical features of DCCS. **(A)** Diffuse multinuclear tumor giant cells were dispersed in sarcoma components (HE, 200×). **(B)** The tumor cells showed characteristics of striated muscle differentiation with enriched cytoplasm (HE, 300×). **(C)** The sarcoma component was conventional osteosarcoma (HE, 300×). **(D)** Osteosarcoma tissue showed perivascular arrangement (HE, 200×). **(E)** Intravascular emboli showed a giant cell-rich structure (HE, 100×). **(F)** The sarcoma component showed epithelioid angiosarcoma differentiation (HE, 300×).

27 patients showed no evidence of recurrence and survived disease free.

DISCUSSION

In 1971, Dalin and Beabout first fully described the dedifferentiation of low-grade chondrosarcomas, which is rare, and reported a combination of well-differentiated chondrosarcoma of the ordinary type and juxtaposed zones of anaplastic fibrosarcoma or osteogenic sarcoma. The incidence of peripheral DCS has ranged between 8.9 and 13.7% of all DCS cases (15). Staals et al. (16) found 109 central DCS cases out of 784 central chondrosarcomas (13.9%). In our hospital, from 2009 to 2019, 694 cases of chondrosarcoma were treated at our institution. Among them, 57 patients were diagnosed with

DCCS, which accounts for an 8.2% dedifferentiation rate and does not include peripheral DCS. DCCS usually affects the long bones, such as the proximal femur, humerus and tibia. The femur was involved twice as often as the pelvis in DCCS, and there were slightly more males than females at the Razzoli Institute (17). However, in our series, the pelvis was a more common location than the femur, and there were more females than males. These differences may be explained by the selection bias associated with more complicated lesions at the Orthopedic Oncologic Center.

The biphasic pattern is the most characteristic feature of imaging and is appreciated more clearly on contrast-enhanced CT images and MRI than on radiography. Plain radiography has a poor ability to assess the soft tissue mass of the aggressive part. MRI has been investigated well in DCCS and proved to be a useful imaging modality. On MR fluid-sensitive sequences such as

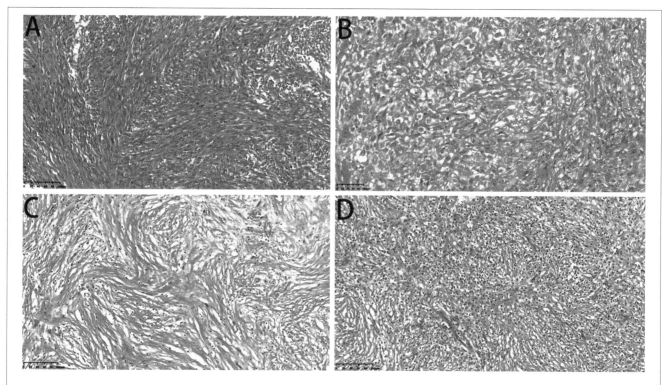

FIGURE 6 | Microscopic features of DCCS. **(A)** The spindle cells were arranged in a bundle-like fibrosarcoma (HE, 200×). **(B)** The sarcoma component resembled sclerotic epithelioid fibrosarcoma (HE, 300×). **(C)** Low-grade sarcoma components showed storiform structures (HE, 200×). **(D)** Low-grade areas showed inflammatory fibroblastoma morphology (HE, 200×).

T2-weighted or STIR images, chondral tumors are hyperintense, whereas dedifferentiated tumors have reduced signal intensity or heterogeneous signal intensity. Based on our results, CT is a good imaging technique to show matrix calcifications of the underlying chondral tumor and osteoid production by osteosarcoma, and with post-contrast images, the soft tissue mass of dedifferentiated tumors is clearly demonstrated with avid enhancement. Imaging findings of the biphasic pattern are important to help pathologists choose the appropriate areas to observe.

DCCS can take place at the first surgery for endochondroma or low-grade chondrosarcoma, which is called synchronous (primary) DCCS, and can also be found at recurrence after resection of these chondrogenic tumors, which is called metachronous (secondary) DCCS. When recurrence occurs at the same site of the chondrosarcoma, the lesion may include the chondrosarcoma structure, which must be combined with the previous pathology to make a precise diagnosis. In addition the dedifferentiated component may be very small; therefore, pathologists should sample cartilaginous tumors thoroughly paying special attention to zones that seem grossly abnormal. For the diagnosis of primary DCCS, due to limitations of biopsy, it is often difficult to obtain both cartilage and dedifferentiated components at the same time, which leads to errors in diagnosis. CT-guided puncture could greatly improve the accuracy of diagnosis. For the diagnosis of secondary DCCS, biopsy combined with history could be easier to diagnose.

The Evans grading system classifies chondrosarcoma into grades I, II, and III (low, intermediate and high grade, respectively) according to nuclear morphology, mitotic activity and the degree of cellularity (18). Similar to reports in the literature, the cartilage components in our case had grade I and II morphology, and no grade III morphology was observed. It should be noted that cells around the grade II cartilage lobules are often densely distributed and should be distinguished from grade III. Moreover, in cases of secondary dedifferentiation, the grade of cartilage components are higher than that in the original case. Myxoid degeneration of cartilage was also common, but it was not a criterion for grading. The dedifferentiation components may show multiple features, and UPS, fibrosarcoma and osteosarcoma were the main types. Rare types, such as small cell osteosarcoma, could also be seen. In many cases of osteosarcoma, osteoid production may occupy a small part and show multiple patterns. We also observed other rare types of histology, including angiosarcoma and rhabdomyosarcoma. Similar to Wick's description (19), in our cases, the dedifferentiated component also showed low-grade spindle cell tumor features, which existed in the form of a storiform structure, with focal lymphocyte infiltration, generating an inflammatory myofibroblastoma-like morphology. Consistent with literature reports of giant cell tumor-like morphology, there were indeed a large number of giant cells in our cases, in either

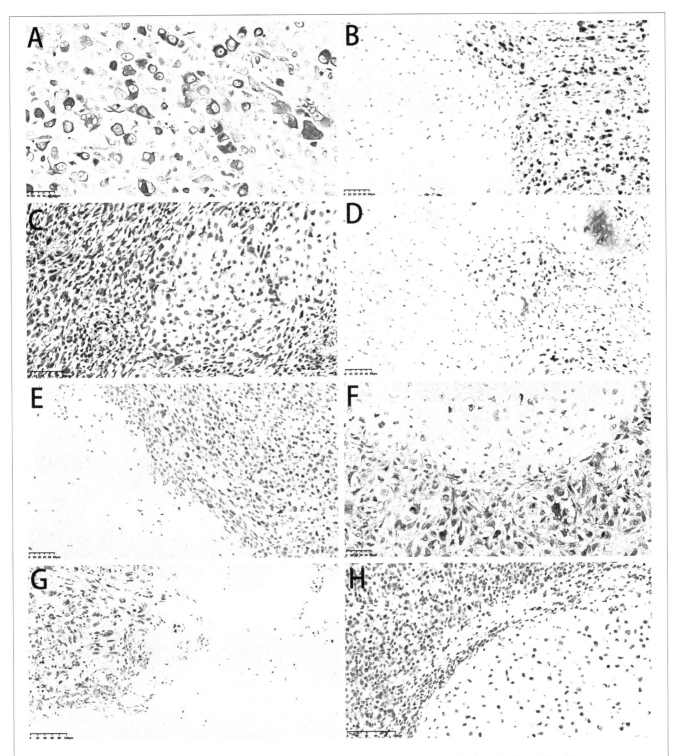

FIGURE 7 | Immunohistochemical features of DCCS. **(A)** Immunohistochemistry showed desmin positivity for striated muscle differentiation. **(B)** Immunohistochemistry showed that Ki-67 was highly expressed in sarcomas. **(C)** Immunohistochemistry showed dense expression of p16 in cartilage and sarcomas. **(D)** Immunohistochemistry showed p53 expression in sarcomas. **(E)** Immunohistochemistry showed Cyclin D1 expression in sarcomas. **(F)** Immunohistochemistry showed that both cartilage and sarcoma components expressed CDK4. **(G)** Immunohistochemistry showed RB expression in sarcoma. **(H)** Immunohistochemistry showed that H3K27me3 was expressed in both the cartilage and sarcoma components.

giant cell-rich undifferentiated sarcomas or giant cell-rich osteosarcomas, especially in the latter, where the focal lesion may present low-grade features similar to those of giant cell tumors of bone. These giant cells were all benign and behaved differently from tumor giant cells in undifferentiated pleomorphic sarcoma.

TABLE 3 | Immunohistochemical results of DCCS.

	Negative (–) n (%)		Focal positive (+) n (%)		Diffuse positive (++) n (%)	
	Chondrogenic	Sarcoma	Chondrogenic	Sarcoma	Chondrogenic	Sarcoma
Desmin	57 (100)	54 (94.7)	0	3 (5.3)	0	0
Myogenin	57 (100)	54 (94.7)	0	3 (5.3)	0	0
S-100	0	57 (100)	0	0	57 (100)	0
RB	57 (100)	15 (26.3)	0	23 (40.4)	0	19 (33.3)
CDK4	45 (78.9)	29 (50.9)	12 (21.1)	20 (35.1)	0	8 (14.0)
Cyclin D1	54 (94.7)	40 (70.2)	3 (5.3)	14 (24.6)	0	3 (5.3)
p53	56 (98.2)	31 (54.4)	1 (1.7)	19 (33.3)	0	7 (12.3)
p16	47 (82.4)	45 (78.9)	4 (7.0)	6 (10.5)	6 (10.5)	6 (10.5)
H3k27me3	0	0	0	6 (10.5)	57 (100)	51 (89.5)

The origin of the dedifferentiation component remains controversial. Sanerkin and Woods (20) suggested that two completely different tumor cell components developed from multipotent mesenchymal stem cells into different cell clones and then differentiated into different neoplastic cell components (collision tumor). In contrast to this theory, more evidence supports the monoclonal origin theory that genomic instability causes a common primitive mesenchymal cell progenitor, which possesses both the ability to develop into a differentiated (chondrocytic features) and a dedifferentiated cell population (high-grade sarcoma features) (21). The fact that chondrocytes were found to have the potential to differentiate into osteoblastic cells supports this theory. Therefore, chondrocyte transition to other tissues may also be possible. The molecular mechanisms of chondrosarcoma dedifferentiation transition also must be further explored.

Morphological observation shows that there is more active mitosis in the sarcoma component than in the cartilage component. Moreover, the Ki-67 proliferation index was significantly increased in sarcoma components by immunohistochemical staining. Therefore, we performed immunohistochemical analysis of cell cycle-related molecules. p53 plays a role in cell cycle regulation, apoptosis, genomic stability, and inhibition of angiogenesis. Studies have shown that p53 mutation is the main mutant gene in high-grade chondrosarcoma (22, 23) and DCS. In DCS, p53 mutation or loss of heterozygosity (LOH) was detected only in the advanced dedifferentiated components (24). It has been reported that p53 is overexpressed in dedifferentiated areas, while chondrosarcoma areas have only focal weakly positive or negative expression 25). Bovée et al. (26) found that p53 was expressed in both chondrosarcoma and dedifferentiated regions. These differences were thought to be due to the different cartilage grades; grade II cartilage is more likely to be p53 positive than grade I cartilage. According to these findings, in our one case, p53 was weakly positive in grade II cartilage; the other cases were negative in the cartilage area, but p53 was positive to varying degrees in the sarcoma area of 26 cases. Another study confirmed the role of the p53 pathway in the high-grade progression of chondrosarcoma

(27). Therefore, we believe that p53 may be related to the malignant transformation of chondrosarcoma dedifferentiation.

The retinoblastoma (RB) protein controls E2F-mediated gene transcription activation and is a key factor for cells entering S phase and cell cycle progression. Loss of RB function is an essential step in tumorigenesis. The LOH of RB is associated with high-grade cartilage tumors and is thought to occur only in the anaplastic component (28, 29). We found that the expression of RB occurs in dedifferentiated components without exception and that the cartilage components are all negative. Therefore, we hypothesized that abnormal expression of RB could induce cartilage tumor stem cells to accelerate cell cycle progression and combine with p53 gene mutation to lead to the development of sarcoma.

Amary et al. (30) showed that p16 copy number variation could be found in high-grade chondrosarcoma (GII, GIII and dedifferentiated) and may be associated with tumor progression. Analysis of a DCS cell line suggests that deletion of the p16 gene plays a major role in the malignant phenotype of DCS (31). p16 regulates the cell cycle by inhibiting CDK4 and Cyclin D1. We found that in most cases, p16 showed a loss of expression in cartilage and dedifferentiated components, which may suggest that the inhibition of CDK4 and Cyclin D1 was reduced, prompting tumor cells to enter the cell cycle progression. Therefore, p16 may also play a role in the high-grade progression of chondrosarcoma.

Our immunohistochemical results showed that positive cells were often located at the junction of cartilage nodules and dedifferentiated components—that is, cells around the cartilage lobules. We believe that the cells surrounding the cartilage lobules are germinal cells or tumor stem cells of cartilage tumors, which could generate new chondrocytes and differentiate in different directions. This expression suggests that these cells terminally differentiate into dedifferentiated sarcoma components. In other words, the cartilage component and the sarcoma components are from the same source. However, the mechanism by which cartilage tumor stem cells differentiate into sarcoma cells remains unknown.

H3K27me3 deficiency was found in 34–75% of malignant peripheral nerve sheath tumors (MPNSTs), and the loss of H3K27me3 expression by immunohistochemical staining could provide a diagnostic clue for MPNSTs (32). The histology of DCS that was deficient in H3K27me3 was different from that of DCS that fully expressed H3K27me3 because the former exhibited characteristics of malignant peripheral nerve sheath tumors (33). In our study, six cases showed a dispersed reduction in H3K27me3 expression, and the morphologies were spindle cell tumors. Nevertheless, the basis for the diagnosis of MPNST is insufficient.

The tumors must be differentiated from other cartilaginous tumors and non-chondroid mesenchymal tumors, which may be confused on clinical and roentgenologic grounds. Occasional high-grade chondrosarcoma, which has dense spindle cells around the periphery of cartilaginous lobules, could be explained as the primitive multipotential stem cell of chondrosarcoma, but dedifferentiation does not occur. In mesenchymal chondrosarcoma, there is also relatively well-differentiated cartilage, but the compact proliferated cells adjacent to the cartilage are composed of round or oval primitive cells, and a perivascular structure may exist. However, in DCCS, the high-grade non-chondroid component showed more variable features. In chondroblastic osteosarcoma, the cartilage is usually grade II or grade III, and there is either a gradual rather than rapid transition between the cartilage and the high-grade osteosarcoma zones or a mixing of the two components. Other non-chondroid mesenchymal tumors, such as UPS or fibrosarcoma of bone, may be mixed with secondary DCS without cartilage areas. Therefore, careful sampling combined with patient history is important.

CONCLUSIONS

We reported histological and immunohistochemical characteristics of a large institutional series of DCCS. Immunohistochemical analysis showed that p53 and RB may be related to malignant transformation of DCCS. Because of its rareness, DCCS should be diagnosed carefully and differentiated from other primary malignant sarcomas. Recognizing DCCS is important because of its aggressive clinical behaviors, frequency of recurrence and poor prognosis.

AUTHOR CONTRIBUTIONS

L-HG and YD conceived the study and designed the experiments. L-HG, WZ, and R-FD performed the experiments. Y-BS and W-FL collected and analyzed the radiology data. X-QS and MZ collected the immunohistochemical data. All authors read and approved the final manuscript.

REFERENCES

1. WHO Classification of Tumours Editorial Board eds. *World Health Organization Classification of Soft Tissue and Bone Tumours.* 5th ed. Lyon: IARC Press (2020).
2. Mitchell AD, Ayoub K, Mangham DC, Grimer RJ, Carter SR, Tillman RM. Experience in the treatment of dedifferentiated chondrosarcoma. *J Bone Joint Surg Br.* (2000) 82:55–61. doi: 10.1302/0301-620X.82B1.0820055
3. Pring ME, Weber KL, Unni KK, Sim FH. Chondrosarcoma of the pelvis. A review of sixty-four cases. *J Bone Joint Surg Am.* (2001) 83-A:1630–42. doi: 10.2106/00004623-200111000-00003
4. Franchi A, Baroni G, Sardi I, Giunti L, Capanna R, Campanacci D. Dedifferentiated peripheral chondrosarcoma: a clinicopathologic, immunohistochemical, and molecular analysis of four cases. *Virchows Arch.* (2012) 460:335–42. doi: 10.1007/s00428-012-1206-2
5. Okada K, Hasegawa T, Tateishi U, Endo M, Itoi E. Dedifferentiated chondrosarcoma with telangiectatic osteosarcoma-like features. *J Clin Pathol.* (2006) 59:1200–2. doi: 10.1136/jcp.2005.029629
6. Capanna R, Bertoni F, Bettelli G, Picci P, Bacchini P, Present D, et al. Dedifferentiated chondrosarcoma. *J Bone Joint Surg Am.* (1988) 70:60–9. doi: 10.2106/00004623-198870010-00010
7. Akahane T, Shimizu T, Isobe K, Yoshimura Y, Kato H. Dedifferentiated chondrosarcoma arising in a solitary osteochondroma with leiomyosarcomatous component: a case report. *Arch Orthop Trauma Surg.* (2008) 128:951–3. doi: 10.1007/s00402-008-0567-0
8. Bisceglia M, D'Angelo VA, Guglielmi G, Dor DB, Pasquinelli G. Dedifferentiated chordoma of the thoracic spine with rhabdomyosarcomatous differentiation. Report of a case and review of the literature. *Ann Diagn Pathol.* (2007) 11:262–73. doi: 10.1016/j.anndiagpath.2006.09.002
9. Ishida T, Dorfman HD, Habermann ET. Dedifferentiated chondrosarcoma of humerus with giant cell tumor-like features. *Skeletal Radiol.* (1995) 24:76–80. doi: 10.1007/BF02425959
10. Estrada EG, Ayala AG, Lewis V, Czerniak B. Dedifferentiated chondrosarcoma with a noncartilaginous component mimicking a conventional giant cell tumor of bone. *Ann Diagn Pathol.* (2002) 6:159–63. doi: 10.1053/adpa.2002.33905
11. Knösel T, Werner M, Jung A, Kirchner T, Dürr HR. Dedifferentiated chondrosarcoma mimicking a giant cell tumor. Is this low grade dedifferentiated chondrosarcoma? *Pathol Res Pract.* (2014) 210:194–7. doi: 10.1016/j.prp.2013.12.003
12. Huang J, Jiang Z, Yang Q, Zhang H. Benign looking giant cell component in dedifferentiated chondrosarcoma: benign or malignant? A case report. *Int J Surg Pathol.* (2013) 21:48–53. doi: 10.1177/1066896912451322
13. Akisue T, Kishimoto K, Kawamoto T, Hara H, Kurosaka M. Dedifferentiated chondrosarcoma with a high-grade mesenchymal component mimicking a gastrointestinal stromal tumor. *Open J Pathol.* (2012) 2:90–5. doi: 10.4236/ojpathology.2012.23017
14. Gambarotti M, Righi A, Frisoni T, Donati D, Vanel D, Sbaraglia M, et al. Dedifferentiated chondrosarcoma with "adamantinoma-like" features: a case report and review of literature. *Pathol Res Pract.* (2017) 213:698–701. doi: 10.1016/j.prp.2017.04.019
15. Bertoni F, Present D, Bacchini P, Picci P, Pignatti G, Gherlinzoni F, Campanacci M. Dedifferentiated peripheral chondrosarcomas. A report of seven cases. *Cancer.* (1989) 63:2054–9. doi: 10.1002/1097-0142(19890515)63:10<2054::AID-CNCR2820631030>3.0.CO;2-V
16. Staals EL, Bacchini P, Mercuri M, Bertoni F. Dedifferentiated chondrosarcomas arising in preexisting osteochondromas. *J Bone Joint Surg Am.* (2007) 89:987–99. doi: 10.2106/JBJS.F.00288
17. Staals EL, Bacchini P, Bertoni F. Dedifferentiated central chondrosarcoma. *Cancer.* (2006) 106:2682–91. doi: 10.1002/cncr.21936
18. Evans HL, Ayala AG, Romsdahl MM. Prognostic factors in chondrosarcoma of bone. A clinicopathologic analysis with emphasis on histologicgrading.

Cancer. (1977) 40 818-831 doi: 10.1002/1097-014240:2<818::AID--CNCR2820400234>3.0.CO;2-B

19. Wick MR, Siegal GP, Mills SE, Thompson RC, Sawhney D, Fechner RE. Dedifferentiated chondrosarcoma of bone. An immunohistochemical and lectin-histochemical study. *Virchows Arch A Pathol Anat Histopathol.* (1987) 411:23–32. doi: 10.1007/BF00734510

20. Sanerkin NG, Woods CG. Fibrosarcomata and malignant fibrous histiocytoma arising in relation to enchondromata. *J Bone Jt Surg.* (1979) 61B:366–72. doi: 10.1302/0301-620X.61B3.225333

21. Bridge JA, DeBoer J, Travis J, Johansson SL, Elmberger G, Noel SM, et al. Simultaneous interphase cytogenetic analysis and fluorescence immunophenotyping of dedifferentiated chondrosarcoma. Implications for histopathogenesis. *Am J Pathol.* (1994) 144:215–20.

22. Terek RM, Healey JH, Garin-Chesa P, Mak S, Huvos A, Albino AP. p53 mutations in chondrosarcoma. *Diagn Mol Pathol.* (1998) 7:51–6. doi: 10.1097/00019606-199802000-00009

23. Dobashi Y, Sugimura H, Sato A, Hirabayashi T, Kanda H, Kitagawa T, et al. Possible association of p53 overexpression and mutation with high-grade chondrosarcoma. *Diagn Mol Pathol.* (1993) 2:257–63. doi: 10.1097/00019606-199300020-00037

24. Simms WW, Ordóñez NG, Johnston D, Ayala AG, Czerniak B. p53 expression in dedifferentiated chondrosarcoma. *Cancer.* (1995) 76:223–7. doi: 10.1002/1097-0142(19950715)76:2<223::AID-CNCR2820760210>3.0.CO;2-4

25. Coughlan B, Feliz A, Ishida T, Czerniak B, Dorfman HD. p53 expression and DNA ploidy of cartilage lesions. *Hum Pathol.* (1995) 26:620–4. doi: 10.1016/0046-8177(95)90166-3

26. Bovée JV, Cleton-Jansen AM, Rosenberg C, Taminiau AH, Cornelisse CJ, Hogendoorn PC. Molecular genetic characterization of both components of a dedifferentiated chondrosarcoma, with implications for its histogenesis. *J Pathol.* (1999) 189:454-62. doi: 10.1002/(SICI)1096-9896(199912)189:4<454::AID-PATH467>3.0.CO;2-N

27. Meijer D, de Jong D, Pansuriya TC, van den Akker BE, Picci P, Szuhai K, et al. Genetic characterization of mesenchymal, clear cell, dedifferentiated chondrosarcoma. *Genes Chromosomes Cancer.* (2012) 51:899–909. doi: 10.1002/gcc.21974

28. Röpke M, Boltze C, Meyer B, Neumann HW, Roessner A, Schneider-Stock R. Rb-loss is associated with high malignancy in chondrosarcoma. *Oncol Rep.* (2006) 15:89–95. doi: 10.3892/or.15.1.89

29. Sakamoto A. The molecular pathogenesis of dedifferentiated chondrosarcoma *Indian J Orthop.* (2014) 48:262–5. doi: 10.4103/0019-5413.132506

30. Amary MF, Ye H, Forbes G, Damato S, Maggiani F, Pollock R, et al. M Flanagan (2015) isocitrate dehydrogenase 1 mutations (IDH1) and p16/CDKN2A copy number change in conventional chondrosarcomas. *Virchows Arch.* 466:217–22 doi: 10.1007/s00428-014-1685-4

31. Yang L, Chen Q, Zhang S, Wang X, Li W, Wen J, et al. A novel mutated cell line with characteristics of dedifferentiated chondrosarcoma. *Int J Mol Med.* (2009) 24:427–35. doi: 10.3892/ijmm_00000249

32. Prieto-Granada CN, Wiesner T, Messina JL, Jungbluth AA, Chi P, Antonescu CR. Loss of H3K27me3 expression is a highly sensitive marker for sporadic and radiation-induced MPNST. *Am J Surg Pathol.* (2016) 40:479–89. doi: 10.1097/PAS.0000000000000564

33. Makise N, Sekimizu M, Konishi E, Motoi T, Kubo T, Ikoma H, et al. H3K27me3 deficiency defines a subset of dedifferentiated chondrosarcomas with characteristic clinicopathological features. *Mod Pathol.* (2019) 32:435–5. doi: 10.1038/s41379-018-0140-5

2

Female Presidents of the "Royal College of Pathologists": Their Achievements and Contributions

Sarah E. Coupland[1,2]*, Lance N. Sandle[3] and Michael Osborn[4]

[1] Department of Molecular and Clinical Cancer Medicine, University of Liverpool, Liverpool, United Kingdom, [2] Liverpool Clinical Laboratories, Liverpool University Hospitals NHS Foundation Trust, Liverpool, United Kingdom, [3] The Royal College of Pathologists, London, United Kingdom, [4] Department of Cellular Pathology, Charing Cross Hospital, North West London Pathology Hosted at Imperial College NHS Trust, London, United Kingdom

*Correspondence:
Sarah E. Coupland
s.e.coupland@liverpool.ac.uk

The Royal College of Pathologists (RCPath) celebrates its Diamond Jubilee in 2022 since its opening by Her Majesty Queen Elizabeth II in 1962. One of the main remits of RCPath is the overseeing of the training of pathologists and scientists working in pathology's 17 different specialties within the United Kingdom and across the globe. During its 60 years, three female Presidents have been elected: Dame Barbara Clayton (1984–1987), Dr. Suzannah (Suzy) Lishman CBE (2014–2017), and Prof. Joanne (Jo) Martin (2017–2020). Whilst Clayton specialised in Chemical Pathology and its relevance to public health, both Lishman and Martin are diagnostic cellular histopathologists with differing areas of expertise. This article reviews the contributions of these three distinguished and inspirational female pathologists to Pathology ("the science behind the cure"), to healthcare, public health and education, medical research, and to teaching. It highlights their qualities as leaders and mentors for those not only in medicine but in other career settings.

Keywords: Royal College of Pathologists, Chemical Pathology, diagnostic histopathology, Dame Barbara Clayton, Dr. Suzy Lishman, Prof. Jo Martin, leadership in Pathology

INTRODUCTION

The Royal College of Pathologists (RCPath) is celebrating its 60th anniversary in 2022. The College was founded on June 21st, 1962. It received its Royal Charter in February 1970. Its first substantive premises were at two Carlton House Terrace, a Grade I listed Georgian Townhouse located in the heart of Westminster, London. It was opened on 16th December that year by its Royal patron, Her Majesty Queen Elizabeth II. In November 2018, RCPath moved to its new premises, a bespoke award-winning building designed by Bennetts Associates in Alie Street, Aldgate, East London.

The College is a charity with over 11,000 members worldwide. RCPath oversees the training of pathologists and scientists working in 17 different specialties, including cellular pathology, clinical biochemistry, haematology, medical microbiology and virology, immunology, forensic, and veterinary pathology. Most members are medical, scientific, dental, or veterinary practitioners working mainly in United Kingdom hospitals and universities. The Trustee Board of the College includes its Honorary Officers, comprising amongst others the elected President of the College and three Vice-Presidents (Communications; Teaching and Learning; and Professionalism). The President and Vice-Presidents have 3-year terms, and they undertake these unremunerated roles in addition to their routine diagnostic work. The first President of the College was Sir Roy Cameron, from 1962 to 1966. During its 60 years, three female Presidents have been elected: *Dame Barbara Clayton* (1984–1987), *Dr. Suzannah (Suzy) Lishman CBE* (2014–2017), and *Prof. Joanne (Jo) Martin* (2017–2020). The aim of the following article is to review the contributions of these three distinguished female pathologists to Pathology ("the science behind the cure"), to healthcare, and to medical research and teaching.

DAME BARBARA EVELYN CLAYTON (1984–1987)

Prof. Dame Barbara Clayton was born in Liverpool, United Kingdom, on September 2nd, 1922, to her parents Constance Evelyn (née Caine) and William Clayton, who then moved to Orpington, London (1). Her father was a food scientist who is renowned for inventing salad cream. Dame Barbara was educated at St Nicholas Preparatory School in Orpington, and subsequently at nearby Bromley County School for Girls, where she was head girl. She then studied medicine at the University of Edinburgh and the Edinburgh Royal Infirmary, qualifying in 1946. Following graduation, she commenced a Ph.D. in the Medical Research Council Clinical Endocrinology Unit in Edinburgh, on the topic of oestrogens (1, 2). After completing this in 1949, Clayton returned to London and became the Holden Research Fellow at St Thomas's Hospital Medical School for 7 years, before she was promoted to Clinical Lecturer in Chemical Pathology. Her research on hormones – e.g., adrenocorticotropic hormone (ACTH), parathyroid hormone and its interactions with Vitamin D, as well as ascorbic acid metabolism – and the development of new biochemical techniques – brought her well-deserved recognition.

In 1959, she moved to Great Ormond Street Hospital (GOSH) where she was a consultant pathologist and continued to do research, particularly in the genetic metabolic disorders suffered by newborn babies. She pursued a passion for improving childrens' healthcare and was renowned for her expertise in the diagnosis of phenylketonuria – the special diet that Clayton designed continues to be in common use today (3, 4).

In 1964, Prof. Clayton and others were very concerned with the high levels of lead found in some children's blood, and this led to her writing a landmark paper entitled "Lead poisoning in children" in 1964 (5), highlighting the detrimental effects lead has on the growth and development of their nervous systems. Whilst a member of the "Royal Commission on Environmental Pollution" in the 1980s, she campaigned for and lobbied the United Kingdom government to enforce a ban on lead in petrol, paint, and other products.

In 1978, after the sudden death of her husband (William [Bill] Klyne), Clayton moved to the new medical school at the University of Southampton as Prof. of Chemical Pathology and Human Metabolism (*its first female Prof.*) and honorary

consultant chemical pathologist at the University hospital. She was Dean of Medicine at the University from 1983 to 1986, and honorary consultant chemical pathologist at the Southampton General Hospital. Appointed Emeritus Prof. in 1987, she continued her work on nutrition, but this time looking at the needs of the elderly, particularly those in care homes, about which there was little information and under resourcing.

Over her career, Clayton published about 200 academic papers, which addressed basic and translational research as well as hospital-based and community screening/care of metabolic disorders. She also served on more than 30 expert committees, several of which she chaired. These included the British Nutrition Foundation, the Association of Clinical Biochemists, the Biomedical Sciences Section of the British Association for the Advancement of Science, the Society for the Study of Inborn Errors of Metabolism, the British Nutrition Foundation, and the medical/scientific panel of the Leukaemia Research Fund. Clayton served on Royal Commission on Environmental Pollution from 1981 to 1996 and chaired the enquiry into the Camelford water pollution incident in 1988. The latter dealt with the inadvertent addition of aluminium sulphate to the water supply, raising the concentration to 3,000 times the then admissible level.

Relevant to this article, *Clayton was the first female President of the Royal College of Pathologists* her term being 1984–1987. Her College portrait now located in the new RCPath building in Alie Street shows her not with microscope or a learned tome on her lap but with a simple cup of tea – a symbol of her convivial personality and her ability to solve problems with diplomacy (**Figure 1**). She was also President of the National Society for Clean Air and Pollution (1995–1997) and the British Dietetic Association (1989–2008).

She received several Honours including a CBE in 1983 and DBE in 1988 for "outstanding contributions on the importance of diet and nutrition and in Chemical Pathology." In 1999, she was awarded the "British Medical Association's Gold Medal" for distinguished merit (a rarely awarded honour), and was conferred an Honorary Fellow of the Institute of Biology as well as an Honorary Fellow of the Royal College of Paediatrics and Child Health.

Dame Barbara Clayton was an inspiration and believed that women just had to be better than men to succeed. She was both sociable and private, never shouting about her own achievements.

DR. SUZANNAH (SUZY) CLAIRE LISHMAN, CBE (2014–2017)

Dr. Suzy Lishman was born in 1967 into a medical family (grandfather and father, both GPs; aunt, respiratory physician; mother and both grandmothers, all nurses), in Beverley in the East Riding of Yorkshire and was educated at Wakefield Girls' High School, The King's School Ely and the Neale Wade Community College in March, Cambridgeshire (6). She grew up in Yorkshire and the Fens in England. She was inspired by her aunt Angela, who showed her that women can have good careers in medicine, and so she followed her footsteps to Girton College,

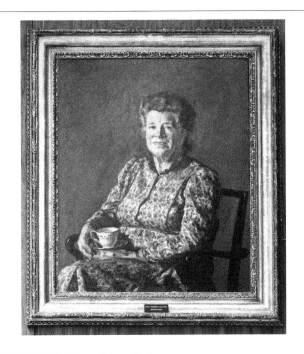

FIGURE 1 | Prof. Dame Barbara Clayton.

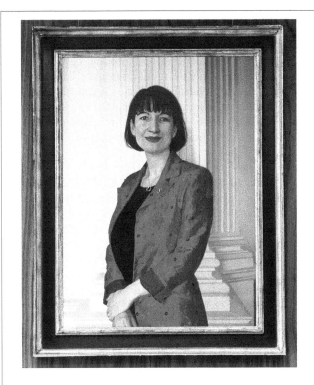

FIGURE 2 | Dr. Suzy Lishman, CBE.

Cambridge and the London Hospital Medical College to study Medicine, qualifying in 1992. After completing house jobs in East London, Lishman applied to University College Hospital to specialise in histopathology; she completed this specialist training in 1999. Her first consultant job was at Hinchingbrooke Hospital in Huntingdon, and she moved to Peterborough District Hospital in 2006. The hospitals merged in 2017 to form North West Anglia NHS Foundation Trust. Lishman is currently a consultant cellular pathologist and lead medical examiner at this Trust. She has an interest in colorectal pathology and is pathology lead for the Bowel Cancer Screening Programme.

Lishman was involved with the College very early even as a Trainee in Histopathology, attending trainees' committee meetings. Between 2005 and 2017, she held every honorary office of the Royal College of Pathologists (except Treasurer), as Assistant Registrar (2005–2009), Registrar (2009–2011), Vice-President (Communications; 2011–2014), and President (2014–2017) (**Figure 2**). During this time, Dr. Lishman raised the profile of the speciality tremendously by introducing public engagement initiatives such as National Pathology Week and International Pathology Day. She has closely collaborated with the Science Museum, Royal Institution, Royal Society, and Cheltenham Science Festival, amongst many other venues and organisations. She has also contributed to numerous television documentaries, talking on a range of topics from the health of Henry VIII to the hidden dangers in the Tudor, Victorian, and Edwardian home. Lishman is active on social media with the Twitter and Instagram handles of "@ilovepathology." She uses various media to achieve outreach: in particular, Lishman is renowned for the development of "Living Autopsy" events, which involve a talk and simulation about what happens during a post-mortem examination. The format employs a "living model," who "acts" as a dead body whilst the pathologist talks through how they would perform an autopsy, showing the real instruments used and then drawing on the chest of the model's body to explain where incisions are made, the location of major organs and what tests would be carried out. The aim of the 60–90 min demonstration is to give a scientifically accurate and sensitive account of this important medical examination. The film of Dr. Lishman performing "The Living Autopsy" has received well over a million views on the RCPath YouTube channel (7). Dr. Lishman has often adapted her Living Autopsy demonstration to incorporate various themes of cultural and local interest. Previous events have explored the bubonic plague, Richard III's death, and what would happen if one died in space. Her public engagement work led to some amusing situations, including "being filmed for television demonstrating the effect of wearing a tight corset on a male model at Griff Rhys Jones' London home; performing a virtual brain autopsy at Latitude Festival (complete with blancmange brain); and being interviewed by actor Larry Lamb about the pathology faced by soldiers in WWI trenches). In 2013, she was named one of the fifty most inspirational women in healthcare by the "Health Service Journal," which described her as the "public face of pathology" and "the most outward facing person from that specialism." Dr. Lishman was awarded the Royal College of Pathologists' Medal in 2010 and the Royal Society Kohn Award in 2012 for her public engagement work.

Ultimately, Dr. Lishman was elected President of the Royal College of Pathologists, commencing in November 2014, *as the College's second female (and youngest) president.* As

President, she passionately represented the views of members, working closely with other specialist societies, and forging links with parliamentarians and other policy makers to ensure that pathology is considered in health-related discussions. She continued performing her living autopsies and talking to school groups in between presidential duties. A quote from Lishman is: "One of the joys of being a College officer is working with a diverse group of people from different regions, specialties and professional backgrounds for the benefit of members and patients."

Following her Presidential term, Dr. Lishman was appointed to (and remains) Chair of the RCPath Medical Examiners' Committee and national training lead for medical examiners. Medical examiners are senior medical doctors, who are trained in the legal and clinical elements of death certification processes. The Committee overseas a national system of medical examiners that is currently being rolled out in England and Wales to provide much-needed support for bereaved families and to improve patient safety. Dr. Lishman has delivered training to over 1400 medical examiners so far and is currently co-chairing joint training sessions for medical examiners and coroners and organising the second annual medical examiners conference. She is also one of the editors of the first textbook for medical examiners, which will be published in 2022.

In addition to her work on death certification reform, Dr. Lishman is a member of Council of the Royal Veterinary College and chairs their Ethics and Welfare Committee. She has chaired the Scientific Advisory Committee of the charity Bowel Cancer United Kingdom since 2017 and is a trustee of National Enquiry into Patient Outcome and Death (NCEPOD) and the Association for Art History. She has served as a non-executive director of the Medical Protection Society and is on the national Lynch Syndrome Steering group. Dr. Lishman regularly gives talks to schools through "Speakers for Schools" and "Inspiring the Future" and mentors disadvantaged students through the Social Mobility Foundation. She is a regular contributor to several leadership courses, particularly for women.

Dr. Lishman has won several awards: she was nominated one of the top 100 Pathologists of the Power List in 2015 (8, 9) and 2018. In 2018, she also received a CBE for services to pathology. She has an honorary doctorate (DSc) from Swansea University, is an honorary member of the Royal Colleges of Physicians of London, Edinburgh, and Ireland and is an honorary fellow of Girton College, Cambridge. Dr. Lishman was appointed to the David Jenkins memorial Chair in Forensic and Legal Medicine in 2019 and is an honorary fellow of that organisation.

PROF. JOANNE (JO) ELIZABETH MARTIN (2017–2020)

Prof. Jo Martin was born into a modest background, with a stimulating, happy family in Hertfordshire. Her education was supported by a county scholarship to the local girls' school. She moved to Uppingham School for A levels for the science teaching, and she applied to Cambridge University for Medicine and was accepted. She was the first of her family to

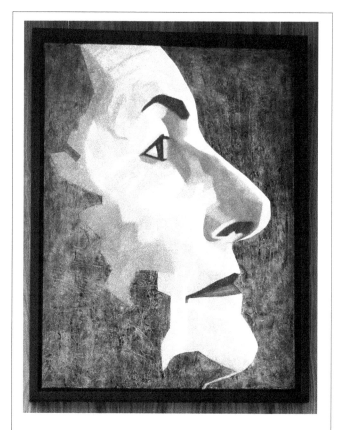

FIGURE 3 | Prof. Jo Martin.

go to university. She qualified *via* Cambridge University and the London Hospital Medical College in 1984 and, following House appointments at Guy's and then St Thomas' Hospitals, she returned to the London Hospital to train in pathology. Martin was awarded an MRC Training Fellowship in 1988, an MRC Fellowship in 1990 and Wellcome Trust Advanced Research Training Fellowship in 1991. She gained her MRCPath (as it was then) in 1993. She was awarded a Ph.D at the University of London in 1997 in "The cellular pathology of the lower motor neuron in motor neuron disease," before becoming established at Queen Mary University of London. She was appointed Clinical Senior Lecturer/Consultant Histopathologist in 1996 and subsequently, Prof. of Neuropathology in 1997 at Queen Mary University of London. She was the only clinician in a major international programme of genetics related to neurodegeneration and neurological disorders, and as part of this designed the "SHIRPA" protocol which has been used in models ever since (10). She has published over 130 papers, including in Nature group and Science journals. She is a practising histopathologist, with a particular expertise in neuromuscular disease of the gut and renal pathology.

Prof. Martin has wide experience of healthcare management and leadership in a range of positions, including Acting Medical Director (January–June 2010), Deputy Medical Director (June 2010–December 2011), Interim Chief Medical Officer (July 2015–January 2016), and Director of Academic Health Sciences at

Barts Health NHS Trust. She negotiated the entry of Barts and Queen Mary into UCLPartners, an Academic Health Science partnership, as founding partners. She was Executive lead for both the Clinical Research Network North Thames, and the Collaboration for Leadership in Applied Health Research and Care (CLAHRC) North Thames, involving multiple acute, primary care and third sector organisations and higher education establishments across a very wide complex organisational region. She led education and research across Barts Health NHS Trust, and created App-based training tools for staff, students, patients, and carers, including eCPD which has delivered over 50,000 free modules. She also acquired further degrees at University of London Master's degree in Leadership (2005), and as part of her involvement in pathology benchmarking, became an Honorary Lecturer in Healthcare Management, Keele University. Additionally, from 2013 to 2016, Prof. Martin was National Clinical Director for Pathology for NHS England.

Prof. Martin was elected the third female President of the Royal College of Pathologists from November 2017 until November 2020 (**Figure 3**). During her Presidency, she worked across programmes and projects in all the 17 pathology disciplines within the College including genetics, transfusion, digital pathology, data, networks, and with many professional bodies and patient groups. She also visited labs all over the United Kingdom to meet pathologists and learn about their needs and expertise. In particular, she championed expansion of, and support for, workforce, and investment into laboratory information management systems, many of which are obsolete, and roll out of digital pathology. All three of these programmes are now funded and being rolled out, with her support from NHSE/I as National Speciality Advisor, as she Chairs the National Pathology Board and Pathology Workforce Board.

Since March 2021, she has been Director of the Blizard Institute, part of the Whitechapel campus of The Faculty of Medicine and Dentistry of Queen Mary University London and is a world class biomedical research institute that integrates all stages of research from basic science through to clinical studies across a diverse range of fields including genomics, cell biology, translational immunology, neuroscience, and trauma. She has chaired the Research Advisory Board of the Motor Neurone Disease Association since 2018, with involvement in that organisation dating back to 1997. In 2021, she took up post as the Deputy Vice Principal Health at Queen Mary University London.

Finally, Prof. Martin is RCPath lead in a partnership with Health Education England on the innovative Pathology Portal project. The Pathology Portal, to be formally launched in June 2022, will deliver a platform to host high-quality training materials in all pathology disciplines that can be customised to individual needs covering flexible training, return-to-work training, and testing to support learning. The aim is to expand the platform to cover all pathology specialties, providing trainees with an adaptive learning approach, to support development of proficiency in general and specialist areas and to provide flexible and equitable access to content.

For her dedication to Pathology, exceptional service to healthcare, research, and education, Prof. Martin has received numerous awards, including Innovation Trust of the Year NHSIL (2012); Innovation of the Year, Barts Health NHS Trust (2018); she was nominated to be one of the top 100 Pathologists of the Power List in 2018 and was number 3 on this list (11). Her eCPD app won the Education App of the year 2019 at the United Kingdom App awards. She has received the Israel Doniach Lifetime Achievement Award Pathological Society (2018) (12); IBMS Honorary Fellowship (2020; a rare and prestigious honour); Honorary Fellowship of the Royal College of Physicians of Ireland (2020) and Honorary Fellowship of the Faculty of Public Health (2021), in recognition of her work during the COVID pandemic.

SUMMARY

Each of RCPath's former female Presidents represent inspirational and formidable women, each having differing strengths, contributing in differing ways to Pathology, healthcare, medical teaching, and research, all with steely determination, stamina, and great leadership skills. Their lifepaths were/are ones of commitment and determination, where they have made the absolute best of the "cards they had been dealt" at each stage and have created clearer paths for those following behind them. They are mentors for future generations of women in not only a career in medicine, but one in all areas of life. In the **Box 1** below is a quote from each of them, which may provide guidance for future generations.

As part of the College's 60th Birthday year, we celebrate what Clayton, Lishman, and Martin have achieved as Leaders and what they have contributed to this speciality.

AUTHOR CONTRIBUTIONS

All authors listed have made a substantial, direct, and intellectual contribution to the work, and approved it for publication.

ACKNOWLEDGMENTS

The authors thank Mr. Shane Johns for providing the photos (www.shanejohns.com).

REFERENCES

1. Richmond, C. *Lancet Obituary.* (2011) 377:23–9.

2. Munksroll. *Munks Roll Details for Barbara Evelyn (Dame) Clayton.* London: The Roll of the Royal College of Physicians (2018).

3. Casemore DP, Armstrong M, Jackson B, Gordon Nichols, Thom BT. Screening for cryptosporidium in stools. *Lancet.* (1984) 1:734–5. doi: 10.1016/s0140-6736(84)92245-1

4. Clayton BE. Phenylketonuria. *J Med Genet.* (1971) 8:37–40. doi: 10.1136/jmg.8.1.37

5. Moncrieff AA, Koumides OP, Clayton BE, Patrick AD, Renwick AG, Roberts GE. Lead poisoning in children. *Arch Dis Child.* (1964) 39:1–13.

6. Suzy Lishman: grateful to the air bubble. *BMJ.* (2015) 351:h3458. doi: 10.1136/bmj.h3458

7. Youtube. *Living Autopsy | Dr Suzy Lishman | Discovery Day at Home.* (2020). Available online at: https://www.youtube.com/watch?v=rGwJQuKZjpI (accessed Sep 26, 2020).

8. The Pathologist. *The Power List.* (2015). Available online at: https://thepathologist.com/power-list/the-power-list-2015/7-suzy-lishman (accessed January 25, 2022).

9. Government Digital Service. *"New Year's Honours 2018" (PDF).* London: Government Digital Service (2017). p. 17.

10. Rogers DC, Fisher EM, Brown SD, Peters J, Hunter AJ, Martin JE. Behavioral and functional analysis of mouse phenotype: SHIRPA, a proposed protocol for comprehensive phenotype assessment. *Mamm Genome.* (1997) 8:711–3.

11. The Pathologist. *The Power List.* (2018). Available online at: https://thepathologist.com/power-list/2018/3-jo-martin (accessed January 25, 2022).

12. Pathological Society. *Chronological list of Doniach Lecturers.* Edinburgh: Pathological Society (2011).

3

Syphilitic Hepatitis–A Rare and Underrecognized Etiology of Liver Disease with Potential for Misdiagnosis

Hiba A. Al Dallal[1†], Siddharth Narayanan[2†], Hanah F. Alley[3], Michael J. Eiswerth[4],
Forest W. Arnold[5], Brock A. Martin[1] and Alaleh E. Shandiz[1]*

[1] Department of Pathology and Laboratory Medicine, University of Louisville, Louisville, KY, United States, [2] Department of
Pediatrics, Nationwide Children's Hospital, Columbus, OH, United States, [3] Department of Neurology, University of Louisville,
Louisville, KY, United States, [4] Department of Internal Medicine, University of Louisville, Louisville, KY, United States, [5] Division
of Infectious Diseases, University of Louisville, Louisville, KY, United States

*Correspondence:
Alaleh E. Shandiz
alaleh.shandiz@louisville.edu

† These authors share first authorship

Syphilitic hepatitis (SH) in adults is a rare condition that can be easily misdiagnosed. Clinical and histopathologic manifestations of SH can mimic other infectious and non-infectious conditions, and the diagnosis should be considered in all at-risk patients with abnormal liver function tests. We present an unusual case of SH presenting with seizures and multiple liver lesions. This case report, in line with other newly published reports, promotes awareness of SH as a rare manifestation of treponemal infection and highlights the importance of including SH in the differential diagnosis for patients at risk for sexually transmitted infections and presenting with liver enzyme abnormalities. From a hospital quality control and socioeconomic perspective, our case adds to the growing body of evidence that demonstrates an increasing incidence of patients suffering from venereal diseases and injection drug use disorders, and the burden these conditions place on the healthcare system. Recognition of the clinicopathologic features of SH is required to prevent missed diagnosis and to foster systematic crosstalk between healthcare staff and public health personnel managing this problem.

Keywords: syphilis, drug abuse, hepatitis, seizure, liver enzymes, infection

INTRODUCTION

Syphilis is a disease caused by the non-hepatotropic bacterium *Treponema pallidum* and is associated with high-risk sexual activity. The stages of syphilis are well-defined, but the clinical manifestations can greatly vary between these stages (1, 2). In comparison to the first two stages (primary/secondary), untreated tertiary syphilis can present years after initial infection to cause devastating multi-organ system manifestations (3). While the overall incidence of syphilitic hepatitis (SH) is low, SH may occur in an estimated 3% of secondary syphilis cases (1). The incidence of tertiary syphilis presenting as SH is much less common.

Syphilitic hepatitis is usually asymptomatic or presents with non-specific symptoms. Non-hepatic manifestations of secondary syphilis, such as a characteristic diffuse maculopapular rash, are usually more helpful in pointing to the diagnosis than any hepatic signs or symptoms. The diagnosis of SH typically requires biochemical evidence of liver injury in the setting of confirmed treponemal serology, after exclusion of alternative causes of hepatic dysfunction (4). The pattern

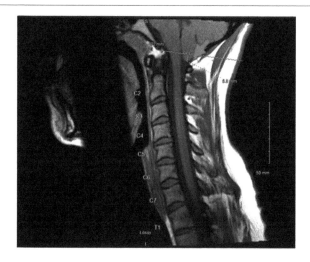

FIGURE 1 | A magnetic resonance imaging of the cervical spine showing a Chiari I malformation (red arrow) with a 5.8 mm displacement of the cerebellar vermis through the foramen magnum.

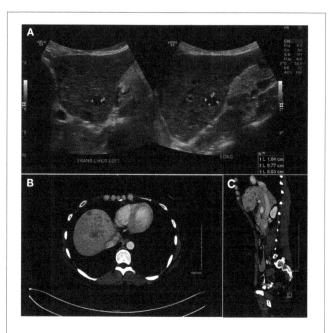

FIGURE 2 | (A) Liver ultrasound showing multiple hypo-echoic lesions ranging between 0.5 and 3.3 cm. **(B)** A liver computerized tomography scan showing multiple hypo-echoic lesions with peripheral rim of increased enhancement. **(C)** A magnetic resonance imaging (sagittal view) showing same as **(A,B)**.

of liver enzyme abnormalities is often cholestatic with altered alkaline phosphatase (ALP) levels and mildly elevated transaminases and bilirubin. Liver biopsy is often not required for diagnosis as response to antimicrobial therapy serves as a useful confirmatory finding.

We present an unusual case of an incarcerated adult female with a history of injection drug use (IDU) and multiple sexual partners who presented to our hospital with a constellation of neurological deficits and multiple liver lesions on imaging. After a comprehensive workup, she was diagnosed with tertiary SH with hepatic gummatous lesions but left against medical advice after only completing 4 days of penicillin treatment.

CASE REPORT

A 36-year-old incarcerated female with a history of polysubstance abuse and multiple sexual partners was found exhibiting seizure-like activity in her cell. On arrival at our hospital, she was unresponsive with convulsions of all extremities. Upon physical examination, she had upper motor neuron symptoms, including dilated pupils, rigidity of the lower extremities, and clonus, and a rectal temperature of 103°F. The patient was administered benzodiazepine to control the convulsions and intubated for airway protection. A computerized tomography (CT) scan of her head and neck was unremarkable, and magnetic resonance imaging (MRI) of the cervical spine demonstrated Chiari I malformation (**Figure 1**). An electroencephalogram of the brain confirmed seizure activity. Chest radiographs showed no evidence of an acute pulmonary process. Based on the initial presentation, a broad differential diagnosis was considered, including drug/toxin-induced neurological manifestations, infection, paraneoplastic syndrome, and metabolic (e.g., vitamin B12) deficiency.

An extensive workup was performed that included complete blood count, liver function tests, toxicology screens, and testing for multiple infectious diseases. Her white blood cell count was highly elevated (16×10^9 cells/L). Liver function tests revealed mildly elevated aspartate aminotransaminase (35 units/L, normal 8–34 units/L), alanine aminotransaminase (47 units/L, normal 7–24 units/L), and alkaline phosphatase (112 units/L, normal 25–105 units/L) with normal bilirubin. Vitamin B12 level was within the normal range. Urine toxicology was positive for cannabinoids, amphetamines, and benzodiazepines. An HIV screen was negative; however, the patient tested positive for *Treponema pallidum* antibodies (titer of 1:1,024) as well as hepatitis B surface antigen and DNA (PCR confirmation). A lumbar puncture for a cerebrospinal fluid culture and analysis was deferred due to the risk of herniation because of her Chiari I malformation.

Empiric treatment with intravenous penicillin G was initiated for a presumed diagnosis of neurosyphilis. However, the patient continued to exhibit unexplained, medically refractory severe nausea and vomiting, prompting abdominal imaging. An ultrasound assessment revealed multiple bilobar hypoechoic hepatic lesions (**Figure 2A**) which were confirmed as multiple hypoenhancing lesions on subsequent abdominal CT and MRI (**Figures 2B,C**). These additional imaging results raised consideration for atypical hepatic abscesses vs. metastatic malignancy, and a targeted liver core biopsy was performed.

Histologic sections of the biopsy showed involvement of the liver parenchyma by a dense mixed lymphoplasmacytic and granulocytic inflammatory infiltrate associated with

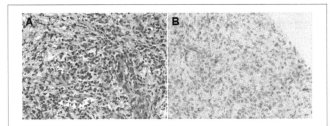

FIGURE 3 | (A) A H&E stain of the liver biopsy (400 X) showing mixed inflammatory infiltrate composed predominantly of lymphocytes and plasma cells and smaller numbers of neutrophils and eosinophils. The bile duct (red arrows) and portal vessel (yellow arrows) are highlighted. **(B)** An Anti-*Treponema pallidum* immunohistochemical staining confirmed the presence of spirochetes and highlighted numerous microorganisms having an epitheliotropic and vasculotropic pattern. The IHC was performed on the same tissue area as for the H&E stain.

TABLE 1 | Liver biochemical profile of our patient before and after antimicrobial treatment.

Liver function test	Hospital: Day 0	Hospital: Day 13 (discharge)
ALP (normal: 25–105 units/L)	112	84
AST (normal: 8–34 units/L)	35	29
ALT (normal: 7–24 units/L)	47	47
Albumin (normal: 3.4–4.8 g/dL)	2.7	3.1
Total bilirubin (normal: 0.2–1.1 mg/dL)	0.6	0.5

ALP, alkaline phosphatase; AST, aspartate transaminase; ALT, alanine transaminase.

reactive fibrosis (**Figure 3A**), foci of necrosis, and clusters of epithelioid histiocytes, consistent with inflammatory pseudo-tumor. In addition, foci of vascular and biliary inflammatory injury were present (**Figure 3A**). While a Warthin-Starry stain on the sample was negative, immunohistochemistry for treponemal organisms confirmed the presence of *Treponema pallidum* (Biocare APA 135 AA) and the diagnosis of tertiary stage SH with hepatic gummas (**Figure 3B**). The patient's liver function tests were monitored daily and showed initial improvement (**Table 1**); however, she left against medical advice following completion of only 4 days of the recommended 10–14-day course of intravenous penicillin for neurosyphilis.

DISCUSSION

Syphilis constantly challenges healthcare providers due to its multi-organ involvement, overlapping clinical stages, protean presentation, and it is an under-recognized etiology of liver dysfunction. In a retrospective study, liver enzyme abnormalities were common in patients with early syphilis (39%), yet only a small fraction (2.7%) were diagnosed with SH (5). Some authors have previously proposed clinical diagnostic criteria for SH (6), although diagnosis is still limited by the known clinical heterogeneity and lack of specific features of the disease (7).

The clinical manifestations of SH tend to be non-specific in adults. Common symptoms including low-grade fever, abdominal pain, sore throat, headache, weight loss, arthralgia or myodynia, splenomegaly, lymphadenopathy, and uveitis (7). Moderate elevations in liver enzymes, as well as markedly increased ALP and gamma-glutamyl transpeptidase levels, are reported in patients with SH (1, 2, 4). While the classic symmetric maculopapular rash of secondary syphilis, which involves the trunk and extremities including palms and soles, is a strong clue to the diagnosis of SH as a cause of liver enzyme abnormalities (8), it is not uniformly observed in all patients. Liver involvement represents spirochete dissemination (9) but can occur at any stage of the disease. In a systematic review of SH, the vast majority of patients (88.9%) presented with early stage (i.e., primary or secondary) disease; whereas, a small minority presented with latent (4.9%) or tertiary (6.3%) stage disease (10) when classic signs and symptoms of syphilis may be less apparent.

The histopathologic features of SH are likewise non-specific. Cases typically show mixed lymphoplasmacytic and granulocytic portal inflammation with variable bile duct injury and associated granulomas (9). A vasculotropic and epitheliotropic pattern of inflammation may be seen in some cases, but this is not etiologically specific and overlaps with other, more common inflammatory liver diseases. Although identification of spirochetes in the tissue by special stain or immunohistochemistry is diagnostic in the appropriate setting (11), false negative staining is not uncommon in the setting of disseminated treponemal disease, reaffirming the need for close clinicopathologic correlation to make the diagnosis in most cases. In the absence of known or reported risk factors for SH, the diagnosis is likely to be missed. Furthermore, potentially misleading clinical and imaging findings may prompt consideration and additional testing for other infectious, autoimmune, or neoplastic diseases, leading to delayed or misdiagnosis.

Our case emphasizes the importance of maintaining a broad differential diagnosis for hepatic enzyme abnormalities, including a comprehensive review of patient risk factors for common and uncommon causes of hepatitis. Despite an initial presentation with only mild liver enzyme elevations and multiple confounding and potentially misleading clinical and imaging findings, careful clinicopathologic correlation and appropriate diagnostic investigation eventually facilitated a conclusive diagnosis of tertiary SH.

Most cases of SH resolve with antibiotic medications for treponemal infection. Heightened clinical awareness and recognition of patients at risk for the disease are necessary to facilitate timely diagnosis and treatment. Risk factors including unprotected sexual activity, polysubstance abuse and IDU attribute to notably high rates of coinfection, increased hospital costs and a massive burden on the healthcare system (2, 12, 13). The incidence of primary and secondary syphilis are on the rise (1), and the identification and treatment of syphilis cases prevents progression to tertiary syphilis in affected individuals and the spread to other individuals.

Therefore, increased attention to the diagnosis of SH by care providers and pathologists is essential for achieving positive patient outcomes as well as hospital quality control and socioeconomic goals.

CONCLUSIONS

SH can be easily overlooked and misdiagnosed because of non-specific signs and symptoms at the presentation and mild hepatic manifestations, in addition to non-specific and overlapping histopathologic findings. The diagnosis of tertiary SH is particularly problematic as other clinical signs and symptoms of disseminated treponemal disease may be absent or inapparent. Given the availability of effective treatment, timely diagnosis can greatly decrease morbidity and mortality associated with this condition. Even in the absence of non-hepatic manifestations, SH should be considered in high-risk patients with altered liver function tests. Multi-disciplinary efforts from healthcare and regulatory bodies are needed to reduce its growing incidence.

AUTHOR CONTRIBUTIONS

HAA collected the data and interpreted the diagnosis. SN analyzed the literature and wrote the manuscript. HFA and ME helped in collecting the data and edited the manuscript. FA, BM, and AS provided framework for the study, reviewed, and edited the manuscript. All authors have read and agreed to the final version of the manuscript.

REFERENCES

1. Alemam A, Ata S, Shaikh D, Leuzzi B, Makker J. Syphilitic hepatitis: a rare cause of acute liver injury. *Cureus.* (2021) 13:e14800. doi: 10.7759/cureus.14800

2. Narang N, Al-Jashaami L, Patel N. Spirochetes in the liver: an unusual presentation of a common STI. *Case Rep Med.* (2019) 2019:1012405. doi: 10.1155/2019/1012405

3. Ghanem KG, Ram S, Rice PA. The modern epidemic of syphilis. *N Engl J Med.* (2020) 382:845–54. doi: 10.1056/NEJMra1901593

4. Horn CL, Jalali S, Abbott J, Stein M. A surprising diagnosis: syphilitic gastritis and hepatitis. *Am J Med.* (2018) 131:1178–81. doi: 10.1016/j.amjmed.2018.03.023

5. Adachi E, Koibuchi T, Okame M, Sato H, Kikuchi T, Koga M, et al. Liver dysfunction in patients with early syphilis: a retrospective study. *J Infect Chemother.* (2013) 19:180–2. doi: 10.1007/s10156-012-0440-5

6. Mullick CJ, Liappis AP, Benator DA, Roberts AD, Parenti DM, Simon GL. Syphilitic Hepatitis in HIV-Infected Patients: A Report of 7 Cases and Review of the Literature. *Clin Infect Dis.* (2004) 39:e100–5. doi: 10.1086/425501

7. Huang J, Lin S, Wang M, Wan B, Zhu Y. Syphilitic hepatitis: a case report and review of the literature. *BMC Gastroenterol.* (2019) 19:191. doi: 10.1186/s12876-019-1112-z

8. Kaya A, Kaya SY. Management of syphilitic hepatitis. *BMC Gastroenterol.* (2020) 20:379. doi: 10.1186/s12876-020-01496-5

9. Pizzarossa AC, Rebella M. Hepatitis in patients with syphilis: an overlooked association. *BMJ Case Rep.* (2019) 12:226918. doi: 10.1136/bcr-2018-226918

10. Huang J, Lin S, Wan B, Zhu Y. A systematic literature review of syphilitic hepatitis in adults. *J Clin Transl Hepatol.* (2018) 6:306–9. doi: 10.14218/JCTH.2018.00003

11. Hoang MP, High WA, Molberg KH. Secondary syphilis: a histologic and immunohistochemical evaluation. *J Cutan Pathol.* (2004) 31:595–9. doi: 10.1111/j.0303-6987.2004.00236.x

12. Elnazeir M, Narayanan S, Badugu P, Hussain A, Stephens CB, Bhagat R, et al. Neurological manifestations associated with synthetic cannabinoid use–a case series. *Open Neurol J.* (2020) 14:53–8. doi: 10.2174/1874205X0201401 0053

13. Al Dallal HA, Narayanan S, Jones CM, Lockhart SR, Snyder JW. First case report of an unusual fungus (sporopachydermia lactativora) associated with a pulmonary infection in a drug injection user. *Clin Pathol.* (2021) 14:2632010X211029970. doi: 10.1177/2632010X21102 9970

4

Lymphatic Vessel Invasion in Routine Pathology Reports of Papillary Thyroid Cancer

Costanza Chiapponi[1]*, Hakan Alakus[1], Matthias Schmidt[2], Michael Faust[3], Christiane J. Bruns[1], Reinhard Büttner[4], Marie-Lisa Eich[4] and Anne M. Schultheis[4]

[1] Department of General, Visceral, Cancer and Transplant Surgery, University Clinic of Cologne, Cologne, Germany, [2] Department for Nuclear Medicine, University Clinic of Cologne, Cologne, Germany, [3] Policlinic for Endocrinology, Diabetes and Prevention Medicine, University Clinic of Cologne, Cologne, Germany, [4] Institute for Pathology, University Clinic of Cologne, Cologne, Germany

*Correspondence:
Costanza Chiapponi
costanza.chiapponi@uk-koeln.de

Purpose: It is not mandatory to report lymphatic vessel invasion in pathology reports of papillary thyroid cancer (PTC) according to the current Union for International Cancer Control (UICC) TNM (tumor, nodes, and metastases) classification. However, there is some evidence for its correlation with lymph node metastasis (LNM) and prognosis. The aim of this study was to explore the clinical implication of lymphatic vessel invasion documentation of PTC because pathology reports play a pivotal role in postsurgical clinical decision-making in endocrine tumor boards.

Methods: Patients undergoing postoperative radioiodine treatment for PTC at the University Hospital of Cologne, Germany between December 2015 and March 2020 were identified. Pathology reports were screened for documentation of lymphatic vessel invasion. Demographics and clinicopathologic data of patients documented, including lymphatic vessel invasion and lymph nodal involvement were analyzed.

Results: A total of 578 patients were identified and included. Lymphatic vessel invasion was reported in pathology reports of 366 (63.3%) and omitted in 112 (36.7%) patients. Positive lymphatic vessel invasion (L1) was diagnosed in 67 (18.3%) of 366 patients and was documented as absent (L0) in 299 (81.7%) patients. Lymph nodal (N) status was positive (N+) in 126 (45.6%) and negative (N0) in 150 (54.3%) of these patients. In 54 (80.6%) L1 cases N+ status and in 137 (65.6%) L0 cases N0 status was diagnosed. In 13 (19.4%) cases with L1 status, there were no LNMs (L1 N0). In total, 72 (34.4%) patients had LNM despite L0 status (L0 N+). The sensitivity and specificity of LVI reporting for LNM were 0.42 and 0.91, respectively.

Conclusion: In routine pathology reports of PTC used for indication to postoperative radioiodine treatment by a German endocrine tumor board, lymphatic vessel invasion was found to be reported inconsistently and mostly as L0. L1 diagnoses, however, reliably correlated with reported LNM and might, thus, be relevant for clinical decision-making. For this reason, we advocate for standardized pathologic reassessment of lymphatic vessel invasion, in particular for cases where lymph nodes are not included in the pathologic specimen and if L0 is documented.

Keywords: papillary thyroid cancer, lymph node metastasis, lymph vascular invasion, nodal involvement of papillary thyroid cancer, L0, L1, lymph vessel

INTRODUCTION

Papillary thyroid cancer (PTC) has a very good prognosis. For this reason, the extent of surgery and prophylactic lymphadenectomy are controversial issues. The European Society of Endocrine Surgery (ESES) recommends prophylactic lymphadenectomy in patients with tumor stages T3 or T4, in patients older than 45 years or younger than 15 years, of the male gender, with bilateral or multifocal tumors, and known involved lateral lymph nodes (1). The British Thyroid Association (BTA) advocates for it in aggressive histopathological subtypes, in patients older than 44 years, with multifocality and tumors sized >4 cm at their largest diameter (2). Also, according to the American Thyroid Association (ATA) "prophylactic central-compartment neck dissection (ipsilateral or bilateral) should be considered in patients with papillary thyroid carcinoma with clinically uninvolved central neck lymph nodes (cN0) who have advanced primary tumors (T3 or T4) or clinically involved lateral neck nodes (cN1b), or if the information will be used to plan further steps in therapy" (3). The European Society of Medical Oncologists (ESMO) underlines that it facilitates the precise staging of the disease and guides subsequent treatment and follow-up, although there is controversial evidence supporting the improvement of recurrence or mortality rate (4). Moreover, the Japanese Association of Endocrine Surgeons (JAES) recommends it for all patients with PTC, excluding papillary microcarcinoma of the thyroid (5). Personalized approaches are required, taking into account the context of the patient, the tumor biology, the experience of the thyroid surgeon, and the benefit/risk ratio (6). In a recent meta-analysis including 9,369 PTCs, lymph node metastasis (LNM) was identified in 31.7% of patients (7). Significant risk factors were age (<45 years), gender (male), multifocality, tumor size (>1 cm), tumor location (upper third of the thyroid), capsular invasion, and extrathyroidal extension (ETE) (7). However, not negligible rates of LNM have been reported for pT1a tumors (8, 9). The clinical significance of lymph nodal involvement in pT1a and pT1b tumors is controversial. Although a recent study reports rates of 11% for PTCs incidentally diagnosed during autopsy (10), there is also some evidence for an increased risk of recurrence (11) and for compromised overall survival in patients with nodal involvement (12), making this issue very relevant for young patients. For this reason, the diagnosis of LNM leads to radioiodine treatment and suppressive TSH treatment during follow-up, even in pT1a patients in Germany. Since pT1a or even pT1b tumors can be diagnosed incidentally in patients undergoing thyroidectomy for multinodular goiter, many of these patients do not undergo lymphadenectomy.

Lymphatic vessel invasion (LVI) has been shown to correlate with LNM and with patients' prognoses in several tumor entities (13–16). In a recent study, it was found to be the only independent prognostic factor of disease free survival (DFS) in patients with lymph node-negative superficial esophageal squamous cell carcinoma (17). Even its documented absence (L0) might play some predictive role: a multicenter retrospective analysis found that no LNMs were identified in women with low-risk cervical cancer and no LVI. L0 was suggested as a possible argument for omitting prophylactic lymphadenectomy in these patients (18). Although there is some evidence that LVI in PTC correlates with LNMs (19–22) and with outcomes of patients (6, 23, 24), LVI does not play any concrete role in clinical decision-making. Vascular invasion instead is included among those crucial histologic variables for initial risk stratification and clinical management of PTC, alongside ETE, margin status (R), and the number of metastatic lymph nodes (pN-status) (25–27). LVI (L-status; L1 = invasion and L0 = no invasion) is not regularly included in pathology reports in PTC in Europe, as it is not mandatory to report LVI according to the current TNM classification (28). One possible explanation is that LVI in PTC is often not easily identified in thyroid parenchyma (**Figure 1**) (29).

Lymphatic vessel invasion is defined as "*tumor deposits within lymphatic spaces*" that may manifest "*as psammoma bodies alone within these spaces*" (27, 30, 31). However, often the invaded lymph vascular channels are overgrown by the tumor, as evidenced by the absence of lymphatic channels in the central part of most PTCs with lymph node metastases (29). The thin walls of the lymphatic vascular channels and the invasive nature of the tumors are factors, which can make LVI detection challenging (**Figure 1**). In addition, LVI assessment is not sufficiently standardized in our experience: for the most part, only representative tumor sections are embedded and H&E staining of representative sections are deemed sufficient for reporting the lack of LVI (L0). However, LVI is not only limited to the tumor itself and tumor interface but could be manifested by the spread of PTC in the ipsilateral and even contralateral lobe seen as psammomas and/or (usually subcapsular) "tumor seeds." Additional immunohistochemical stains or additional tissue sectioning might help detect LVI. Both, generally, are not routinely performed in the clinical setting (**Supplementary Figure 1**).

The aim of this study was to critically question the LVI documentation in routine pathology reports of papillary thyroid cancer. Tumors that were deemed worth treating with radioiodine therapy by the multidisciplinary endocrine tumor board of the university were included and the impact of LVI documentation on clinical and pathological parameters was explored. We also investigated if LVI documentation might be helpful for identifying nodal involvement in pT1a tumors.

METHODS

Patients

Patients who underwent postoperative radioiodine therapy between December 2015 and March 2020 (4 years and 3 months) for PTC as judged by the interdisciplinary tumor board for endocrine tumors at the University Hospital Cologne, Germany were identified and included. In Germany, national guidelines advise for radioiodine therapy in PTC pT1b and higher, and in selected cases of pT1a (e.g., unfavorable histology, lymph node involvement, etc.). Postoperative tumor board recommendations are generally based on pathology reports besides clinical information delivered by the presenting physician.

Surgery was performed as thyroidectomy with or without central lymph node dissection depending on the time of

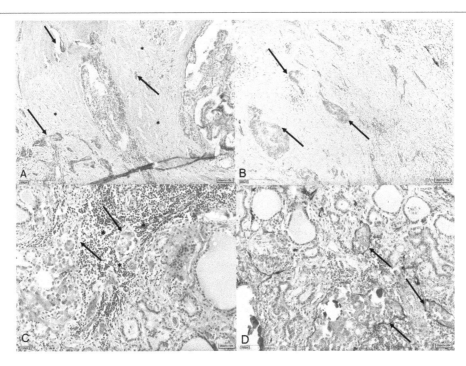

FIGURE 1 | (A) Papillary thyroid carcinoma (PTC) displaying significant stromal desmoplasia (*) with small tumor foci surrounded by slit-like spaces (→) indicating vascular invasion. **(B)** Immunohistochemical staining for Podoplanin/D2-40 shows that slit-like spaces lack circumferential staining for D2-40 (→) indicating the presence of retraction artifacts and not lymphatic vessel invasion (LVI). **(C)** Different tumor areas of the same PTC show small tumor nodules with discrete slit-like spaces (→) surrounded by lymphocytes (*). **(D)** Circumferential D2-40-positivity confirming LVI (→).

diagnosis (pre- or postoperatively) and the experience of surgeon, as recommended by the German Guidelines (32). In some cases, lateral lymph node dissection was also performed, when the preoperative radiologic diagnosis suggested lymph node involvement, according to the current German Guidelines (32).

Histopathology

In our pathologic institute, the resected specimens were fixed in 4% phosphate-buffered formalin and embedded in Paraffin. For each cm of the tumor (largest diameter), one tumor section was embedded. A 3-cm large tumor would be analyzed using three tumor sections, ideally comprising one entire diametrical section of the tumor. Three micron thick sections were cut and stained with H&E. Diagnoses were made according to the, at that time, current (2009 and 2017) WHO classification of Tumors of Endocrine Organs. Shortly, H&E-stained sections were routinely screened for signs of LVI. These included the presence of tumor tissue and/or psammoma bodies in lymphatic spaces, including lymphatic spaces within the tumor, but also at the periphery of the tumor, or somewhere else in the resection specimen, as described by Mete et al. (27) and Wittekind (28). Additional immunohistochemical staining was not routinely performed, but only in a subset of cases, which were deemed unclear. Staging, including the assessment of the Nodal Status and LVI, was performed according to the 2018 International Union Against Cancer (UICC) TNM classification system (28). In addition to the number of the resected and metastatic lymph nodes, the number of metastatic lymph nodes with extracapsular extension (ece+) was also determined.

In instances where patients were only referred for radioiodine treatment to our University Hospital, only pathology reports were obtained and included.

Additionally, in order to find out if LVI identification might be helpful for identifying nodal involvement in pT1a tumors, 22 specimens of papillary microcarcinomas with confirmed nodal involvement were retrospectively reassessed with H&E and D2-40 immunohistochemistry (IHC) by two experienced pathologists, according to the criteria defined above (28) (presence of tumor tissue and/or psammoma bodies in lymphatic spaces, including lymphatic spaces within the tumor, but also at the periphery of the tumor, or somewhere else in the resection specimen).

Data Collection, Analysis, and Ethic

Electronic and paper data of the University Hospital of Cologne were retrospectively collected and analyzed. Data were analyzed using Excel 365 and IBM SPSS Statistics for Windows, Version 25.0, Armonk, NY, USA. This study was approved by the ethics committee of the University Hospital Cologne (Approval ID 20-1724).

RESULTS

Characteristics of Patients

Between December 2015 and March 2020, 740 patients received radioiodine treatment at our institution. Forty (5.4%) cases were excluded due to incomplete data. Five hundred and seventy-eight (82.6%) reports described papillary thyroid carcinomas (PTC) and were included in the present analysis. They corresponded to 175 (30.2%) males and 403 (69.8%) females. The median age of male patients was 50 years (range 17–82 years) and that of female patients 47 years (range 11–85 years) ($p < 0.05$). Advanced tumor stages (pT3/T4) were diagnosed more frequently ($p < 0.05$) in men (42 of 175 cases, 42%) than in women (63 of 403, 15.6%).

Lymphatic Vessel Invasion Report

In 366 (63.3%) of 578 pathology reports, the LVI status was described. The frequency of LVI reporting was not associated with gender of patients ($p = 0.54$), age ($p = 0.37$), tumor size ($p = 0.11$), PTC variant ($p = 0.57$), or pT status ($p = 0.66$). LVI status was more often reported in patients without N-reporting (Nx, $p < 0.05$) (**Table 1**).

Lymphatic Vessel Invasion Status

Lymphatic vessel invasion absence (L0) was documented in 299 (81.7%) and positive lymph vascular invasion (L1) in 67 (18.3%) of 366 pathology reports. Lymph vascular invasion (L1) was more frequently detected in male patients ($p = 0.01$), greater tumor size ($p < 0.05$), higher pT- ($p < 0.01$), and pN-status ($p < 0.01$). Whereas, lymph vascular invasion (L1) was seen in only 5% of patients with a pT1a status, the frequency of L1 increased to 23.5% in pT2, 32% in pT3 and 66.7% in pT4 ($p < 0.01$). Similarly, lymph vascular invasion (L1) was reported in only 8.7% patients with pN0 and in 42.8% patients with pN+ ($p < 0.01$). In Nx patients L1 was reported in only 4.4% of cases ($p < 0.01$) (**Table 2**).

Lymphatic Vessel Invasion and Lymph Node Metastasis (LNM)

In 454 (78.5%) of 578 PTC pathology reports the N-status was reported either as negative 256 (N0, 56.4%) or positive 198 (N+, 43.6%). In 276 (60.8%) reports, a LVI and a pN-status were also documented (**Table 2**).

Patients with nodal involvement showed significantly more often an L1 diagnosis (80.6 vs. 19.4%, $p < 0.01$) and an advanced pT status (pT4 88.9 vs. 11.1%, $p < 0.05$) in their pathology report (**Supplementary Table 1**). They were significantly more frequently male (63.8 vs. 36.2%; $p < 0.01$), younger (median age 41 years, range 11–84 vs. 51, range 18–85; $p < 0.01$) and had a higher number of harvested lymph nodes (21.3 ± 15.8 vs. 14.5 ± 13.9, $p < 0.01$) (**Supplementary Table 1**). The independent variables LVI, pT status, gender, age, and the number of harvested lymph nodes, which were significant in univariate analysis, were then entered into the regression model for multivariate logistic regression analysis. The results showed that LVI, male gender, younger age, a larger number of harvested lymph nodes were significant risk factors for LNM (**Supplementary Table 2**).

Positive LVI (L1) was described in 67 (24.3%) patients. Among them, 54 (80.6%) also had positive pN-status (L1pN+) and 13 (19.4%) had a pN0-status (L1pN0).

L0 was documented in 209 (57.1%) patients. Among them, 137 (65.6%) had a pN0-status (L0pN0), whereas in 72 (34.4%) patients a pN+ status was documented (L0pN+). Most L0pN+

TABLE 1 | Lymphatic vessel invasion (LVI) report and clinicopathologic variables (*p-values are calculated for LVI reported vs. non-reported).

		LVI report		
	Σ\n$n = 578$	LVI reported\n$n = 366$\n(81.7%)	LVI non-reported\n$n = 212$\n(18.3%)	p^*
Age				
Median (range)	47.5 (11–85)	48 (11–85)	49 (18–82)	n.s.
Gender				
Male	175 (30.3%)	113 (64.6%)	62 (35.4%)	n.s.
Female	403 (69.7%)	253 (62.7%)	150 (37.3%)	
Tumor size				
Median (mm)	18.5 (11–79)	20 (11–75)	18 (11–79)	n.s.
PTC variant				
Conventional	495 (85.6%)	315 (63.6%)	180 (36.3%)	
Follicular	7 (12.6%)	45 (61.6%)	28 (38.4%)	
Tall cell	6 (1.0%)	3 (50.0%)	3 (50.0%)	n.s.
Columnar	3 (0.5%)	3 (100.0%)	0	
Cribriform morular	1 (0.2%)	0	1 (100.0%)	
pT status				
1a	135 (23.3%)	79 (58.6%)	56 (41.4%)	
1b	205 (35.4%)	127 (62.0%)	78 (38.0%)	
2	133 (23%)	98 (73.7%)	35 (26.3%)	n.s.
3	88 (15.2%)	53 (60.2%)	35 (39.8%)	
4	17 (2.9%)	9 (53.0%)	8 (47.0%)	
pN category				
N0	256 (44.3%)	150 (58.6%)	106 (41.4%)	
N+	198 (34.2%)	126 (63.6%)	72 (36.3%)	<0.05
No lymph nodes resected	124 (21.4%)	90 (72.6%)	34 (27.4%)	

Tumor size was calculated for the non-pT1a tumors. Next to the median values, the ranges are reported. n.s., non-significant.

cases were found in pT1b (39.2%), followed by pT2 (24.3%) and pT1a (17.5%).

Additionally, 22 pT1a tumors with nodal involvement were reassessed using H&E and D2-40 IHC (**Supplementary Figure 1**). They had been diagnosed as L0 in 13 (61.9%) cases and as L1 in 2 (9%) cases. In 7 (31.8%) cases, L status was not documented. Retrospective reassessment using both H&E and D2-40 IHC performed by two independent, experienced pathologists delivered no tumor tissue and/or psammoma bodies in lymphatic spaces, including lymphatic spaces within the tumor, but also at the periphery of the tumor, or somewhere else in the resection specimen, and L0 was reassessed according to this definition in all cases (**Supplementary Table 2**).

Predictive Value of LVI Report for Lymph Node Metastasis

The positive assessment of LVI (L1) correlated in 80.6% of cases with lymph node metastases. The documented absence of LVI (L0) was correlated in 65.5% of cases with tumor-free lymph nodes. The sensitivity and specificity of the LVI report for lymph nodal involvement in this study were 0.41 and 0.92, respectively.

TABLE 2 | LVI presence (L1) and absence (L0) and clinicopathologic variables (*p-values are calculated for L0 vs. L1).

		LVI status		
	Σ n = 366	L0 n = 299 (75.7%)	L1 n = 67 (24.3%)	p*
Age				
Median (range)	48 (11–85)	48 (17–85)	46 (11–76)	n.s.
Gender				
Male	113 (30.9%)	84 (74.3%)	29 (25.7%)	<0.01
Female	253 (69.1%)	215 (84.9%)	38 (15.0%)	
Tumor size				
Median (mm)	20 (11–75)	18 (11–64)	25.5 (11–75)	<0.05
PTC variant				
Conventional	315 (81.4%)	255 (80.9%)	60 (19%)	
Follicular	45 (12.2%)	41 (91.1%)	4 (8.9%)	
Tall cell	3 (0.8%)	2 (66.7%)	1 (33.3%)	
Columnar	3 (0.8%)	1 (33.3%)	2 (66.7%)	n.s.
Cribriform morular	0 (0.0%)	0	0	
pT status				
1a	79 (21.5%)	75 (94.9%)	4 (5.0%)	
1b	127 (34.6%)	110 (86.6%)	17 (13.4%)	
2	98 (26.8%)	75 (76.5%)	23 (23.5%)	<0.01
3	53 (14.5%)	36 (68.0%)	17 (32.0%)	
4	9 (2.5%)	3 (33.3%)	6 (66.7%)	
pN category				
N0	150 (41.0%)	137 (91.3%)	13 (8.7%)	
N+	126 (34.4%)	72 (57.2%)	54 (42.8%)	<0.01
No lymph nodes resected	90 (24.6%)	86 (95.6%)	4 (4.4%)	

Tumor size was calculated for the non-pT1a tumors. Next to the median values, the ranges are reported. n.s., non-significant.

The positive and the negative predictive value were 0.80 and 0.65, respectively.

As described above, reported LVI was a significant independent risk factor for LNM in the multivariate analysis ($p = 0.001$, **Supplementary Table 2**).

DISCUSSION

In several tumor entities, LVI has been shown to correlate with LNMs and with prognoses of patients (13–18). Similar data are available for PTC (6, 19–24). However, LVI does not play a role in clinical decision-making according to all major guidelines and is not mandatory in pathology reports of PTC according to the current TNM classification (28). In Australia, it has been shown to be routinely reported and is only omitted in 15.8% of cases (33). In this study, the data of a German academic endocrine center were explored in order to identify the extent of LVI documentation in routine pathology reports of papillary thyroid cancer and estimate its role as a possible predictor for LNM, especially in cases that

generally do not require lymphadenectomy like microcarcinomas <1 cm.

Lymphatic vessel invasion was reported in 63.3% of pathology reports of patients with PTCs, who underwent postoperative radioiodine treatment at our institute. The presence of LVI increased expectedly alongside with higher stage, from 5% in pT1a, 13.4% in pT1b, 23.5% in pT2, 32% in pT3 to 66.7% in pT4 (**Table 2**). Similarly, the rate of LNM rose from 42.5% in pT1a, 40.8% in pT1b, 44.2% in pT2, 53.5% in pT3, to 88.9% in pT4 (**Supplementary Table 1**).

Our data confirm that L1 documented in pathology report quite reliably correlated with a diagnosis of lymph node metastases (pN+). A total of 54 (80.6%) patients with reported positive LVI also had a diagnosis of LNM. On the other hand, 13 (19.4%) patients with positive LVI (L1) had a pN0-status in the initial histopathologic report. These L1pN0 cases might be due to the fact that the surgeon performing a prophylactic lymphadenectomy might have missed deeper or lateral lymph nodes, in order to avoid complications in a procedure performed for a cancer, which generally has an excellent prognosis. Eleven (84.6%) of these 13 patients achieved biochemical and radiological cure in a mean follow-up of 27.6 ± 16 months after radioiodine treatment. One 59-year-old woman with a pT1b pN0 (0/1), L1 tumor, and a 31-year-old woman with a pT2 pN0 (0/1), L1 tumor instead have not been cured by initial surgery and radioiodine therapy (RAIT). In the first case, there are elevated and slowly increasing thyroglobulin levels with currently no evidence of structural disease in repeated iodine and PET-CT scan. The second patient underwent repeated cervical surgery delivering eight PTC metastases in 40 resected lymph nodes.

In 72 (34.4%) cases, LNM was reported despite L0 status indicating a concrete risk of lymph node involvement even in L0 reporting. Thirteen of these patients had a pT1a tumor. Pathologic reassessment of 22 specimens including 13 L0, 2 L1, and seven tumors with no LVI documentation was performed by two independent, experienced pathologists. No cases showed LVI diagnosis according to the current definition [presence of tumor tissue and/or psammoma bodies in lymphatic spaces, including lymphatic spaces within the tumor, but also at the periphery of the tumor, or somewhere else in the resection specimen (29)], despite nodal involvement. Two cases, which had originally been reported as L1 (**Supplementary Table 3**), could not be confirmed as L1. This underlines the difficulty of diagnosing lymph vessel invasion especially in smaller tumors, even with the additional use of IHC.

In the interpretation of the data presented in this study, the reliability of pathology reports needs to be discussed. The thin walls of the lymphatic vascular channels and the invasive nature of the tumors are likely elements masking the evidence of lymphatic invasion (30). Xu and Ghossein recently pointed out that features separating lymphatic from vascular invasion based on histology alone can be difficult (34). Lymphatic invasion is generally assessed by H&E staining method only. One major challenge of this method is to distinguish lymphatic invasion from the retraction artifacts caused by tissue handling and fixation (29) (**Figure 1**). The use of IHC staining methods can support the diagnosis: a meta-analysis on lymphatic invasion in breast cancer showed detection rates ranging from 10 to 49% for H&E and a narrower range from 21 to 42% for IHC (35). In the daily practice, moreover, only representative parts of the tumor are sectioned and examined, and IHC is not used routinely, indicating a possibility of underdiagnosis of lymphatic invasion (**Supplementary Figure 1**). Since the CAP 2021 considers LVI as a core reporting element (27), the clear criteria for diagnosis, including direct and indirect LVI signs, should be more broadly implemented in routine pathologic protocols for PTC.

Another issue to consider is the variability in the number of harvested lymph nodes in lymph node dissections. Some pathology reports included only one lymph node and cases were signed out as "pN0" based on this singular, possibly unintended resected node. In several cases lymphadenectomy had not been performed, according to the German guidelines stating that the benefit of prophylactic lymphadenectomy is unclear and should be performed only by experienced thyroid surgeons, weighing the risk of morbidity and the possible benefit for the patient. If lymphadenectomy is performed, there are three main aspects influencing lymphadenectomy results. There are individual patient-associated anatomic aspects, like the normal number of lymph nodes in the central neck compartment varying between 2 and 44 lymph nodes (36). There are also technical aspects, which are relevant to the surgeons and some which are relevant to the pathologist. The surgeon must make sure that the extent of resection does not unnecessarily increase morbidity and the pathologist must be aware that smaller lymph nodes may be hard to detect within large dissection specimens and ideally embed the complete specimen (36). A retrospective Surveillance, Epidemiology, and End Results (SEER) analysis, including the results of 5,107 central lymphadenectomies for PTC, reported an average total number of lymph nodes removed of 4 (37). The significantly higher number reported in this study is possibly due to the fact that most patients receiving lymphadenectomy had been operated in specialized clinics. Additionally, according to the German guidelines, lateral lymphadenectomy is also warranted if the lymph nodes appear sonographically enlarged or suspicious. While evidence of LNMs can help the nuclear medicine specialist in correct staging and for adjusting the radioiodine activity to administer (38), a diagnosis of four tumor-free lymph nodes, instead, can hardly rule out lymph node involvement.

Several studies agree that LVI has a positive correlation with LNMs (19–22), and a negative impact on outcomes of patient (6, 23, 24), although single studies report no significant association with response to therapy (39). In this study, the positive correlation with LNMs can be confirmed. An additional finding is the remarkably high percentage of LNM (34.4%) in L0 tumors, which is also confirmed by the data of Pontius et al. (32.5%) (23). Given this high rate of LNMs, despite the lack of LVI and given the limits of the currently widely used methods (H&E staining of representative parts of the tumors only), the L0 report appears of poor clinical significance.

Some shortcomings of this study must be mentioned. First, the reference standard consisted of pathology reports, thus conclusions might be affected by the individual bias of pathologists, who initially signed out the specimens. So far, we did not routinely reassess specimens of patients referred for postoperative treatment at our institution. Based on the data presented, we plan to reassess lymph vessel invasion in the future, in order to investigate if this information might impact clinical decision-making. Second, long-term follow-up data for some of these patients are not included, hence we did not analyze systematically which of these patients developed metastases in the course of their disease or even radioiodine refractory disease. Finally, the patients included in this study were treated or referred to a university center (40). It also needs to be mentioned that active surveillance for low-risk PTC has shown to be safe and feasible in certain populations. However, in Europe and especially in the time lapse of this study, it is currently limited to clinical trials. Moreover, to the best of our knowledge, there are no data on active surveillance of nodal involvement.

CONCLUSION

We conclude that the presence of LVI (L1) documented in routine pathology reports delivers important information, as it likely correlates with LNM. The reported absence of LVI (L0) however, with the widely used H&E staining of a representative section of the tumor, does not reliably correlate with the absence of LNM and might suggest wrong assumptions. In the absence of lymph nodes in the surgical specimen, standardized pathologic reassessment of L0 diagnosis included in routine pathology reports might be helpful for better assessment of the risk of nodal involvement.

AUTHOR CONTRIBUTIONS

CC and AS designed the study, together with CJB and RB. CC, M-LE, and AS collected the data. CC, HA, M-LE, MS, MF, and AS contributed to the interpretation of the results. MS, HA, CJB, RB, and MF contributed critical feedback and helped shape the research, analysis, and manuscript. CC and AS wrote the first draft of the manuscript. All authors critically revised the manuscript, approved the final version of the manuscript, decided to submit this study, and agreed to be accountable for all aspects of the work as recommended by the International Committee of Medical Journal Editors (ICMJE) authorship criteria.

ACKNOWLEDGMENTS

We would like to thank Mrs. Caitlin Czarniecki for language editing.

SUPPLEMENTARY MATERIAL

Supplementary Figure 1 | Representative cases of papillary thyroid carcinoma depicting the need for standardized LVI evaluation. **(A)** Papillary thyroid carcinoma (PTC; pT1b) without evidence of lymphovascular invasion (LVI) on H&E-stained section of the primary tumor. However, psammoma bodies can be appreciated ( )

sometimes surrounded by slit-like spaces. No additional staining was performed. The case was signed out as L1 as a lymph node metastasis was detected [pN1 (4/5)]. **(B)** Hereinafter performed Podoplanin (D2-40) immunohistochemistry (IHC) showed very few lymphovascular channels (→) at the periphery of the tumor; no evidence for LVI. **(C)** PTC (pT1a) with small tumor nodules at the periphery, some of which are surrounded by slit-like-spaces potentially suggesting LVI on HE stained sections. The case was signed out as L0 without further analysis and

showed lymph node metastases [pN1 (2/33)]. **(D)** Subsequently performed D2-40 staining depicts vascular channels at the periphery of the tumor without tumor cell invasion supporting the absence of LVI. **(E)** PTC (pT1b) with small foci of tumor nodules surrounded by slit-like spaces at the periphery (∗) suggesting LVI. The case was signed out as L1. No lymph node metastases were detected [pN0 (0/6)]. **(F)** LVI could not be confirmed by D2-40 staining.

Supplementary Table 1 | Patients with L- and N status. Lymph nodal involvement was significantly more frequent in younger patients, in men and in patients with a higher number of harvested lymph nodes, higher pT status, and lymphatic vessel invasion (LVI) documented in the pathology report. Tumor size was not significant ($p = 0.47$).

Supplementary Table 2 | Results of a multivariate analysis including the independent variables gender, age, pT status, LVI and number of harvested lymph nodes, which had been found significant in **Supplementary Table 1**. The results showed that LVI, gender, age, and a number of harvested lymph nodes were significant risk factors for lymph node metastasis. B, β coefficient; SIG, statistical significance, p-value.

Supplementary Table 3 | Pathology reassessment of 22 cases of pT1a pN1 papillary thyroid carcinoma (PTCs), including 13 L0, 2 L1, and 7 cases in which LVI had not been documented. LVI could not be diagnosed in any case, also in the two cases in which it had been reported.

REFERENCES

1. Sancho JJ, Lennard TWJ, Paunovic I, Triponez F, Sitges-Serra A. Prophylactic central neck dissection in papillary thyroid cancer: a consensus report of the European Society of Endocrine Surgeons (ESES), Langenbecks. *Arch Surg.* (2014) 399:155–63. doi: 10.1007/s00423-013-1152-8
2. Perros P, Boelaert K, Colley S, Evans C, Evans RM, Gerrard Ba G, et al. Guidelines for the management of thyroid cancer. *Clin Endocrinol.* (2014) 81(Suppl 1):1–122. doi: 10.1111/cen.12515
3. Haugen BR, Alexander EK, Bible KC, Doherty GM, Mandel SJ, Nikiforov YE, et al. 2015 American Thyroid Association Management Guidelines for adult patients with thyroid nodules and differentiated thyroid cancer: the American Thyroid Association Guidelines Task Force on thyroid nodules and differentiated thyroid cancer. *Thyroid.* (2016) 26:1–133. doi: 10.1089/thy.2015.0020
4. Filetti S, Durante C, Hartl D, Leboulleux S, Locati LD, Newbold K, et al. Thyroid cancer: ESMO Clinical Practice Guidelines for diagnosis, treatment and follow-up. *Ann Oncol.* (2019) 30:1856–83. doi: 10.1093/annonc/mdz400
5. Ito Y, Onoda N, Okamoto T. The revised clinical practice guidelines on the management of thyroid tumors by the Japan Associations of Endocrine Surgeons: core questions and recommendations for treatments of thyroid cancer. *Endocr J.* (2020) 67:669–717. doi: 10.1507/endocrj.EJ20-0025
6. Sun W, Lan X, Zhang H, Dong W, Wang Z, He L, et al. Risk factors for central lymph node metastasis in CN0 papillary thyroid carcinoma: a systematic review and meta-analysis. *PLoS ONE.* (2015) 10:e0139021. doi: 10.1371/journal.pone.0139021
7. Luo Y, Jiang H, Xu W, Wang X, Ma B, Liao T, et al. Clinical, pathological, and molecular characteristics correlating to the occurrence of radioiodine refractory differentiated thyroid carcinoma: a systematic review and meta-analysis. *Front Oncol.* (2020) 10:549882. doi: 10.3389/fonc.2020.549882
8. Medas F, Canu GL, Cappellacci F, Boi F, Lai ML, Erdas E, et al. Predictive factors of lymph node metastasis in patients with papillary microcarcinoma of the thyroid: retrospective analysis on 293 cases. *Front Endocrinol.* (2020) 11:551. doi: 10.3389/fendo.2020.00551
9. Huang Y, Yin Y, Zhou W. Risk factors for central and lateral lymph node metastases in patients with papillary thyroid microcarcinoma: retrospective analysis on 484 cases. *Front Endocrinol.* (2021) 12:640565. doi: 10.3389/fendo.2021.640565
10. Robenshtok E, Neeman B, Reches L, Ritter A, Bachar G, Kaminer K, et al. Adverse histological features of differentiated thyroid cancer are commonly found in autopsy studies: implications for treatment guidelines. *Thyroid.* (2021) 32:37–45. Online ahead of print. doi: 10.1089/thy.2021.0268
11. Kluijfhout WP, Drake FT, Pasternak JD, Beninato T, Vriens MR, Shen WT, et al. Incidental positive lymph nodes in patients with papillary thyroid cancer is independently associated with recurrent disease. *J Surg Oncol.* (2017) 116:275–80. doi: 10.1002/jso.24680
12. Adam MA, Pura J, Goffredo P, Dinan MA, Reed SD, Scheri RP, et al. Presence

and number of lymph node metastases are associated with compromised survival for patients younger than age 45 years with papillary thyroid cancer. *J Clin Oncol.* (2015) 33:2370–5. doi: 10.1200/JCO.2014.59.8391
13. Wakayama A, Kudaka W, Matsumoto H, Aoyama H, Ooyama T, Taira Y, et al. Lymphatic vessel involvement is predictive for lymph node metastasis and an important prognostic factor in endometrial cancer. *Int J Clin Oncol.* (2018) 23:532–8. doi: 10.1007/s10147-017-1227-6
14. Moy AP, Mochel MC, Muzikansky A, Duncan LM, Kraft S. Lymphatic invasion predicts sentinel lymph node metastasis and adverse outcome in primary cutaneous melanoma. *J Cutan Pathol.* (2017) 44:734–9. doi: 10.1111/cup.12969
15. Ishikawa Y, Aida S, Tamai S, Akasaka Y, Kiguchi H, Akishima-Fukasawa Y, et al. Significance of lymphatic invasion and proliferation on regional lymph node metastasis in renal cell carcinoma. *Am J Clin Pathol.* (2007) 128:198–207. doi: 10.1309/0FT8WTDKREFHHP4P
16. Lee YJ, Huh JW, Shin JK, Park YA, Cho YB, Kim HC, et al. Risk factors for lymph node metastasis in early colon cancer. *Int J Colorectal Dis.* (2020) 35:1607–13. doi: 10.1007/s00384-020-03618-7
17. Oguma J, Ozawa S, Kazuno A, Yamamoto M, Ninomiya Y, Yatabe K, Makuuchi H, Ogura G. Prognostic impact of lymphovascular invasion in lymph node-negative superficial esophageal squamous cell carcinoma. *Dis Esophagus.* (2019) 32:doz001. doi: 10.1093/dote/doz001
18. Minig L, Fagotti A, Scambia G, Salvo G, Patrono MG, Haidopoulos D, et al. Incidence of lymph node metastases in women with low-risk early cervical cancer (<2 cm) without lymph-vascular invasion. *Int J Gynecol Cancer.* (2018) 28:788–93. doi: 10.1097/IGC.0000000000001236
19. So YK, Kim MJ, Kim S, Son YI. Lateral lymph node metastasis in papillary thyroid carcinoma: A systematic review and meta-analysis for prevalence, risk factors, and location. *Int J Surg.* (2018) 50:94–103. doi: 10.1016/j.ijsu.2017.12.029
20. Aydin Buyruk B, Kebapci N, Yorulmaz G, Buyruk A, Kebapci M. An evaluation of clinicopathological factors effective in the development of central and lateral lymph node metastasis in papillary thyroid cancer. *J Natl Med Assoc.* (2018) 110:384–90. doi: 10.1016/j.jnma.2017.07.007
21. Lim II, Hochman T, Blumberg SN, Patel KN, Heller KS, Ogilvie JB. Disparities in the initial presentation of differentiated thyroid cancer in a large public hospital and adjoining university teaching hospital. *Thyroid.* (2012) 22:269–74. doi: 10.1089/thy.2010.0385
22. Sun W, Zheng B, Wang Z, Dong W, Qin Y, Zhang H. Meta-analysis of risk factors for CCLNM in patients with unilateral cN0 PTC. *Endocr Connect.* (2020) 9:387–95. doi: 10.1530/EC-20-0058
23. Pontius LN, Youngwirth LM, Thomas SM, Scheri RP, Roman SA, Sosa JA. Lymphovascular invasion is associated with survival for papillary thyroid cancer. *Endocr Relat Cancer.* (2016) 23:555–62. doi: 10.1530/ERC-16-0123
24. Shin CH, Roh JL, Song DE, Cho KJ, Choi SH, Nam SY, et al. Prognostic value of tumor size and minimal extrathyroidal extension in papillary thyroid

carcinoma. *Am J Surg.* (2020) 220:925–31. doi: 10.1016/j.amjsurg.2020. 02.020

25. Haddad RI, Nasr C, Bischoff L, Busaidy NL, Byrd D, Callender G, et al. NCCN guidelines insights: thyroid carcinoma, version 2.2018. *J Natl Compr Canc Netw.* (2018) 16:1429–40. doi: 10.6004/jnccn.2018.0089

26. Leenhardt L. et al., 2013 European Thyroid Association Guidelines for cervical ultrasound scan and ultrasound-guided techniques in the postoperative management of patients with thyroid cancer. *Eur Thyroid J.* (2013) 2:147–59. doi: 10.1159/000354537

27. Mete O, Seethala RR, Asa SL, Bullock MJ, Carty SE, Hodak SP, et al. *College of American Pathologists: Protocol for the Examination of Specimens From Patients With Carcinomas of the Thyroid Gland.* (2019). Available online at: https://documents.cap.org/protocols/cp-endocrine-thyroid-19-4200.pdf (accessed January 10, 2022).

28. Wittekind C. *TNM Klassifikation maligner Tumoren.* Berlin: Springer (2020).

29. Mai KT, Truong LD, Ball CG, Olberg B, Lai CK, Purgina B. Lymphatic endothelial cancerization in papillary thyroid carcinoma: hidden evidence of lymphatic invasion. *Pathol Int.* (2015) 65:220–30. doi: 10.1111/pin.12272

30. Kovacevic B, Vucevic D, Cerovic S, Eloy C. Peripheral versus intraparenchymal papillary thyroid microcarcinoma: different morphologies and PD-L1 expression. *Head Neck Pathol.* (2021). doi: 10.1007/s12105-021-01337-1

31. Cheng SP, Lee JJ, Chien MN, Kuo CY, Jhuang JY, Liu CL. Lymphovascular invasion of papillary thyroid carcinoma revisited in the era of active surveillance. *Eur J Surg Oncol.* (2020) 46:1814–9. doi: 10.1016/j.ejso.2020.06.044

32. Dralle H, Musholt TJ, Schabram J, Steinmüller T, Frilling A, Simon D, et al. German Association of Endocrine Surgeons practice guideline for the surgical management of malignant thyroid tumors. *Langenbecks Arch Surg.* (2013) 398:347–75. doi: 10.1007/s00423-013-1057-6

33. Kahn C, Simonella L, Sywak M, Boyages S, Ung O, O'Connell D. Postsurgical pathology reporting of thyroid cancer in New South Wales, Australia. *Thyroid.* (2012) 22:604–10. doi: 10.1089/thy.2011.0501

34. Xu B. and Ghossein R, Critical prognostic parameters in the anatomic pathology reporting of differentiated follicular cell-derived thyroid carcinoma. *Cancers.* (2019) 11:1100. doi: 10.3390/cancers11081100

35. Zhang S, Zhang D, Yi S, Gong M, Lu C, Cai Y, et al. The relationship of lymphatic vessel density, lymphovascular invasion, and lymph node metastasis in breast cancer: a systematic review and meta-analysis. *Oncotarget.* (2017) 8:2863–73. doi: 10.18632/oncotarget.13752

36. Hu JQ, Wen D, Ma B, Zhang TT, Liao T, Shi X. et al. The extent of lymph node yield in central neck dissection can be affected by preoperative and intraoperative assessment and alter the prognosis of papillary thyroid carcinoma. *Cancer Med.* (2020) 9:1017–24. doi: 10.1002/cam4. 2762

37. Enyioha C, Roman SA, Sosa JA. Central lymph node dissection in patients with papillary thyroid cancer: a population level analysis of 14,257 cases. *Am J Surg.* (2013) 205:655–61. doi: 10.1016/j.amjsurg.2012.06.012

38. Nylén C, Eriksson FB, Yang A, Aniss A, Turchini J, Learoyd D, et al. Prophylactic central lymph node dissection informs the decision of radioactive iodine ablation in papillary thyroid cancer. *Am J Surg.* (2021) 221:886–92. doi: 10.1016/j.amjsurg.2020.08.012

39. Kim Y, Roh JL, Song D, Cho KJ, Choi SH, Nam SY, et al. Predictors of recurrence after total thyroidectomy plus neck dissection and radioactive iodine ablation for high-risk papillary thyroid carcinoma. *J Surg Oncol.* (2020) 122:906–13. doi: 10.1002/jso.26090

40. Alzahrani AS, Moria Y, Mukhtar N, Aljamei H, Mazi S, Albalawi L, et al. Course and predictive factors of incomplete response to therapy in low- and intermediate-risk thyroid cancer. *J Endocr Soc.* (2020) 5:bvaa178. doi: 10.1210/jendso/bvaa178

5

Analysis of Circulating Tumor Cells in a Triple Negative Spindle-Cell Metaplastic Breast Cancer Patient

Tania Rossi [1*], Michela Palleschi [2], Davide Angeli [3], Michela Tebaldi [3], Giovanni Martinelli [4],
Ivan Vannini [1], Maurizio Puccetti [5], Francesco Limarzi [6], Roberta Maltoni [7], Giulia Gallerani [1†]
and Francesco Fabbri [1†]

[1] Biosciences Laboratory, IRCCS Istituto Romagnolo per lo Studio dei Tumori (IRST) "Dino Amadori", Meldola, Italy,
[2] Department of Medical Oncology, IRCCS Istituto Romagnolo per lo Studio dei Tumori (IRST) "Dino Amadori", Meldola, Italy,
[3] Unit of Biostatistics and Clinical Trials, IRCCS Istituto Romagnolo per lo Studio dei Tumori (IRST) "Dino Amadori", Meldola,
Italy, [4] Scientific Directorate, IRCCS Istituto Scientifico Romagnolo per lo Studio dei Tumori (IRST) "Dino Amadori",
Meldola, Italy, [5] Azienda Unità Sanitaria Locale Imola, Imola, Italy, [6] Pathology Unit, Morgagni-Pierantoni Hospital, Forlì, Italy,
[7] Healthcare Administration, IRCCS Istituto Romagnolo per lo Studio dei Tumori (IRST) "Dino Amadori", Meldola, Italy

*Correspondence:
Tania Rossi
tania.rossi@irst.emr.it

[†] These authors have contributed
equally to this work and share last
authorship

Circulating tumor cells (CTCs) are a rare population of cells found in the bloodstream and represent key players in the metastatic cascade. Their analysis has proved to provide further core information concerning the tumor. Herein, we aim at investigating CTCs isolated from a 32-year-old patient diagnosed with triple negative spindle-shaped metaplastic breast cancer (MpBC), a rare tumor poorly responsive to therapies and with a dismal prognosis. The molecular analysis performed on the primary tumor failed to underline effective actionable targets to address the therapeutic strategy. Besides the presence of round-shaped CTCs, cells with a spindle shape were present as well, and through molecular analysis, we confirmed their malignant nature. This aspect was coherent with the primary tumor histology, proving that CTCs are released regardless of their morphology. Copy number aberration (CNA) profiling and variant analysis using next-generation sequencing (NGS) showed that these cells did not harbor the alterations exhibited by the primary tumor (*PIK3CA* G1049A mutation, *MYC* copy number gain). However, despite the great heterogeneity observed, the amplification of regions involved in metastasis emerged (8q24.22–8q24.23). Our findings support the investigation of CTCs to identify alterations that could have a role in the metastatic process. To the best of our knowledge, this is the first examination of CTCs in an MpBC patient.

Keywords: metaplastic breast cancer, circulating tumor cells, next generation sequencing, copy number aberration, metastasis, liquid biopsy

INTRODUCTION

Among all the breast malignancies, metaplastic breast cancer (MpBC) accounts for <1% and has a dismal prognosis, worse than the other BC types. Pathologically, MpBCs are ductal carcinomas composed by one or more cell populations that have undergone metaplastic transformation into a non-glandular pattern, leading to the presence of epithelial (e.g., squamous cells) and sarcomatous (e.g., chondroid, spindle cell, and osseous) elements. The World Health Organization (WHO) further divides MpBCs in subgroups, resulting in a plethora of chemorefractory and aggressive MpBC variants (1–3).

Despite the paucity of MpBC cases, some studies in literature have detected epithelial-to-mesenchymal transition (EMT), phosphoinositide 3-kinase (PI3K) signaling, epidermal growth factor receptor (EGFR) signaling, and others as the major altered pathways in this disease (3). Nevertheless, the lack of actionable targets remains a matter of concern, and conventional regimens of chemotherapy mainstay are the gold standards for treatment together with surgery and radiation therapy (4, 5). However, the poor survival and the high recurrence rates further emphasize the inadequacy of the available treatment options and the imperative need to individuate appropriate therapeutic strategies.

Genetic and phenotypic heterogeneity is a hallmark of MpBC and has important reflections for cancer treatment as the presence of multiple clones may hide cells responsible for relapse (6, 7). In this context, the characterization of circulating tumor cells (CTCs), a rare population of cells considered as pro-metastasis precursors (8), may be helpful in the unraveling of tumor heterogeneity (9).

We report a case of a patient diagnosed with triple negative spindle-cell MpBC for which molecular analysis of the primary tumor failed to highlight valid actionable alterations. We decided to characterize CTCs at both morphological and molecular levels, as they may bring out new alterations to be explored. To the best of our knowledge, this is the first examination of CTCs in a MpBC patient.

CASE PRESENTATION

Here we report the case of a 32-year-old patient (**Figure 1**) who presented, on December 20, 2018, during breastfeeding, a clinical onset of a right breast lump. Ultrasound-guided core biopsy of this right breast mass was performed with histological diagnosis of metaplastic spindle-cell infiltrating carcinoma of the breast, estrogen receptor (ER) = 0%, progesterone receptor (PgR) = 0%, HER2-neu negative (score 0), and Ki-67 = 90%. She had a past history of Crohn's disease, at the time of MpBC diagnosis during treatment with mesalamine. Positron emission tomography-computed tomography (PET-CT) revealed a 40-mm lesion in the right breast without bone or visceral involvement. In January 2019, treatment began with neoadjuvant chemotherapy (NAC) with adryamicin (60 mg/m^2) and cyclophosphamide (600 mg/m^2) intravenous for one cycle. Due to local progression, NAC was switched to docetaxel for one cycle (January 23, 2019), but the patient experienced further local progression.

In February 2019, she underwent right mastectomy with axillary node dissection; the histopathology exam describes a lesion of 65-mm maximum diameter, ypT3 ypN0 M0, ER = 0%, PgR = 0%, HER2-neu negative (score 0), and Ki-67 = 90%. The microscopic photograph (10× magnification) of hematoxylin and eosin staining of the resected tumor is reported in **Figure 2**. On immunostains, the tumor cells were strongly positive for vimentin and showed weak positivity for p63. Cytokeratins (AE1/AE3 clone) and E-cadherin were positive in scattered cells. Moreover, CAM5.2, calponin, SMA, GATA-3, ALK, ER, PR,

and Her2-neu were negative. Expression of programmed death-ligand 1 (PD-L1) was <1%.

From March to June 2019, she received adjuvant weekly paclitaxel (80 mg/m^2) for 12 cycles. From July to August 2019 right chest radiotherapy (total dose 50 Gy) was performed.

In November 2019, PET-CT scan revealed the presence of a 40 × 37-mm lung lesion and other sub-centimeter bilateral lung nodules. Further analyses on primary tumor revealed no BRCA1/BRCA2 alterations.

From November to December 2019, she received two cycles of cisplatin (60 mg/m^2; day 1), vinorelbine (20 mg/m^2; days 1 and 3), and capecitabine (500 mg thrice a day).

In January 2020, PET-CT showed lung, bone, and bilateral ovarian progression. The NGS Oncomine Focus Assay (Thermo Fisher Scientific) on the primary tumor exposed the G1049A PIK3CA mutation and amplification of the MYC locus (copy number: 26 copies).

In January 2020, she received two cycles of eribulin (1.23 mg/m^2), and in February, she underwent bilateral ovariectomy and wedge liver resection. The histopathology exam described triple negative metaplastic BC metastases. Moreover, several subcutaneous metastases on the scalp, neck, and chest arise, other than bilateral lung nodules. After multidisciplinary meeting, in consideration of the absence of valid therapeutic alternatives, physicians decided to start an "off-label" treatment regimen: doxorubicin (30 mg/m^2) plus bevacizumab (15 mg/kg every 3 weeks) plus everolimus (7.5 mg daily) (10).

In February 2020, she started the first cycle (without bevacizumab due to recent surgery), with a clinically stable disease, improvement on pain, and reduction of all subcutaneous nodules. Before chemotherapy administration, CTC investigation was performed.

In March 2020, she received the second cycle (including bevacizumab). She had a clinical benefit in terms of the disappearance of most subcutaneous metastases, no pain, and a good quality of life until April 2020 when she complained of fever, cough, and low blood pressure. Therefore, she was hospitalized for the appropriate treatment with antibiotics and steroids without benefit, and she died on April 21, 2020 due to respiratory failure.

ISOLATION OF CIRCULATING TUMOR CELLS AND ANALYSES

To investigate the features of CTCs, approximately 9 ml of peripheral blood was collected in a PAXGene Blood ccfDNA tube before the administration of the off-label therapy. CTCs were enriched from whole blood by immunomagnetic negative selection. In order to identify the highest number of CTCs, we opted for antibody cocktails for the detection of each phenotype, instead of a single target for each channel. EpCAM, CKs, and E-cadherin antibodies were used to identify epithelial phenotype (phycoerythrin, PE channel), and N-cadherin, ABCG2, CD44v6, and CD133 were used to identify stem/mesenchymal phenotype (allophycocyanin, APC channel). Hoechst 33342 (DAPI channel) was used for nuclear staining

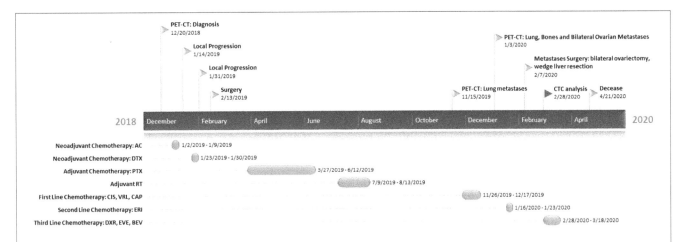

FIGURE 1 | Patient's timeline. At the top, we reported the milestones of her clinical course, while on the bottom the treatment regimens administered to the patient. PET-CT, positron emission tomography-computed tomography; AC, adryamicin-cyclophosphamide; DTX, docetaxel; PTX, paclitaxel; CIS, cisplatin; VRL, vinorelbine; CAP, capecitabine; ERI, eribulin; DXR, doxorubicin; EVE, everolimus; BEV, bevacizumab; CTC, circulating tumor cell.

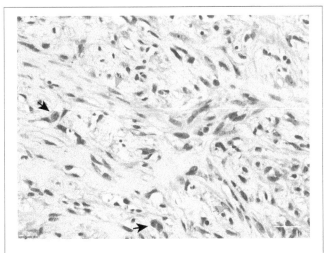

FIGURE 2 | Microscopic hematoxylin and eosin photograph of metaplastic breast carcinoma (MpBC) with coexisting spindled (green arrows) and oval (black arrows) cells. Scale bar: 50 μm.

and anti-CD45 Alexafluor488 antibody (FITC channel) as leukocyte marker for CTC negative selection. CTC identification and analysis were performed by DEPArray NxT platform (**Figure 3A**). To set up the auto-fluorescence signal detected in FITC channel, we used MCF7 cell line (CD45−) and leukocytes (CD45+) (**Supplementary Figure 1**).

We identified non-canonical cells positive for both epithelial and stem/mesenchymal targets with a spindle-shaped morphology ($n = 14$) and CTCs with a round-shaped morphology ($n = 184$). CTC clusters ($n = 5$) were present as well (**Supplementary Figure 2**). Due to the high amount of debris into the sample, we successfully sorted one single spindle-shaped cell (ID: 793) and two 10-CTC pools (Pool 1 and Pool 2).

Next, we aimed at assessing the molecular characteristics of the MpBC patient's CTCs isolated through DEPArray and to

establish the nature of the spindle-shaped cell. To do this, we massively amplified the genome of the samples using Ampli1 WGA kit (Menarini-Silicon Biosystems) to obtain evaluable genetic material, then we proceeded with library construction and sequencing for copy number aberrations (CNAs) and single nucleotide variant (SNV) analyses.

For CNAs, libraries were prepared using the Ampli1 LowPass kit for Ion Torrent (Menarini-Silicon Biosystems).

After Ion 520 chip loading was performed on Ion Torrent Chef (Thermo Fisher Scientific), sequencing was carried out on an Ion S5 System (Thermo Fisher Sc.), and CNAs were called with Control-FREEC (11). Through this technique, we were able to unequivocally establish the tumor nature of the unconventional spindle-shaped CTC (ID: 793), since it was characterized by an aneuploid genome with an altered CNA profile (**Figure 3B**). Through intersection bioinformatic analysis, we observed that the greatest part of the entire genome was not comparable among the three samples, suggesting high heterogeneity levels. We detected only three mutual aberrant regions (4p16.1, 8q24.22–8q24.23, and 22q12.3) shared among the samples, which were always in gain. The genes within the mentioned regions are reported in **Supplementary Table 1**. We did not observe the gain of *MYC* gene, which was observed in the primary tumor molecular characterization. Moreover, after whole genome amplification, we assessed the mutational status of 60 cancer-related genes. Libraries were prepared using the Ampli1 OncoSeek kit (Menarini Silicon Biosystems) and run on a 300-cycle V2 cartridge on the miSeq instrument (Illumina Inc.). We did not observe the *PIK3CA* mutation G1049A, which emerged at primary tumor NGS analysis. The single CTC 793 harbored the homozygous *RET* I602V and heterozygous M249V variant of gene *MAP2K1*. Interestingly, we also found a heterozygous synonymous C50C variant of *TP53* that, although not responsible for the amino acid change in protein structure, may be associated with gene expression regulation as it occurs in the noncoding exon 1 (12). Concerning the 10-CTC pools, in Pool 1, we found the variants *KRAS* S17I (frequency 80%),

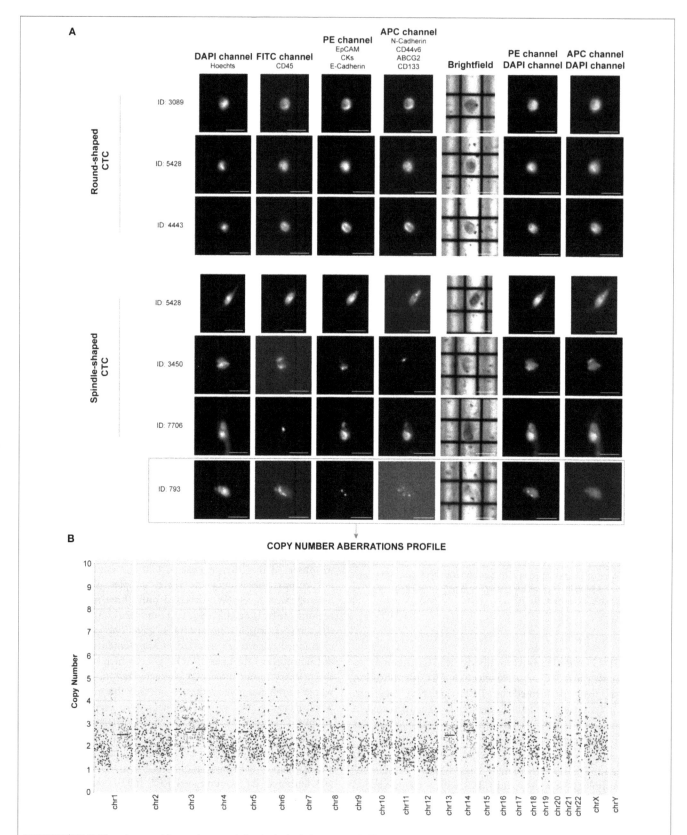

FIGURE 3 | (A) DEPArray images of the most representative single circulating tumor cells (CTCs) of the patient based on their shape (round- and spindle-shaped). The DAPI channel was used for nuclear staining using Hoechst 33342, PE channel for epithelial tag [anti-EPCAM, anti-cytokeratins (CKs) and anti-E-cadherin antibodies],

(Continued)

PIK3CA W498C (20%), *PTEN* A34T (16%), *MET* T835N (14%), *PIK3CA* L1026I (14%), *SMAD4* Q249R (10%), *KIT* G534V (10%), *MAP2K1* G131A and N122K (10%), and *PTEN* M35T (10%). Pool 2 harbored the *HRAS* frameshift deletion I46fs (20%) and the non-synonymous SNV of *RB1* R556G (10%). None of the detected variants were already described as pathogenic in literature, and no variants were identified in common among the samples. However, frequencies of some alterations found in samples Pool 1 and Pool 2 reveal that more than one cell within each pool harbor certain mutations.

DISCUSSION

Here, we report a case of a 32-year-old patient diagnosed with triple-negative spindle-cell MpBC, a rare disease with marked tendency to metastasize to secondary organs. Because of the paucity of cases, few is known about the molecular mechanisms underlying its aggressiveness, and no druggable targets have been identified yet.

Investigation of the primary tumor performed through an NGS-based approach detected alterations that are not uniquely ascribable to MpBC and failed to underline effective actionable targets to address the therapeutic strategy. Indeed, *MYC* copy number gain (13, 14) and *PIK3CA* mutation (15, 16) are widely described in the literature to be involved in many cancer types, including BC (17, 18). Herein, by exploiting a liquid biopsy approach, we emphasize that the characterization of CTCs, rare cells with a crucial role in the metastatic cascade, could be worthwhile to guide the investigation of the molecular mechanisms underlying rare tumors. However, this study has some weaknesses. First, due to the high amount of debris in the sample, it was not possible for us to recover, for downstream analysis, all the CTCs found. Moreover, the primary tumor and metastatic tissue specimens were not available, making impossible the comparison with CTCs, except for clinical reports. Conversely, to the best of our knowledge, this is the first investigation of CTCs in an MpBC case and could have a strong impact in the improvement of personalized medicine in the future. In fact, the investigation of CTCs has the potential to unmask the intra-tumor heterogeneity of MpBC, revealing the presence of under-represented clones from the primary tumor. Simultaneously, longitudinal molecular profiling of CTCs could reveal acquired resistance mechanism, helping to address the therapeutic strategy (19).

Our analysis revealed a high count of CTCs expressing both epithelial and mesenchymal markers in the peripheral blood of the MpBC patient. CTC enumeration and evaluation have been performed in a delayed period after removal of the primary tumor. Therefore, in the absence of their major source, CTCs are likely to come from secondary homing sites such as bone marrow or other occult niches (9, 20).

The first criterion concerned the different morphology of CTCs retrieved in the bloodstream of the patient. Along with the canonical round CTCs, we found unconventional cells characterized by a spindle morphology, whose nature was confirmed to be cancerous due to the presence of CNAs along the genome. A study by Yu et al., conducted on non-metaplastic BC patients, demonstrates that besides the presence of round-shaped CTCs with unconventional morphology associated with EMT initiation, therapy failure and tumor progression were present as well (21). However, it is not clear whether the presence of both round- and spindle-shaped CTCs in this MpBC case assumes the same meaning as in non-metaplastic BC, or is consistent with tumor histology solely. Indeed, the cytopathology of CTCs detected in this MpBC case is coherent with primary tumor histology, in which oval and spindle-shaped cells were shown to coexist. Thorough analysis on the metastatic site specimens would provide further information about the role of CTC morphology in MpBC tumor progression.

Concerning molecular analyses, we found that CTCs did not harbor primary tumor-specific alterations (*MYC* copy number gain and G1049A *PIK3CA* mutation). In addition, CTC samples had discordant CNAs and SNVs compared with each other, suggesting molecular heterogeneity as well. These results are consistent with the presence of circulating heterogeneous subclones with a potential role in tumor progression and resistance to therapies. Accordingly, in the HR-positive metastatic BC patient, CTCs could circulate as heterogeneous subclones and harbor molecular alterations that could drive to different mechanisms of resistance to endocrine therapies (22). Together with our data, these findings support the need to increase the application of CTCs in the clinical practice to gain further complementary information concerning the tumor evolution, including therapy resistance.

CNA profiling revealed the existence of three amplified genomic regions (4p16.1, 8q24.22–8q24.23, and 22q12.3) shared among the CTC samples. Among these, region 8q24.22–8q24.23 turned out to be highly attractive.

Amplification of chromosome 8q regions has been described in numerous cancer types, such as hepatocellular carcinoma (23), gastric cancer (24), clear cell renal carcinoma (25), and BC (26). In particular, in BC, 8q is considered a hotspot site of amplification associated with unfavorable prognosis (27) and, accordingly in our study, poor response to NAC (28), in part due to the location of c-myc locus in 8q24.1, near 8q24.22–8q24.23. However, the tendency to drive metastasis is not only imputable to *MYC* solely, but other genes have been hypothesized to enhance the metastatic process, as reported by Han and collaborators (28). Accordingly, investigation of CTCs revealed that several cancer-associated genes were found altered, but not *MYC*.

For instance, *WISP1* codifies for WNT1-inducible signaling pathway protein 1 (WISP1/CCN4), a member of the CCN family that acts as an oncogene in BC. It has been shown to stimulate EMT and metastasis, and to modulate the expression of the tumor suppressor N-myc downstream-regulated gene 1 (NDRG1) in BC cell lines. This modulation occurs through the NDGR1 gene promoter, which is located within the 8q24.23 site (29). However, the role of this tumor-suppressor protein is controversial, as recent data highlighted that NDRG1 expression is a predictor of worse prognosis in inflammatory BC patients receiving adjuvant radiotherapy (30). Both *WISP1* and *NDGR1* loci are included within the regions that we found in gain in all the CTC samples.

Another gene located in the 8q22.2 locus that recently emerged as a metastasis driver is the Otoconin 90 (*OC90*) gene. Although it is normally expressed in the cochlea for appropriate otolith development, its expression and gene amplification were observed in different cancer types, such as breast, prostate, and lung cancer. In TNBC cell lines, *OC90* overexpression was shown to increase invasion, and knockdown reduced cellular viability and invasiveness (31).

Taken together, despite high levels of heterogeneity, we observed that the analysis of CTCs at the molecular level can potentially drive to the discovery of chromosomal regions that may have a role in the metastatic cascade. In the future, this aspect could be helpful to deepen the knowledge regarding MpBC and to address new therapeutic strategies.

AUTHOR CONTRIBUTIONS

TR, MPa, GM, IV, GG, and FF contributed to the conceptualization and design of the study. TR and MPa wrote the first draft. DA and MT performed bioinformatic analysis. TR, MPa, MPu, FL, RM, and GG contributed to data collection. GG and FF reviewed the final draft before submission. All authors contributed to the manuscript revision, and read and approved the submitted version.

REFERENCES

1. Pezzi CM, Patel-Parekh L, Cole K, Franko J, Klimberg VS, Bland K. Characteristics and treatment of metaplastic breast cancer: analysis of 892 cases from the national cancer data base. *Ann Surg Oncol.* (2006) 14:166–73. doi: 10.1245/s10434-006-9124-7

2. Tray N, Taff J, Adams S. Therapeutic landscape of metaplastic breast cancer. *Cancer Treat Rev.* (2019) 79:101888. doi: 10.1016/j.ctrv.2019.08.004

3. Reddy TP, Rosato RR, Li X, Moulder S, Piwnica-Worms H, Chang JC. A comprehensive overview of metaplastic breast cancer: clinical features and molecular aberrations. *Breast Cancer Res.* (2020) 22:121. doi: 10.1186/s13058-020-01353-z

4. Chen IC, Lin CH, Huang CS, Lien HC, Hsu C, Kuo WH, et al. Lack of efficacy to systemic chemotherapy for treatment of metaplastic carcinoma of the breast in the modern era. *Breast Cancer Res Treat.* (2011) 130:345–51. doi: 10.1007/s10549-011-1686-9

5. Al-Hilli Z, Choong G, Keeney MG, Visscher DW, Ingle JN, Goetz MP, et al. Metaplastic breast cancer has a poor response to neoadjuvant systemic therapy. *Breast Cancer Res Treat.* (2019) 176:709–16. doi: 10.1007/s10549-019-05264-2

6. Geyer FC, Weigelt B, Natrajan R, Lambros MB, de Biase D, Vatcheva R, et al. Molecular analysis reveals a genetic basis for the phenotypic diversity of metaplastic breast carcinomas. *J Pathol.* (2010) 220:562–73. doi: 10.1002/path.2675

7. Kim C, Gao R, Sei E, Brandt R, Hartman J, Hatschek T, et al. Chemoresistance evolution in triple-negative breast cancer delineated by single-cell sequencing. *Cell.* (2018) 173:879–93.e13. doi: 10.1016/j.cell.2018.03.041

8. Yu T, Wang C, Xie M, Zhu C, Shu Y, Tang J, et al. Heterogeneity of CTC contributes to the organotropism of breast cancer. *Biomed Pharmacother.* (2021) 137:111314. doi: 10.1016/j.biopha.2021.111314

9. Rossi T, Gallerani G, Angeli D, Cocchi C, Bandini E, Fici P, et al. Single-cell NGS-based analysis of copy number alterations reveals new insights in circulating tumor cells persistence in early-stage breast cancer. *Cancers.* (2020) 12:2490. doi: 10.3390/cancers12092490

10. Basho RK, Yam C, Gilcrease M, Murthy RK, Helgason T, Karp DD, et al. Comparative effectiveness of an mTOR-based systemic therapy regimen in advanced, metaplastic and nonmetaplastic triple-negative breast cancer. *Oncologist.* (2018) 23:1300–9. doi: 10.1634/theoncologist.2017-0498

11. Boeva V, Popova T, Bleakley K, Chiche P, Cappo J, Schleiermacher G, et al. Control-FREEC: a tool for assessing copy number and allelic content using next-generation sequencing data. *Bioinformatics.* (2012) 28:423–5. doi: 10.1093/bioinformatics/btr670

12. Hainaut P, Pfeifer GP. Somatic TP53 mutations in the era of genome sequencing. *Cold Spring Harb Perspect Med.* (2016) 6:a026179. doi: 10.1101/cshperspect.a026179

13. Lee KS, Kwak Y, Nam KH, Kim D-W, Kang S-B, Choe G, et al. c-MYC copy-number gain is an independent prognostic factor in patients with colorectal cancer. *PLoS ONE.* (2015) 10:e0139727. doi: 10.1371/journal.pone.0139727

14. Ribeiro FR, Henrique R, Martins AT, Jerónimo C, Teixeira MR. Relative copy number gain of MYC in diagnostic needle biopsies is an independent prognostic factor for prostate cancer patients. *Eur Urol.* (2007) 52:116–25. doi: 10.1016/j.eururo.2006.09.018

15. Mei ZB, Duan CY, Li CB, Cui L, Ogino S. Prognostic role of tumor PIK3CA mutation in colorectal cancer: a systematic review and meta-analysis. *Ann Oncol.* (2016) 27:1836–48. doi: 10.1093/annonc/mdw264

16. Seo AN, Kang BW, Bae HI, Kwon OK, Park KB, Lee SS, et al. Exon 9 mutation of PIK3CA associated with poor survival in patients with Epstein-Barr virus-associated gastric cancer. *Anticancer Res.* (2019) 39:2145–54. doi: 10.21873/anticanres.13328

17. Nedeljković M, Tanić N, Dramićanin T, Milovanović Z, Šušnjar S, Milinković V, Vujović I, et al. Importance of copy number alterations of FGFR1 and C-MYC genes in triple negative breast cancer. *J Med Biochem.* (2019) 38:63–70. doi: 10.2478/jomb-2018-0012

18. Keraite I, Alvarez-Garcia V, Garcia-Murillas I, Beaney M, Turner NC, Bartos C, et al. PIK3CA mutation enrichment and quantitation from blood and tissue. *Sci Rep.* (2020) 10:17082. doi: 10.1038/s41598-020-74086-w

19. Alix-Panabières C, Pantel K. Clinical applications of circulating tumor cells and circulating tumor DNA as liquid biopsy. *Cancer Discov.* (2016) 6:479–91. doi: 10.1158/2159-8290.CD-15-1483

20. Banys M, Krawczyk N, Becker S, Jakubowska J, Staebler A, Wallwiener D, et al. The influence of removal of primary tumor on incidence and phenotype of circulating tumor cells in primary breast cancer. *Breast Cancer Res Treat.* (2012) 132:121–9. doi: 10.1007/s10549-011-1569-0

21. Yu M, Bardia A, Wittner BS, Stott SL, Smas ME, Ting DT, et al. Circulating breast tumor cells exhibit dynamic changes in epithelial and mesenchymal composition. *Science.* (2013) 339:580–4. doi: 10.1126/science.1228522

22. Paoletti C, Cani AK, Larios JM, Hovelson DH, Aung K, Darga EP, et al. Comprehensive mutation and copy number profiling in archived circulating breast cancer tumor cells documents heterogeneous resistance mechanisms. *Cancer Res.* (2018) 78:1110–22. doi: 10.1158/0008-5472.CAN-17-2686

23. Zhao K, Zhao Y, Zhu J-Y, Dong H, Cong W-M, Yu Y, et al. A panel of genes identified as targets for 8q24.13-24.3 gain contributing to unfavorable overall survival in patients with hepatocellular carcinoma. *Curr Med Sci.* (2018) 38:590–6. doi: 10.1007/s11596-018-1918-x

24. Kang JU. Chromosome 8q as the most frequent target for amplification in early gastric carcinoma. *Oncol Lett.* (2014) 7:1139–43. doi: 10.3892/ol.2014.1849

25. Klatte T, Kroeger N, Rampersaud EN, Birkhäuser FD, Logan JE, Sonn G, et al. Gain of chromosome 8q is associated with metastases and poor survival of patients with clear cell renal cell carcinoma. *Cancer.* (2012) 118:5777–82. doi: 10.1002/cncr.27607

26. Ching HC, Naidu R, Seong MK, Har YC, Taib NAM. Integrated analysis of copy number and loss of heterozygosity in primary breast carcinomas using high-density SNP array. *Int J Oncol.* (2011) 39:621–33. doi: 10.3892/ijo.2011.1081

27. Zhang Y, Martens JWM, Yu JX, Jiang J, Sieuwerts AM, Smid M, et al. Copy number alterations that predict metastatic capability of human breast cancer. *Cancer Res.* (2009) 69:3795–801. doi: 10.1158/0008-5472.CAN-08-4596

28. Han S, Park K, Shin E, Kim H-J, Kim JY, Kim JY, et al. Genomic change of chromosome 8 predicts the response to taxane-based neoadjuvant chemotherapy in node-positive breast cancer. *Oncol Rep.* (2010) 24:121–8. doi: 10.3892/or_00000836

29. Chiang K-C, Yeh C-N, Chung L-C, Feng T-H, Sun C-C, Chen M-F, et al. WNT-1 inducible signaling pathway protein-1 enhances growth and tumorigenesis in human breast cancer. *Sci Rep.* (2015) 5:8686. doi: 10.1038/srep08686

30. Villodre ES, Gong Y, Hu X, Huo L, Yoon EC, Ueno NT, et al. NDRG1 expression is an independent prognostic factor in inflammatory breast cancer. *Cancers.* (2020) 12:3711. doi: 10.3390/cancers12123711

31. Pearlman A, Rahman MT, Upadhyay K, Loke J, Ostrer H. Ectopic Otoconin 90 expression in triple negative breast cancer cell lines is associated with metastasis functions. *PLoS ONE.* (2019) 14:e0211737. doi: 10.1371/journal.pone.0211737

6

Long-Term Persisting SARS-CoV-2 RNA and Pathological Findings: Lessons Learnt from a Series of 35 COVID-19 Autopsies

Umberto Maccio[1], Annelies S. Zinkernagel[2], Reto Schuepbach[3], Elsbeth Probst-Mueller[4], Karl Frontzek[5], Silvio D. Brugger[2], Daniel Andrea Hofmaenner[3], Holger Moch[1] and Zsuzsanna Varga[1]*

[1] Department of Pathology and Molecular Pathology, University Hospital of Zürich, University of Zurich, Zurich, Switzerland, [2] Department of Infectious Diseases and Hospital Epidemiology, University Hospital of Zürich, University of Zurich, Zurich, Switzerland, [3] Institute of Intensive Care, University Hospital Zurich, University Hospital of Zürich, Zurich, Switzerland, [4] Department of Immunology, University Hospital of Zürich, Zurich, Switzerland, [5] Institute of Neuropathology, University Hospital Zurich, Zurich, Switzerland

*Correspondence:
Zsuzsanna Varga
zsuzsanna.varga@usz.ch

Background: Long-term sequelae of coronavirus disease 2019 (COVID-19), including the interaction between persisting viral-RNA and specific tissue involvement, pose a challenging issue. In this study, we addressed the chronological correlation (after first clinical diagnosis and postmortem) between severe acute respiratory syndrome coronavirus 2 (SARS-CoV-2) RNA and organ involvement.

Methods: The presence of postmortem SARS-CoV-2 RNA from 35 complete COVID-19 autopsies was correlated with the time interval between the first diagnosis of COVID-19 and death and with its relationship to morphologic findings.

Results: Severe acute respiratory syndrome coronavirus 2 (SARS-CoV-2) RNA can be evident up to 40 days after the first diagnosis and can persist to 94 hours after death. Postmortem SARS-CoV-2 RNA was mostly positive in lungs (70%) and trachea (69%), but all investigated organs were positive with variable frequency. Late-stage tissue damage was evident up to 65 days after initial diagnosis in several organs. Positivity for SARS-CoV-2 RNA in pulmonary swabs correlated with diffuse alveolar damage ($p = 0.0009$). No correlation between positive swabs and other morphologic findings was present. Cerebral ($p = 0.0003$) and systemic hemorrhages ($p = 0.009$), cardiac thrombi ($p = 0.04$), and ischemic events ($p = 0.03$) were more frequent in the first wave, whereas bacterial pneumonia ($p = 0.03$) was more prevalent in the second wave. No differences in biometric data, clinical comorbidities, and other autopsy findings were found.

Conclusions: Our data provide evidence not only of long-term postmortem persisting SARS-CoV-2 RNA but also of tissue damage several weeks after the first diagnosis of SARS-CoV-2 infection. Additional conditions, such as concomitant bacterial pulmonary superinfection, lung aspergillosis, thromboembolic phenomena, and hemorrhages can further worsen tissue damage.

Keywords: **COVID-19, long-COVID, SARS-CoV-2 RNA PCR, postmortal swabs, pulmonary superinfections, histopathology, autopsy**

INTRODUCTION

Coronavirus disease 2019 (COVID-19), caused by the beta coronavirus severe acute respiratory syndrome coronavirus 2 (SARS-CoV-2), has been spreading dramatically worldwide since first being reported in Wuhan, China in December 2019 (1).

More than 1 year and a half after the beginning of the pandemic, long-term health consequences of COVID-19 due to persisting SARS-CoV-2 and tissue damage represent an emerging problem, although the pathogenetic mechanisms and the epidemiology of the phenomenon are still largely unknown (2, 3).

COVID-19 can occur with a varying degree of severity (4, 5). Approximately, 33% of patients are asymptomatic (4). Of those who develop symptoms, around 81% experience mild disease, 14% a more severe disease (with respiratory distress), whereas a subset of around 5% of patients progresses to a critical condition (with respiratory insufficiency and/or multi-organ dysfunction) (5). Although the respiratory tract is the most commonly involved organ system (6), patients can also develop cardiovascular complications (7), thromboembolic phenomena (8) including thromboangiitis obliterans (9), several neurologic complications (10), gastroenterological symptoms (11), exuberant inflammatory manifestations (12, 13), and secondary infections (14–17), suggesting that COVID-19 is a systemic disease. The general infection fatality rate is estimated to be 0.68% (18), but it is strongly variable across studies and increases with age and underlying comorbidities (such as arterial hypertension and diabetes) (19, 20).

Long-COVID, in general, used to describe the persistence of symptoms in patients who have recovered from COVID-19, and which cannot be explained by an alternative diagnosis, is thought to occur in up to 10% of cases (21). However, proposals for new classifications aiming to differentiate between acute post-COVID, long post-COVID, and persistent long-COVID are emerging (22).

The pathogenesis of COVID-19 is not fully understood. The angiotensin-converting enzyme 2 (ACE2) and transmembrane protease serine 2 (TMPRSS2) have been shown to be the main receptor and the cofactor for the entry of the virus into the cells (23), but also basigin (CD147) as a receptor (24) and furin as a cofactor (25) play a pivotal role. After the viral attack, complex interplays between humoral and cellular immunity complement activation, cytokines, and coagulation-induced organ damage (26–29). As possible explanations for Long-COVID, several pathogenetic mechanisms, including persistent inflammatory damage, direct viral toxicity in tissues, and post-intensive care syndrome, have been proposed (3, 21).

Autopsies of patients who died from COVID-19 are crucial to gain a better understanding of how SARS-CoV-2 induces damage in human tissues and to consequently improve patient management and therapeutic strategies (30). At the beginning of the pandemic, only few autopsies were performed due to concerns about aerosolization and infectivity of the virus (31). More recently, in compliance with biosafety recommendations of several international regulatory agencies, including the World Health Organization (32), the Centers for Disease Control and Prevention (CDC) (33), and the European Center for Disease Prevention and Control (34), rapidly expanding autopsy literature has become available (35). Nevertheless, although some reports of late histological findings of patients with COVID-19 in the form of single case studies exist, to our knowledge, no autopsy-based studies focusing on the persistence of tissue damage and long-term consequence of SARS-CoV-2 infection have been reported (36).

Additionally, although some clinical studies comparing the first and the second waves of the COVID-19 pandemic exist (37, 38), no detailed autopsy-based studies analyzing the clinical and morphologic differences between the patients who died from COVID-19 in the first compared to the second pandemic wave have been published yet. Moreover, the use of postmortem swabs for detecting the presence of SARS-CoV-2 RNA in autoptic tissues, the postmortem viral distribution, their correlation with the time interval between diagnosis and death, as well as their correlation with morphologic findings have not been extensively studied (39–42).

In view of the foregoing, the aims of our study are: (1) To describe morphologic findings in different organs and tissues and investigate their prevalence. (2) To detect the prevalence of pulmonary superinfection caused by bacteria, viruses, or fungi in patients who died from COVID-19. (3) To analyze possible differences in all those findings between patients who died during the first or second wave of the pandemic. (4) To describe the distribution of SARS-CoV-2 RNA in different organs through postmortem swabs. (5) To correlate the positivity of the postmortem swabs with the time interval between diagnosis of SARS-CoV-2 and death, the incidence of the autoptic morphologic findings with the time interval between diagnosis and death, and the morphologic findings with the positivity of the swabs in the corresponding organs.

MATERIALS AND METHODS

Autopsy Cohort

Overall, 35 autopsies of patients with pre-mortem PCR-confirmed COVID-19 disease were performed at the Department of Pathology and Molecular Pathology of the University Hospital of Zürich, Switzerland.

Seven autopsies (7/35, 20%) were performed during the "first wave" of the COVID-19 pandemic, corresponding to deaths between March 2020 and May 2020. No COVID-19 autopsy was performed between June 2020 and September 2020. The other 28 autopsies (28/35, 80%) were performed during the "second wave" of the COVID-19 pandemic, corresponding to deaths from October 2020 to April 2021. This arbitrary distinction between first and second waves was based on the official classification of the Swiss Federal Office of Public Health and is currently used for comparative purposes by other studies (43, 44).

No cases attributable to any variants of concerns of SARS-CoV-2 according to the WHO definition belonged to this autopsies cohort (45).

Consent to perform the autopsy was given in all cases and the institutional review board (Department of Pathology and Molecular Pathology of the University Hospital Zurich, Switzerland) approved the study. Ethical aspects of research on autopsy tissue of deceased patients, postmortem diagnostics, and molecular analyses were covered in accordance with the Swiss Federal Research Regulations (BASEC Nr. 2020.1316).

Postmortem Examination and Swabs

All postmortem examinations were conducted in a biosafety Level 3 postmortem facility within an average of 33 hours after death (range, 3–93 hours). After a careful macroscopic examination and photographic documentation, several tissue sites were systematically sampled using a standardized protocol for histological, immunohistochemical, immunofluorescence, and ultrastructural examinations.

Samples for histology and immunohistochemistry were routinely taken from the brain, lungs, heart, liver, spleen, gut, kidney, bone marrow, testicle or ovary, and endocrine organs (pituitary, thyroid, and adrenal glands) and immediately fixed in 4% buffered formalin for 24 hours. Of one patient of the second wave, the brain was not examined according to the declared will of the corresponding relatives.

After paraffin inclusion and microtome sectioning, every histologic sample was processed with conventional stain (hematoxylin and eosin, H&E). Subsequently, the samples were independently examined by two experienced pathologists (U.M. and Z.V.) for major morphological alterations (e.g., inflammation type and distribution, distribution and type of thrombi, infarcts or ischemic changes, signs of superinfection, such as fungal elements or nuclear inclusion suspect of viral infection, major reactive changes, such as metaplasia or hyperplasia of pneumocytes type 2). There was perfect agreement between the two pathologists for every finding in all examined samples (Cohen's kappa coefficient = 1).

During autopsies of the "second wave," postmortem swabs for SARS-CoV-2-RNA PCR assays from different organs were performed. Postmortem swabs were obtained from a predefined selection of organs: one swab from tracheal secretions, two from the lung parenchyma (one per each lower lobe), one from the myocardium (left ventricle), one from the liver, one from the kidney, one from the small intestine, one from the spleen, and one from the testicles or ovaries. Of one patient, no postmortem swabs were performed, and of another patient only swabs from the lung, heart, and liver were available.

Additional postmortem swabs from the brain (superior frontal gyrus, right) of six patients and from the lamina cribrosa of four patients were available.

During the gross examination, the swabs were taken from each organ after a small sterile incision prior to the dissection of the organ. Access to tracheal fluid was obtained through a small sterile incision of the membranous tracheal part.

Samples were immediately collected in a viral transport medium (cobas® PCR Media, Roche Nr. 06466281190, serving as a nucleic acid stabilizing transport and a storage medium for human specimens) and transported to the Laboratory of Immunology of the University Hospital Zurich, where the presence of SARS-CoV-2 RNA was assessed via a real-time reverse PCR assay (cobas® SARS-CoV-2, Roche Nr. 09175431190), a fully automated test for nucleic acid extraction and purification followed by real-time PCR (RT-PCR). Together with the nucleic acid from the sample, the added internal control was simultaneously extracted by adding proteinase and lysis reagent. During the PCR, a sequence of the ORF1 a/b, which is unique to SARS-CoV-2, and a conserved region in the envelope E gene were amplified. The product generated can be measured by detecting the fluorescence. In case of a positive result, the Ct-value (cycle threshold) was indicated (**Supplementary Table 1**). The Ct-value refers to the number of cycles needed to amplify the viral RNA to reach the predetermined threshold. The lower the Ct value, the more viral RNA was in the sample. The threshold of Ct-value (ORF1 a/b), under which a sample was interpreted as positive, was 40.

In addition, clinical history (including main comorbidities), biometric data [age, gender (male/female)], and body mass index (BMI, in kg/m^2) of each patient who died during the first and second waves were recorded. Data were obtained from the hospital clinical charts or from the external clinical history submitted to the autopsy (**Table 1**).

Statistical Analyses

Demographic and biometric data from the first and second waves were compared using Student's t-test (for age and body mass index, after having found those data to be normally distributed using the Shapiro-Wilk's test, where $p > \alpha$, setting a significance level [α] of 0.05) or Fisher's exact test (for gender, applying this simple 2 x 2 contingency table with one degree of freedom: first vs. second wave/male vs. female) as statistical hypothesis tests.

A Student's t-test was also performed to compare the time interval between COVID-19 diagnosis and death between patients who died in the first and second waves (after having found the data to be normally distributed using the Shapiro-Wilk's test, where $p > \alpha$, setting a significance level [α] of 0.05).

TABLE 1 | General characteristic, comparison of the two different cohorts (first vs. second wave) and detailed autopsies' findings.

	Patients from first wave of pandemic ($n = 7$)	Patients from second wave of pandemic ($n = 28$)	p-value
Age (years)	69 (range 45–81)	71 (range 22–89)	0.71
M/F	4/7 (57%)	21/28 (75%)	0.38
BMI (kg/m²)	27.9 (21.6–37.8)	27.4 (17.6–43.6)	0.85
Main clinical comorbidities	Cancer (5/7, 71%)	Cancer (9/28, 32%)	0.089
	Arterial hypertension (5/7, 71%)	Arterial hypertension (19/28, 68%)	1.0
	Pulmonary disease (2/7, 28%)	Pulmonary disease (12/28, 43%)	0.68
	Diabetes mellitus (3/7, 43%)	Diabetes mellitus (4/28, 14%)	0.12
	Solid organ transplantation (2/7, 29%)	Solid organ transplantation (2/28, 7%)	0.17
	Bone Marrow transplantation (0/7, 0%)	Bone Marrow transplantation (2/28, 7%)	1.0
	Overweight (3/7, 43%)	Overweight (11/28, 39%)	1.0
	Obesity (2/7, 28%)	Obesity (7/28, 25%)	1.0
Time interval between diagnosis and death (days)	12 (2–20)	18 (1–65)	0.39
DAD	6/7 (86%)	18/28 (64%)	0.39
Bacterial Pneumonia	2/7 (29%)	21/28 (75%)	**0.03**
Lung aspergillosis	0/7 (0%)	6/28 (21%)	0.31
Viral Pneumonia	0/7 (0%)	1/28 (4%) (HSV1+CMV)	1.0
Macroscopic thrombi	General incidence (3/7, 43%)	General incidence (13/28, 46%)	1.0
	Cardiac ventricle (3/7, 43%)	Cardiac ventricle (2/28, 7%)	**0.04**
	Pulmonary central (0/7, 0%)	Pulmonary central (1/28, 4%)	1.0
	Pulmonary paracentral (0/7, 0%)	Pulmonary paracentral (7/28, 25%)	0.30
	Pulmonary peripheral (0/7, 0%)	Pulmonary peripheral (9/28, 32%)	0.1
	Peripheral veins (0/7, 0%)	Major peripheral vessels (3/28, 11%)	1.0
Microscopic fibrin thrombi	General incidence (4/7, 57%)	General incidence (13/28, 46%)	0.69
	Myocardial vessels (1/7, 14%)	Myocardial vessels (2/28, 7%)	0.50
	Pulmonary vessels (2/7, 29%)	Pulmonary vessels (12/28, 43%)	0.68
	Renal (0/7, 0%)	Renal (1/28, 4%)	1.0
	Cerebral vessels (1/7, 14%)	Cerebral vessels (2/28, 7%)	0.5
	Skin (1/7, 14%)	NA	
Leucocytes thrombi	General incidence (3/7, 43%)	General incidence (14/28, 50%)	1.0
	Cardiac (1/7, 14%)	Cardiac (4/28, 14%)	1.0
	Pulmonary (3/7, 43%)	Pulmonary (12/28, 43%)	1.0
	Hepatic (1/7, 14%)	Hepatic (0/28, 0%)	0.20
	Mesenterial (1/7, 14%)	Mesenterial (1/28, 4%)	0.36
Hemorrhages	General incidence (7/7, 100%)	General incidence (12/28, 43%)	**0.009**
	Brain microhemorrhages (6/7, 86%)	Brain microhemorrhages (3/28, 11%)	**0.0003**
	Subarachnoid (1/7, 14%)	Subarachnoid (2/28, 7%)	0.50
	Subdural hematoma (0/7, 0%)	Subdural hematoma (3/28, 11%)	1.0
	Lung (3/7, 43%)	Lung (5/28, 18%)	0.3
Infarcts/Ischemia	General incidence (6/7, 86%)	General incidence (10/28, 36%)	**0.03**
	Cardiac (1/7, 14%)	Cardiac (3/28, 11%)	1.0
	Lung (0/7, 0%)	Lung (5/28, 18%)	0.56
	Small intestine (2/7, 29%)	Small intestine (5/28, 18%)	0.61
	Liver (1/7, 14%)	Liver (8/28, 29%)	0.65
	Cerebral (2/7, 29%)	Cerebral (2/27, 7%)	0.18

M, male; F, female; DAD, diffuse alveolar damage; BMI, body mass index; HSV1, herpes simplex virus 1; CMV, cytomegalovirus; NA, not available. Bold values are the statistically significant results.

Fisher's exact test was also applied to compare the presence of relevant clinical comorbidities (such as cancer history, chronic pulmonary diseases, interstitial lung disease, chronic obstructive pulmonary disorder, pulmonary hypertension, diabetes mellitus, or arterial hypertension) and pathological findings (such as the presence of pulmonary superinfection, cerebral bleedings, etc., as listed in **Table 1**) between the two waves, applying a simple 2 x 2 contingency table with one degree of freedom (first vs. second wave/the presence of a specific pathologic finding vs. the absence of the same).

Point-Biserial Correlation calculator was applied to compare the positivity of postmortem swabs in each analyzed organ with the time interval between diagnosis and death as well as to compare the incidence of morphologic findings with the time interval between diagnosis and death.

Fisher's exact test was performed to correlate the morphologic findings with the positivity of the swabs in the corresponding organs (positive vs. negative swab/the presence of a specific finding in the organ vs. the absence of the same).

Given the exploratory nature of these analyses, no adjustment for multiple testing was performed.

RESULTS

Findings in Patients From the "First Wave"

The average age of the patients was 69 years (range, 45–81 years; standard deviation, 13 years). Four (4/7, 57%) were male, and three (3/7, 43%) were female. The mean time between diagnosis of COVID-19 disease and death was 12 days (range, 2–20 days; standard deviation, 7 days). All patients (7/7, 100%) had one or more chronic comorbidities (arterial hypertension, diabetes mellitus, cancer, overweight, and/or obesity the most common). Two (2/7, 29%) were normal weight (with a BMI between 18.5 and 24.9 kg/m^2, according to the current WHO classification), three (3/7, 43%) were overweight (BMI between 25.1 and 29.9 kg/m^2), one (1/7, 14%) was obese Grade I (BMI between 30 and 34.9 kg/m^2) and one (1/7, 14%) obese Grade II (BMI between 35 and 39.9 kg/m^2). Average BMI was 27.9 kg/m^2 (range, 21.6–37.8 kg/m^2; standard deviation, 5.9 kg/m^2). Two patients (2/7, 29%, all of whom were male) were solid organ transplant recipients (kidney transplantation 7 and 17 years before death, respectively). One patient was diagnosed with SARS-CoV-2-associated pneumonia 2 months before death, and was successfully treated with conservative therapy and did not require oxygen supplementation, but 1 month after the negativity of SARS-CoV-2 PCR developed a reactivation or reinfection with rapid progression to respiratory insufficiency and death.

Regarding neurological manifestations, one patient had a cerebellar hemorrhage during hospitalization (1/7, 14%), one a severe diffuse brain ischemia 2 days before death (1/7, 14%), and one had recurrent seizures 6 months before death (1/7, 14%). The other four patients (4/7, 57%) had no neurological disorders.

Autopsies were performed on average 33 hours after death (range, 18–56 hours).

The cause of death in six patients (6/7, 86%) was diffuse alveolar damage (DAD), whereas the patient with reactivation/reinfection (1/7, 14%) was found to have massive bacterial pneumonia but no DAD.

Altogether, histopathologic findings consistent with bacterial pneumonia were found in two patients (2/7, 29%), but no fungal or viral pneumonia could be demonstrated.

Three patients (3/7, 43%) had intraventricular macroscopic thrombi. Microscopic fibrin thrombi [in the coronary arteries (1/7, 14%), pulmonary capillaries (2/7, 29%), skin capillaries (1/7, 14%), and cerebral capillaries (1/7, 14%)] as well as leukocytes thrombi [in pulmonary (3/7, 43%), cardiac (1/7, 14%),

hepatic (1/7, 14%), and mesenterial capillaries (1/7, 14%)] were also common.

Several patients were also found to have hemorrhages [brain microhemorrhages (6/7, 86%), subarachnoid (1/7, 14%), and pulmonary (3/7, 43%)] and infarcts [small intestine (2/7, 29%) and liver (1/7, 14%)].

Constant adjunctive findings in the lungs were also, to a different degree, endotheliitis of capillaries, alveolar capillary macrophages, prominent hyperplasia of pneumocytes type 2, squamous metaplasia, interstitial edema, lymphocytic and histiocytic inflammation, fibrin-rich alveolar edema, and capillary stasis.

Details are summarized in **Table 1**. Representative images of the most important histopathological findings are shown in **Figures 1**, **2**, and **Supplementary Figure 1**.

Findings in Patients From the "Second Wave"

The average age of patients was 71 years (range, 22–89 years; standard deviation, 15 years). Twenty-one (21/28, 75%) were male, and seven (7/28, 25%) were female. The mean time between diagnosis of COVID-19 disease and death was 18 days (range, 1–65 days; standard deviation, 17 days). All patients (28/28, 100%) had one or more severe chronic comorbidities (arterial hypertension, chronic heart failure, cancer, diabetes mellitus, chronic lung disease [COPD (chronic obstructive pulmonary disease) and idiopathic pulmonary fibrosis], autoimmune diseases, chronic kidney disease, asthma, chronic liver disease, and overweight or obesity the most common).

Concerning neurological disorders, four patients had a history of previous ischemic strokes (4/28, 14%), three Alzheimer's disease or unspecified dementia (3/28, 11%), one mild cognitive impairment (1/28, 4%), two multiple cerebral metastases (2/28, 7%), two developed critical-illness neuromyopathy during hospitalization (2/28, 7%), two had a history of previous brain trauma (2/28, 7%), one developed diffuse hypoxic encephalopathy during hospitalization (1/28, 4%), and thirteen had no neurological disorders (13/28, 46%).

Two patients (2/28, 7%) were underweight (BMI < 18.5 kg/m^2, according to current WHO classification), eight (8/28, 29%) normal weight (BMI between 18.5 and 24.9 kg/m^2), 11 (11/28, 39%) overweight (with a BMI between 25.1 and 29.9 kg/m^2), three (3/28, 11%) obese Grade I (BMI between 30. and 34.9 kg/m^2), one (1/28%, 3%) obese Grade II (BMI between 35. and 39.9 kg/m^2), and three (3/28, 11%) were obese Grade III (BMI > 40 kg/m^2). Average BMI was 27.4 kg/m^2 (range, 17.6–43.6 kg/m^2; standard deviation, 7.2 kg/m^2).

All patients but one (27/28, 96%) were more than 55 years old at the time of death.

Autopsies were performed on average 33 hours after death (range, 3–93 hours).

Most important, autopsy findings in patients who died in the second wave were diffuse alveolar damage (DAD, 18/28, 64%), macrothrombi (general incidence, 13/28, 46%), microscopic fibrin thrombi (general incidence, 13/28, 46%), and leucocyte thrombi (general incidence, 14/28, 50%), hemorrhages

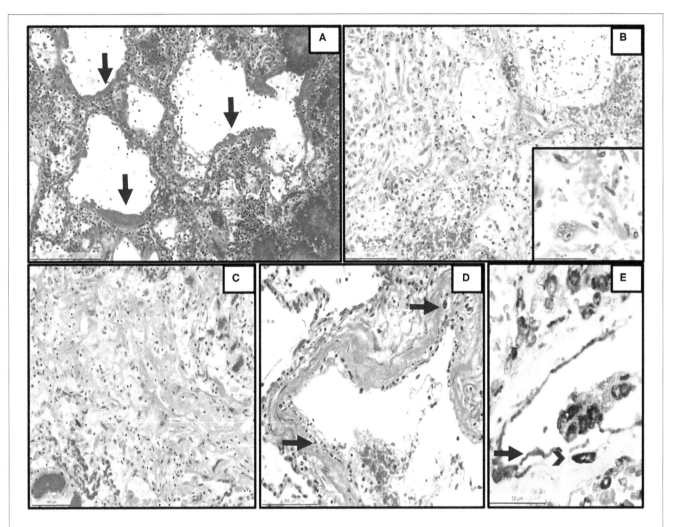

FIGURE 1 | Representative histopathological findings in autopsies from the first wave. **(A)** Lung tissue with diffuse alveolar damage in the exudative phase (hematoxylin and eosin (H&E), magnification 13 x, arrow: hyaline membranes). **(B)** Lung tissue with diffuse alveolar damage in the proliferative phase, which is defined by the presence of organization of the intra-alveolar and interstitial exudate, infiltration with chronic inflammatory cells, and interstitial myofibroblastic reaction. Proliferation and reactive atypias of type II cells are also noted (H&E, magnification 20 x). Inset: reactive pneumocytes type II, magnification 40 x). **(C)** Lung tissue with diffuse alveolar damage in the proliferative phase, showing an excessive collagen deposition (H&E, magnification 20 x). **(D)** Lung arterioles with endotheliitis, which is defined by the presence of subendothelial mononuclear inflammatory infiltrates (arrows) and damage of the endothelium (H&E, magnification 25 x) **(E)** Double immunohistochemistry [red: CD31 (endothelial marker), brown: CD68 (monocytic/macrophage marker)] of another representative case with endotheliitis shows endotheliitis of a venule in the lung with endothelial damage (arrow) and detachment with an associated mononuclear infiltrate (arrowhead) (H&E, magnification 28 x).

(in particular in cerebral parenchyma, subarachnoid and in the lung, with a general incidence of 12/28, 43%), lung infarcts (5/28, 18%), ischemia of small intestine (5/28, 18%, one among those also with angioinvasive candidiasis of the gut as complication), liver necrosis (8/28, 29%), and cerebral infarcts (2/27, 7%). Similar to patients who died in the first wave, constant adjunctive findings in the lungs were also, to a different degree, endotheliitis of capillaries, alveolar capillary macrophages, prominent hyperplasia of pneumocytes type 2, squamous metaplasia, interstitial edema, lymphocytic and histiocytic inflammation, fibrin-rich alveolar edema, and capillary stasis.

Details are summarized in **Table 1**. Representative images of the most important histopathological findings are shown in **Figures 3**, **4**. Additional details of the histopathological findings of this cohort are graphically illustrated in **Figures 5**, **6**.

Postmortem Swabs for SARS-CoV-2 RNA

Altogether, postmortem swabs were positive for SARS-CoV-2 RNA in the following organs/tissues with the following frequencies: trachea (18/26, 69%), lung (19/27, 70%), heart (8/27, 30%), liver (13/27, 48%), spleen (10/26, 38%), gut (9/26, 35%), kidney (13/26, 50%), testicles (9/19, 47%), ovary (1/7, 14%), brain (2/6, 33%), lamina cribrosa (3/4, 75%). Swabs for SARS-CoV-2 RNA were positive up to 39 days after the first diagnosis of COVID-19 (average, 18 days; range, 1–39 days) and up to 93 hours after deaths (average, 30 hours; range, 3–93 hours).

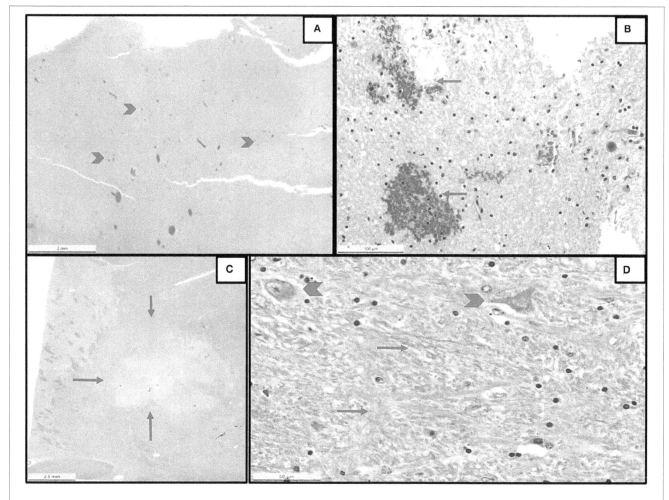

FIGURE 2 | Representative histopathological findings in autopsies from the first wave. **(A)** An overview of multifocal intracerebral microhemorrhages (arrowheads) in a sample from the brain stem (H&E, magnification 1.2 x). **(B)** The detail of image A with microhemorrhages (magnification 25 x, arrows: microhemorrhages). **(C)** An overview of acute brain infarction (arrows) in a sample from basal ganglia (H&E, magnification.62 x). **(D)** Details of image C showing red neurons (arrowheads) and beginning necrosis (arrows) of brain tissue (H&E, magnification 40 x).

Details are graphically shown in **Figures 7–9**, and information on Ct-values is provided in **Supplementary Table 1**.

Comparison Between the Two Waves
Demographic and Biometric Data
No difference concerning age ($p = 0.71$), time interval between diagnosis and death ($p = 0.39$), body mass index ($p = 0.86$), or gender ($p = 0.38$) between patients from the first and second waves could be demonstrated.

Clinical Comorbidities
An important comorbidity in patients who died in the first and second waves was a malignancy. Five patients from the first wave (5/7, 71%) and nine from the second wave (9/28, 32%) had an active or treated oncologic disease. Although cancer prevalence was slightly higher in the patients who died in the first than in the patients who died in the second wave, no statistically significant difference between the two groups could be demonstrated ($p = 0.089$).

A history of arterial hypertension was present in five patients of the first wave (5/7, 71%) and in 19 patients of the second wave (19/28, 68%), without statistically significant differences between the patients of the two waves.

Two patients (2/7, 28%) of the first wave had some form of pulmonary disease (COPD and lung hypertension), whereas 12 patients of the second wave (12/28, 43%) had a positive history of pulmonary disease [COPD, ILD (interstitial lung disease), lung hypertension or asthma)], but no difference in the prevalence of lung diseases between the two waves could be demonstrated ($p = 0.68$).

Three patients of the first wave (3/7, 43%) and four of the second wave (4/28, 14%) had diabetes mellitus. Although diabetes was slightly more common in the patients of the first wave, no statistically significant difference in the prevalence of diabetes between the two waves was found ($p = 0.12$).

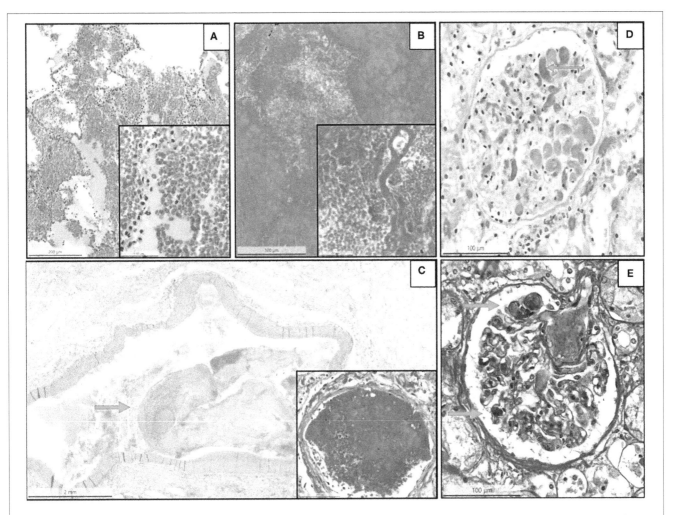

FIGURE 3 | Representative histopathological findings in autopsies from the second wave. **(A)** Acute pulmonary hemorrhage (H&E, magnification 10 x); the inset shows erythrocytes invading alveolar spaces (magnification 40 x). **(B)** Acute hemorrhagic pulmonary infarct (H&E, magnification 5 x); the inset shows a necrotic alveolar septum and hemorrhagic effusion in alveolar space (magnification 40 x). **(C)** Large thrombus (arrow) in a lung arteriole (H&E, magnification 1.4 x); the inset shows a fibrin thrombus in a lung capillary (magnification 28 x). **(D)** Glomerulus (kidney) with fibrin microthrombus (arrow) in a glomerular capillary (H&E, magnification 25 x). **(E)** Acid fuchsin orange G stain (AFOG-stain) shows several fibrin microthrombi (arrows) in the glomerular capillaries (magnification 25 x).

Autopsy Findings

No difference in the time interval between diagnosis of COVID-19 and death could be demonstrated between the patients who died in the first and in the second waves ($p = 0.39$). Moreover, although the finding of DAD was slightly more common in the patients who died in the first wave, no difference between the two cohorts could be identified ($p = 0.39$). Interestingly, the patients of the second wave showed significantly more often (21/28, 75%) bacterial pneumonia (defined histologically by the presence of a granulocytic inflammation with destruction of the lung parenchyma, with or without demonstrable microorganisms through Gram stain) than the patients of the first wave (2/7, 29%) ($p = 0.03$). Another important finding was lung aspergillosis, which was identified in six patients of the second wave (6/28, 21%) but none of the first wave (0/7, 0%), although the difference was not statistically significant ($p = 0.31$).

The general incidence of hemorrhages (independently from the organs considered) was significantly higher in the patients of the first wave (7/7, 100%) than in those of the second wave (14/28, 50%, $p = 0.009$). In more detail, microhemorrhages of the cerebral parenchyma were significantly more frequent among the patients of the first wave ($p = 0.0003$), but no statistically significant difference was observed with regard to hemorrhages in other organs. Similarly, the incidence of ischemic phenomena was significantly higher in the patients of the first wave (6/7, 86%) than in those of the second wave (10/28, 36%) ($p = 0.03$), although no statistically significant differences could be observed if the incidence of ischemic phenomena in the single organs or systems was considered. Intraventricular cardiac thrombi were also more frequent in the patients of the first wave ($p = 0.04$).

Details are demonstrated in **Table 1** and **Figure 10**.

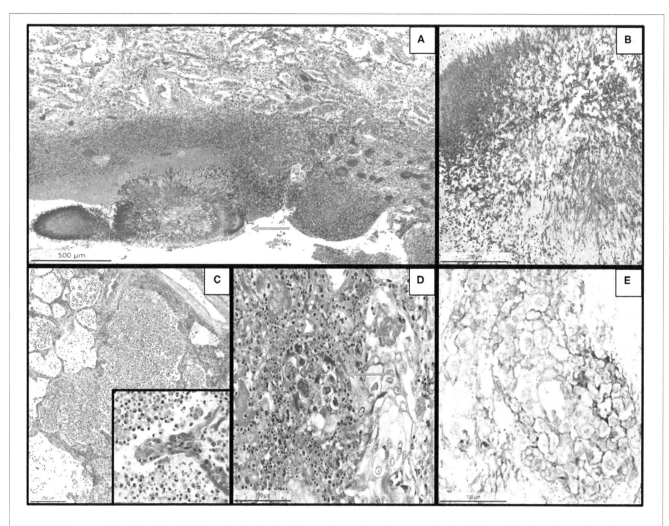

FIGURE 4 | Representative histopathological findings in autopsies from the second wave, illustrating examples of coinfections in the lung of the patients with coronavirus disease 2019 (COVID-19). **(A)** Lung tissue with aspergillosis (arrow) and surrounding acute inflammation (H&E, magnification 10 x). **(B)** Details of image A showing the typical hyphae of Aspergillus *spp*. (PAS, magnification 30 x). **(C)** Acute (bacterial) bronchopneumonia showing granulocytic exudate in the alveolar space and destruction of alveolar septa (H&E, magnification 6 x); the inset illustrates granulocytic inflammation with destruction of a septum (magnification 50 x). **(D)** Herpes simplex pneumonia exhibiting typical herpes-associated nuclear changes (molding, multinucleation, margination of chromatin, see the arrow) (H&E, magnification 25 x). **(E)** Immunohistochemistry for Herpes simplex virus demonstrates a granular cytoplasmic and nuclear positivity along with the typical nuclear changes (magnification 25 x).

Effect of Time Gap Between Diagnosis and Death

In the point-biserial correlation, a negative r between positivity of the postmortem swabs for SARS-CoV-2 RNA and the time interval between diagnosis and death was observed in all examined organs, but only in the lung ($p = 0.001$), trachea ($p = 0.02$), and liver ($p = 0.03$) this association was statistically significant (**Supplementary Table 2**).

A negative association between the time interval between diagnosis and death and the incidence of DAD and general incidence of infarcts (through a negative r in the point biserial correlation) could be demonstrated, although this difference was not statistically significant. In contrast, the association was positive (i.e., with increasing incidence by increasing the time interval between diagnosis and death) for bacterial pneumonia, lung aspergillosis, and general incidence of micro- and macrothrombi, and hemorrhages, but only the association with hemorrhages was statistically significant ($p = 0.012$) (**Supplementary Figure 2** and **Supplementary Table 3**).

The Effect of Positive Postmortem Swabs in Corresponding Organs

The correlation between morphologic findings and the presence of SARS-CoV-2 RNA in the corresponding postmortem tissues was statistically significant only for diffuse alveolar damage ($p = 0.0009$).

We have additionally divided the cases with a postmortem diagnosis of diffuse alveolar damage in two groups, according to the phase of diffuse alveolar damage (exudative vs. proliferative/organizing phase). No statistically significant

Long-Term Persisting SARS-CoV-2 RNA and Pathological Findings: Lessons Learnt from a Series...

47

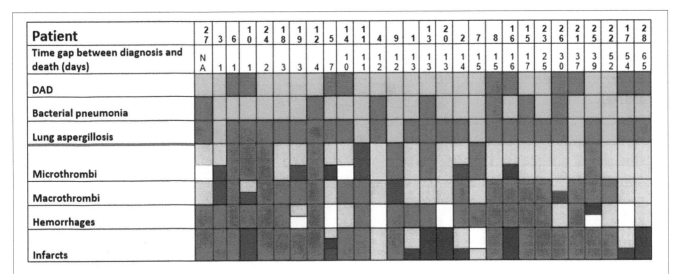

FIGURE 5 | Postmortem findings in the patients of the second wave (green: finding present, red: finding absent. Concerning micro- and macrothrombi, hemorrhages, and infarcts; the following colors to specify the anatomic localization are used: heart and/or major vessels = violet, lung = blue, brain/intracranial = yellow, liver/digestive tract = brown, kidney = orange). The patients are ordered from left to right in a crescent pattern based on the number of days between diagnosis of COVID-19 through nasopharyngeal swab and death. DAD, diffuse alveolar damage; NA, not available.

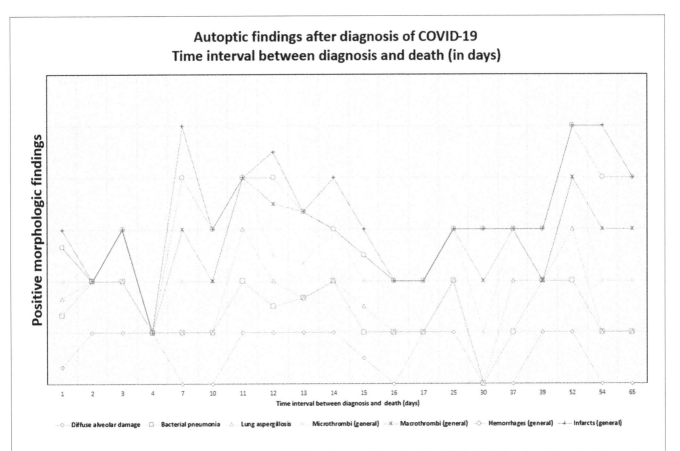

FIGURE 6 | Persistence of histopathologic findings in relation to the time interval between diagnosis and death (in days). The lines do not show absolute percentages but only the relative variation in prevalence of the findings. The different levels of the line along the y-axis are chosen to avoid their overlapping and to facilitate the visual interpretation but do not reflect an absolute percentage, for which we refer the reader to the text.

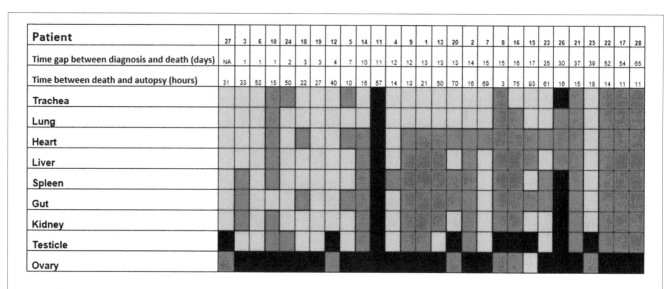

FIGURE 7 | Positivity of the postmortem swabs in the different organs (green: positive, red: negative, black: not available). The patients are ordered from left to right in a crescent pattern based on the number of days between diagnosis of COVID-19 through nasopharyngeal swab and death. Abbreviations: NA, not available.

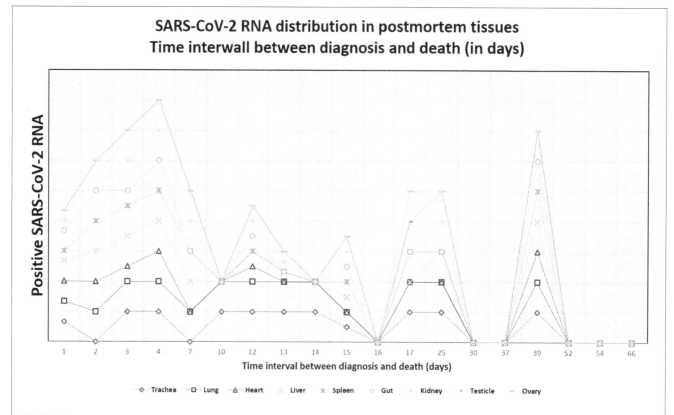

FIGURE 8 | The tendency of positivity of swabs for severe acute respiratory syndrome coronavirus 2 (SARS-CoV-2) RNA in relation to the time interval between diagnosis and death (in days). The lines do not show absolute percentages but only the relative variation in prevalence of the positivity for SARS-CoV-2 RNA. The different levels of the line along the y-axis are selected to avoid their overlapping and to facilitate the visual interpretation but do not reflect an absolute percentage, for which we refer the reader to the text.

association between the phase of diffuse alveolar damage and positivity for SARS-CoV-2 RNA in the lung tissue could be demonstrated (Fisher's exact test, $p = 0.53$). None of those patients had the fibrotic stage of diffuse alveolar damage.

(**Figure 5** and **Supplementary Tables 4, 5**).

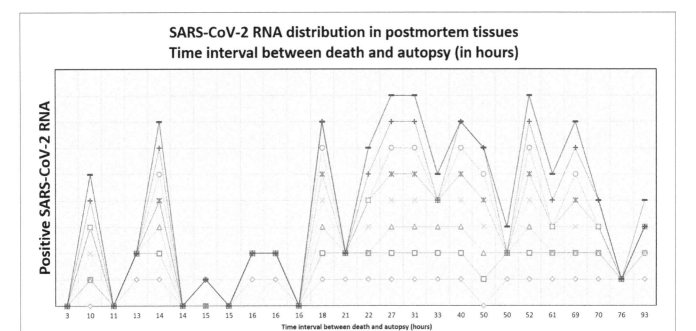

FIGURE 9 | The tendency of postmortem persistence and anatomical distribution of SARS-CoV-2 RNA in relation to the time interval between death and autopsy (postmortem interval, in hours). The lines do not show absolute percentages but only the relative variation in prevalence of the positivity for SARS-CoV-2 RNA. The different levels of the line along the y-axis are chosen to avoid their overlapping and to facilitate the visual interpretation but do not reflect an absolute percentage, for which we refer the reader to the text.

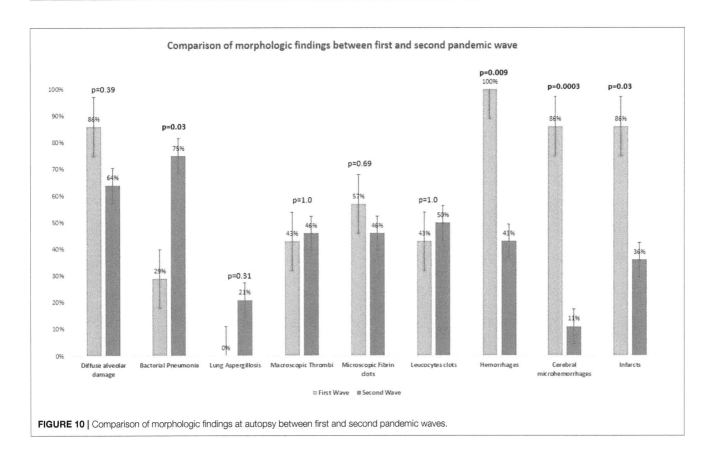

FIGURE 10 | Comparison of morphologic findings at autopsy between first and second pandemic waves.

DISCUSSION

Our data provide evidence of postmortem persisting SARS-CoV-2 RNA up to more than 1 month after the first COVID-19 diagnosis. Moreover, tissue damages, observed in this cohort as diffuse alveolar damage, systemic thromboembolic phenomena, ischemic damages, and hemorrhages, could also be demonstrated up to 2 months after the first diagnosis of SARS-CoV-2 infection. Of note, these morphologic findings can last longer than the persistence of SARS-CoV-2 RNA and can be frequently observed without evidence of SARS-CoV-2 RNA in the affected organs. There is a strong association between persistence of SARS-CoV-2 RNA in the lung and diffuse alveolar damage, but not between the persistence of SARS-CoV-2 RNA and other morphologic findings. In cases of diffuse alveolar damage, no statistically significant difference in the positivity of postmortem swabs for SARS-CoV-2 RNA in the lung could be observed between exudative and proliferative phases. Furthermore, we can show that additional conditions, such as concomitant bacterial pneumonia and lung aspergillosis, can occur at any point after the diagnosis of SARS-CoV-2 infection (ranging from very early, i.e., 1 day after diagnosis, to later, i.e., up to 2 months) and can worsen the tissue damage contributing to mortality and morbidity. Those findings together might suggest that tissue damage is not only and always dependent on direct viral effects but could also be mediated through several inflammatory mechanisms and may, therefore, corroborate the hypothesis of possible long-term persistence of COVID-19 in a subset of patients and thus contribute to the understanding of long-COVID disease. Nevertheless, we acknowledge that 35 autopsies represent a limited cohort compared to the total number of fatal cases of COVID-19 in our country, and that an autopsy-based cohort is exposed to too many biases (such as including just the patients with severe comorbidities in a hospital setting) to draw definitive conclusions on the pathogenesis of long-COVID. Moreover, additional studies are needed to explain how many of those morphologic findings (e.g., hemorrhages or infarcts) are directly related to SARS-CoV-2, to different therapies, or to the clinical settings of critically ill patients, as well as to better characterize harms and benefits of therapies.

This study shows that the most important autoptic findings in the patients who died from COVID-19 were diffuse alveolar damage (24/35, 69%) and concomitant bacterial pneumonia (23/35, 66%). Lung aspergillosis was also a relevant superinfection in many patients of the second wave (6/28, 21%), known as an important cause of death in critically ill patients. In general, the most important cause of death was diffuse alveolar damage, and, according to the interpretation provided in the autopsy report, SARS-CoV-2 was seen as the major responsible factor in death in most cases (26/35, 74%). In all other patients but one, bacterial pneumonia with or without concomitant lung aspergillosis was the main cause of death, and SARS-CoV-2 was a relevant comorbidity (8/35, 23%). Only one patient (1/35, 3%), aged 22, died from the complications of a myocardial infarction, and the concomitant SARS-CoV-2 infection did not contribute to mortality.

The biometric data, prevalence of clinical comorbidities, and morphologic findings of this autopsy-based cohort are in line with those reported in a recently published review by *Caramaschi et al.* on 58 studies on autopsies or biopsies of overall 662 patients with COVID-19, providing further confirmation of the spectrum and characteristics of this new disease (46).

To the best of our knowledge, no previous studies compared biometric and clinical data as well as autoptic findings between the first and second pandemic waves. Of note, only the general incidence of hemorrhages and of brain microhemorrhages was significantly higher among the patients of the first wave compared to those of the second wave (respectively, $p = 0.009$ and $p = 0.0003$). On this point, brain microhemorrhages in COVID-19 are well-known radiologic and autoptic findings (47–51) and are significantly more frequent in the patients with severe disease and in the ICU (intensive care unit) setting (52). According to the literature, their general incidence ranges from 6.9–54% (52), but, to our knowledge, no studies compare the incidence of cerebral microhemorrhages between the two waves. Nevertheless, caution is needed while interpreting these results; the first point to consider is a sampling bias, given the fact that the protocol for brain sampling was not as standardized as for other organs and the quantity of samples varies among autopsies.

Moreover, autopsy findings do not necessarily reflect the situation of critically ill patients, considering that an autoptic examination is performed only in a minor percentage of cases. However, the present result remains interesting and further confirms that COVID-19 is a systemic disease. Cerebral microhemorrhages are indeed a well-known complication in patients with severe COVID-19 and maybe associated with cerebral endotheliitis (35, 53), although they could also be observed in critically ill patients without COVID-19 in the context of critical illness-associated microbleeds (CRAM) (54). Again, those considerations are of utmost importance when evaluating the harms and benefits of different therapies in severe COVID-19.

The association between severe COVID-19 and bacterial superinfection as well as lung aspergillosis has already been reported in the literature, although the incidence varies among studies (55–57). In our cohort, the incidence of bacterial pneumonia was significantly higher in the second wave. Moreover, the patients of the second wave developed lung aspergillosis more frequently, but this difference was not statistically significant. Among others, a possible explication for these differences is the use of dexamethasone as standard therapy in severe COVID-19 during the second pandemic wave. Given the small number of patients of this cohort, only speculations are possible, and larger studies are necessary to validate this hypothesis.

Apart from that, no statistically significant difference between the patients of the first and of the second pandemic wave concerning age, gender prevalence, body mass index, time interval between diagnosis of SARS-CoV-2 and death, prevalence of main comorbidities, and of most autoptic findings was demonstrated. However, due to the small sample size of the entire cohort, no substantial differences between the first and second waves can be drawn and additional studies, in particular, metanalyses might be necessary to better understand the epidemiologic differences between the pandemic waves.

In patients of the second wave, postmortem swabs were most positive in the lung (70%) and the trachea (69%). SARS-CoV-2 RNA could be detected up to 93 hours after death. The persistence of SARS-CoV-2 RNA several hours and even days after death is a described phenomenon in several organs (58–60), and has been detected up to 35 days after death according to one case report (61). A possible limitation in the interpretation of these results might be that positive SARS-CoV-2 RNA does not necessarily reflect the presence of the virus in the tissues. Actually, false-positive results are reported to occur in about 2% of cases in living patients (62), being contamination during collection procedures, extraction or amplification (e.g., through aerosolization in containment hood), or cross-reaction with other viruses (e.g., other Coronaviruses), some of the factors which might contribute to false-positive RT-PCR results (63). Postmortem RT-PCR for SARS-CoV-2 in tissues of the upper respiratory tract has shown a sensitivity of 96.8% and a specificity ranging from 94.2 to 97.5% (64), so that false-positive and false-negative results should be taken into account. Even a true positive result does not always reflect a viable virus. A surrogate estimating virus viability may be the ct-value of the RT-PCR test: a study by *Jaafar et al.* showed that the culture of the virus is successful up to a ct-value of 25 (70%), but at a ct-value of 30, this value drops to 20%, and values above 35 are associated with only a low likelihood of successful culture (3%) (65). In virtue of these considerations, additional studies to assess virus viability from autopsy tissues are needed.

Of note, in the second wave, typical histological signatures of COVID-19, such as endotheliitis, leucocytic- or fibrin-thrombi, could be demonstrated also in organs where no SARS-CoV-2 RNA was detected through postmortem swabs and in the patients in whom SARS-CoV-2 was not the main cause of death. Moreover, in our cohort, apart from diffuse alveolar damage, no significant correlation was found between swabs' positivity and morphologic findings. These findings further support the role of indirect and persisting viral damage rather than a direct viral effect of SARS-CoV-2 (27, 65, 66).

This result partially agrees with an autopsy-based study of *Skok et al.*, where no correlation between viral load and severity of organ damages at autopsy was found (41).

In our cohort, there was an inverse association between the time elapsed from diagnosis and death and the positivity of swabs in the organs (i.e., the more time passes, the less frequent positivity is observed), but this was statistically significant only for the lung, the trachea, and the liver. Despite this tendency, we found positive postmortem swabs in different organs also in the patients who were diagnosed with COVID-19 several days before, and one patient had positive swabs of trachea, lung, heart, gut, liver, and kidney even 39 days after the diagnosis. Importantly, we found a statistically significant correlation between SARS-CoV-2 RNA evidence in swabs in the lungs and the occurrence of diffuse alveolar damage ($p = 0.0009$), but the association between other morphologic findings and positivity of the swabs in the corresponding organs was not statistically significant.

Up to date, postmortem viral tropism and dynamics through swab examinations have not been characterized in detail. Two autopsy-based studies of *Skok et al.* investigated the presence of SARS-CoV-2 RNA on different organs at autopsy and found a systemic distribution of the virus (in the throat, lung, intestine, and brain) and morphologic findings in line with ours (41, 42).

Another autopsy-based study of *Deinhardt-Emmer et al.*, including 11 patients who died from COVID-19, described the viral distribution through postmortem swabs performed in a relatively short time interval after death (mean, 5.6 hours; range, 1.5–15 hours). The authors demonstrated a systemic involvement with the highest viral load in the lungs and hypothesized a topological correlation of viral load and histopathological damage in the lung (39).

In general, our results on postmortem swabs and morphologic findings are in line with the aforementioned autopsy-based studies, providing further confirmation of the systemic nature of COVID-19 and of the tropism of SARS-CoV-2 for different organs. Moreover, the lack of correlation between the presence of SARS-CoV-2 RNA in tissues and morphologic findings seems again to confirm an inflammatory-mediated process, rather than direct viral damage, as already postulated in the literature (66–70).

In summary, SARS-CoV-2 RNA persists in different organs several weeks after the first diagnosis of COVID-19. Macroscopic and histologic pieces of evidence of tissue damage in critically ill patients can be demonstrated up to 2 months thereafter both in organs with and without postmortem evidence of SARS-CoV-2 RNA. Cerebral microhemorrhages were statistically more frequent in the patients of the first pandemic wave. Postmortem SARS-CoV-2 RNA showed a systemic distribution, with the highest prevalence in the lungs and trachea. There is a significant correlation between the presence of SARS-CoV-2 RNA and diffuse alveolar damage in the lungs, but no other correlation with other autoptic findings.

AUTHOR CONTRIBUTIONS

UM designed the study, collected samples, analyzed morphologic data, performed statistical analyses, interpreted clinical and pathological data, and drafted the article. AZ designed the study, interpreted clinical and pathological data, and drafted the article. RS designed the study, interpreted clinical and pathological data, and drafted the article. EP-M performed PCR analyses on postmortem swabs, interpreted clinical and pathological data, and drafted the article. KF, SB, and DH interpreted clinical and pathological data and drafted the article. HM designed the study, analyzed morphologic data, interpreted clinical and pathological data, and drafted the article. ZV designed the study, analyzed morphologic data, interpreted clinical and pathological data, drafted the article, and coordinated the cooperation among the authors. All the authors were involved in critical reading, writing the article, and had final approval of the submitted and published version.

ACKNOWLEDGMENTS

The authors thank the following contributions to the study: Mrs. Daniela Meir, Mrs. Annabelle Marks, and Mr. Fabian Baron for the excellent technical assistance in the postmortem analyses and to all the patients' families who approved performing the autopsies.

SUPPLEMENTARY MATERIAL

Supplementary Figure 1 | Details of **Figures 2C,D** (cerebral tissue from basal ganglia). Inset 1: Luxol-stain demonstrates myelin loss (magnification 25 x). Inset 2: immunostaining for NF70/200 (magnification 25 x) demonstrates loss of axons: as such, myelin loss should be interpreted as secondary to infarction and not as demyelination. Inset 3: Luxol-stain in a control case from the same anatomical region (basal ganglia) without myelin loss. Inset 4: immunostaining for NF70/200 in a control case from the same anatomical region (basal ganglia) without loss of axons.

Supplementary Figure 2 | Comparison between morphologic findings and positivity of postmortem swabs in the corresponding organs. The patients are ordered from up to down in a crescent pattern based on the number of days between diagnosis of COVID-19 through nasopharyngeal swab and death. Interpretation: green = finding present with positive swab; blue = finding present with negative swab; red = finding absent with positive swab; black = finding absent with negative swab. NA, not available; DAD, diffuse alveolar damage; BP, bacterial pneumonia; LA, lung aspergillosis; MiT, microthrombi; MaT, Macrothrombi; LH, lung hemorrhages; LI, lung infarcts; MI, myocardial infarction.

REFERENCES

1. Zhu N, Zhang D, Wang W, Li X, Yang B, Song J, et al. A novel coronavirus from patients with pneumonia in China, 2019. *N Engl J Med.* (2020) 382:727–33. doi: 10.1056/NEJMoa2001017

2. Huang C, Huang L, Wang Y, Li X, Ren L, Gu X, et al. 6-month consequences of COVID-19 in patients discharged from hospital: a cohort study. *Lancet.* (2021) 397:220–32. doi: 10.1016/S0140-6736(20)32656-8

3. Nalbandian A, Sehgal K, Gupta A, Madhavan MV, McGroder C, Stevens JS, et al. Post-acute COVID-19 syndrome. *Nat Med.* (2021) 27:601–15. doi: 10.1038/s41591-021-01283-z

4. Oran DP, Topol EJ. The proportion of SARS-CoV-2 infections that are asymptomatic: a systematic review. *Ann Intern Med.* (2021) 174:655–62. doi: 10.7326/M20-6976

5. Wu Z, McGoogan JM. Characteristics of and important lessons from the coronavirus disease 2019. (COVID-19) outbreak in china: summary of a report of 72314 cases from the chinese center for disease control and prevention. *JAMA.* (2020) 323:1239–42. doi: 10.1001/jama.2020.2648

6. Grant MC, Geoghegan L, Arbyn M, Mohammed Z, McGuinness L, Clarke EL, et al. The prevalence of symptoms in 24,410 adults infected by the novel coronavirus (SARS-CoV-2; COVID-19): A systematic review and meta-analysis of 148 studies from 9 countries. *PLoS ONE.* (2020) 15:e0234765. doi: 10.1371/journal.pone.0234765

7. Wang D, Hu B, Hu C, Zhu F, Liu X, Zhang J, et al. Clinical characteristics of 138 hospitalized patients with 2019 novel coronavirus-infected pneumonia in Wuhan, China. *JAMA.* (2020) 323:1061–9. doi: 10.1001/jama.2020.1585

8. Helms J, Tacquard C, Severac F, Leonard-Lorant I, Ohana M, Delabranche X, et al. High risk of thrombosis in patients with severe SARS-CoV-2 infection: a multicenter prospective cohort study. *Intensive Care Med.* (2020) 46:1089–98. doi: 10.1007/s00134-020-06062-x

9. Luo W YH, Gou J, Li X, Sun Y, Li J, Liu L. Clinical pathology of critical patient with novel coronavirus pneumonia (COVID-19). *Preprints.* (2020).

10. Liotta EM, Batra A, Clark JR, Shlobin NA, Hoffman SC, Orban ZS, et al. Frequent neurologic manifestations and encephalopathy-associated morbidity in Covid-19 patients. *Ann Clin Transl Neurol.* (2020) 7:2221–30. doi: 10.1002/acn3.51210

11. Wiersinga WJ, Rhodes A, Cheng AC, Peacock SJ, Prescott HC. Pathophysiology, Transmission, Diagnosis, and Treatment of Coronavirus Disease 2019. (COVID-19): A Review. *JAMA.* (2020) 324:782–93. doi: 10.1001/jama.2020.12839

12. Huang C, Wang Y, Li X, Ren L, Zhao J, Hu Y, et al. Clinical features of patients infected with 2019 novel coronavirus in Wuhan, China. *Lancet.* (2020) 395:497–506. doi: 10.1016/S0140-6736(20)30183-5

13. Mehta P, McAuley DF, Brown M, Sanchez E, Tattersall RS, Manson JJ, et al. COVID-19: consider cytokine storm syndromes and immunosuppression. *Lancet.* (2020) 395:1033–4. doi: 10.1016/S0140-6736(20)30628-0

14. Bartoletti M, Pascale R, Cricca M, Rinaldi M, Maccaro A, Bussini L, et al. Epidemiology of invasive pulmonary aspergillosis among COVID-19 intubated patients: a prospective study. *Clin Infect Dis.* (2020).

15. Rawson TM, Moore LSP, Zhu N, Ranganathan N, Skolimowska K, Gilchrist M, et al. Bacterial and fungal coinfection in individuals with coronavirus: a rapid review To support COVID-19 antimicrobial prescribing. *Clin Infect Dis.* (2020) 71:2459–68. doi: 10.1093/cid/ciaa530

16. Sepulveda J, Westblade LF, Whittier S, Satlin MJ, Greendyke WG, Aaron JG, et al. Bacteremia and blood culture utilization during COVID-19 surge in New York City. *J Clin Microbiol.* (2020) 58. doi: 10.1128/JCM.00875-20

17. Buehler PK, Zinkernagel AS, Hofmaenner DA, Wendel Garcia PD, Acevedo CT, Gomez-Mejia A, et al. Bacterial pulmonary superinfections are associated with longer duration of ventilation in critically ill COVID-19 patients. *Cell Rep Med.* (2021) 2:100229. doi: 10.1016/j.xcrm.2021.100229

18. Meyerowitz-Katz G, Merone L, A. systematic review and meta-analysis of published research data on COVID-19 infection fatality rates. *Int J Infect Dis.* (2020) 101:138–48. doi: 10.1016/j.ijid.2020.09.1464

19. Zhou F, Yu T, Du R, Fan G, Liu Y, Liu Z, et al. Clinical course and risk factors for mortality of adult inpatients with COVID-19 in Wuhan, China: a retrospective cohort study. *Lancet.* (2020) 395:1054–62. doi: 10.1016/S0140-6736(20)30566-3

20. Onder G, Rezza G, Brusaferro S. Case-Fatality Rate and Characteristics of Patients Dying in Relation to COVID-19 in Italy. *JAMA.* (2020) 323:1775–6. doi: 10.1001/jama.2020.4683

21. Greenhalgh T, Knight M. A'Court C, Buxton M, Husain L. Management of post-acute Covid-19 in primary care. *BMJ.* (2020) 370:m3026. doi: 10.1136/bmj.m3026

22. Fernandez-de-Las-Penas C, Palacios-Cena D, Gomez-Mayordomo V, Cuadrado ML, Florencio LL. Defining post-COVID symptoms (Post-Acute COVID, long COVID, persistent post-COVID): an integrative classification. *Int J Environ Res Public Health.* (2021) 18. doi: 10.3390/ijerph18052621

23. Hoffmann M, Kleine-Weber H, Schroeder S, Kruger N, Herrler T, Erichsen S, et al. SARS-CoV-2 cell entry depends on ACE2 and TMPRSS2 and Is blocked by a clinically proven protease inhibitor. *Cell.* (2020) 181:271–80 e8. doi: 10.1016/j.cell.2020.02.052

24. Wang K, Chen W, Zhang Z, Deng Y, Lian JQ, Du P, et al. CD147-spike protein is a novel route for SARS-CoV-2 infection to host cells. *Signal Transduct Target Ther.* (2020) 5:283. doi: 10.1038/s41392-020-00426-x

25. Walls AC, Park YJ, Tortorici MA, Wall A, McGuire AT, Veesler D. Structure, Function, and Antigenicity of the SARS-CoV-2 Spike Glycoprotein. *Cell.* (2020) 183:1735. doi: 10.1016/j.cell.2020.11.032

26. Chauhan AJ, Wiffen LJ, Brown TP. COVID-19: A collision of complement, coagulation and inflammatory pathways. *J Thromb Haemost.* (2020) 18:2110–7. doi: 10.1111/jth.14981

27. Hu B, Huang S, Yin L. The cytokine storm and COVID-19. *J Med Virol.* (2021) 93:250–6. doi: 10.1002/jmv.26232

28. Lee S, Channappanavar R, Kanneganti TD. Coronaviruses: innate immunity,

inflammasome activation, inflammatory cell death, and cytokines. *Trends Immunol.* (2020) 41:1083–99. doi: 10.1016/j.it.2020.10.005

29. Lo MW, Kemper C, Woodruff TM. COVID-19: Complement, coagulation, and collateral damage. *J Immunol.* (2020) 205:1488–95. doi: 10.4049/jimmunol.2000644

30. Sekhawat V, Green A, Mahadeva U. COVID-19 autopsies: conclusions from international studies. *Diagn Histopathol (Oxf).* (2021) 27:103–7. doi: 10.1016/j.mpdhp.2020.11.008

31. Salerno M, Sessa F, Piscopo A, Montana A, Torrisi M, Patane F, et al. No Autopsies on COVID-19 Deaths: A Missed Opportunity and the Lockdown of Science. *J Clin Med.* (2020) 9. doi: 10.3390/jcm9051472

32. Organisation WH. Infection prevention and control for the safe management of a dead body in the context of COVID-19: interim guidance, 24 March 2020. Available online at: https://appswhoint/iris/handle/10665/331538. (2020).

33. (CDC). CfDCaP. Collection and submission of postmortem specimens from deceased persons with known or suspected COVID-19, March 2020. (Interim guidance) (2020). Available online at: https://wwwcdcgov/coronavirus/2019-ncov/hcp/guidance-postmortem-specimenshtml (2020).

34. Control ECfDPa. Considerations related to the safe handling of bodies of deceased persons with suspected or confirmed COVID-19. Available online at: https://wwwecdceuropaeu/en/publications-data/considerations-related-safe-handling-bodies-deceased-persons-suspected-or (2020).

35. Satturwar S, Fowkes M, Farver C, Wilson AM, Eccher A, Girolami I, et al. Postmortem findings associated with SARS-CoV-2: systematic review and meta-analysis. *Am J Surg Pathol.* (2021) 45:587–603. doi: 10.1097/PAS.0000000000001650

36. Croci GA, Vaira V, Trabattoni D, Biasin M, Valenti L, Baselli G, et al. Emergency lung transplantation after COVID-19: immunopathological insights on two affected patients. *Cells.* (2021) 10. doi: 10.3390/cells10030611

37. Palmieri L, Palmer K, Lo Noce C, Meli P, Giuliano M, Floridia M, et al. Differences in the clinical characteristics of COVID-19 patients who died in hospital during different phases of the pandemic: national data from Italy. *Aging Clin Exp Res.* (2021) 33:193–9. doi: 10.1007/s40520-020-01764-0

38. Soriano V, Ganado-Pinilla P, Sanchez-Santos M, Gomez-Gallego F, Barreiro P, de Mendoza C, et al. Main differences between the first and second waves of COVID-19 in Madrid, Spain. *Int J Infect Dis.* (2021) 105:374–6. doi: 10.1016/j.ijid.2021.02.115

39. Deinhardt-Emmer S, Wittschieber D, Sanft J, Kleemann S, Elschner S, Haupt KF, et al. Early postmortem mapping of SARS-CoV-2 RNA in patients with COVID-19 and the correlation with tissue damage. *Elife.* (2021) 10. doi: 10.7554/eLife.60361

40. Dell'Aquila M, Cattani P, Fantoni M, Marchetti S, Aquila I, Stigliano E, et al. Postmortem swabs in the severe acute respiratory syndrome coronavirus 2 pandemic: report on 12 complete clinical autopsy cases. *Arch Pathol Lab Med.* (2020). 144(11):1298-302. doi: 10.5858/arpa.2020-0362-SA

41. Skok K, Stelzl E, Trauner M, Kessler HH, Lax SF. Post-mortem viral dynamics and tropism in COVID-19 patients in correlation with organ damage. *Virchows Arch.* (2021) 478:343–53. doi: 10.1007/s00428-020-02903-8

42. Skok K, Vander K, Setaffy L, Kessler HH, Aberle S, Bargfrieder U, et al. COVID-19 autopsies: Procedure, technical aspects and cause of fatal course. *Experiences from a single-center Pathol Res Pract.* (2021) 217:153305. doi: 10.1016/j.prp.2020.153305

43. Coronavirus ac. Available online at: https://www.bag.admin.ch/bag/en/home/krankheiten/ausbrueche-epidemien-pandemien/aktuelle-ausbrueche-epidemien/novel-cov.html

44. Wolfisberg S, Gregoriano C, Struja T, Kutz A, Koch D, Bernasconi L, et al. Comparison of characteristics, predictors and outcomes between the first and second COVID-19 waves in a tertiary care centre in Switzerland: an observational analysis. *Swiss Med Wkly.* (2021) 151:w20569. doi: 10.4414/smw.2021.20569

45. WHO. WHO. SARS-CoV-2 variants. (2021). Available online at: https://wwwwhoint/en/activities/tracking-SARS-CoV-2-variants/

46. Caramaschi S, Kapp ME, Miller SE, Eisenberg R, Johnson J, Epperly G, et al. Histopathological findings and clinicopathologic correlation in COVID-19: a systematic review. *Mod Pathol.* (2021). doi: 10.1038/s41379-021-00814-w

47. Chougar L, Shor N, Weiss N, Galanaud D, Leclercq D, Mathon B, et al. Retrospective observational study of brain MRI findings in patients with acute SARS-CoV-2 infection and neurologic manifestations. *Radiology.* (2020)

297:E313–E23. doi: 10.1148/radiol.2020202422

48. Egbert AR, Cankurtaran S, Karpiak S. Brain abnormalities in COVID-19 acute/subacute phase: A rapid systematic review. *Brain Behav Immun.* (2020) 89:543–54. doi: 10.1016/j.bbi.2020.07.014

49. Kantonen J, Mahzabin S, Mayranpaa MI, Tynninen O, Paetau A, Andersson N, et al. Neuropathologic features of four autopsied COVID-19 patients. *Brain Pathol.* (2020) 30:1012–6. doi: 10.1111/bpa.12889

50. Kremer S, Lersy F, de Seze J, Ferre JC, Maamar A, Carsin-Nicol B, et al. Brain MRI findings in severe COVID-19: A retrospective observational study. *Radiology.* (2020) 297:E242–E51. doi: 10.1148/radiol.2020202222

51. Lin E, Lantos JE, Strauss SB, Phillips CD, Campion TR. Jr., Navi BB, et al. Brain imaging of patients with COVID-19: findings at an academic institution during the height of the outbreak in New York City. *AJNR Am J Neuroradiol.* (2020) 41:2001–8. doi: 10.3174/ajnr.A6793

52. Choi Y, Lee MK. Neuroimaging findings of brain MRI and CT in patients with COVID-19: A systematic review and meta-analysis. *Eur J Radiol.* (2020) 133:109393. doi: 10.1016/j.ejrad.2020.109393

53. Kirschenbaum D, Imbach LL, Rushing EJ, Frauenknecht KBM, Gascho D, Ineichen BV, et al. Intracerebral endotheliitis and microbleeds are neuropathological features of COVID-19. *Neuropathol Appl Neurobiol.* (2021) 47:454–9. doi: 10.1111/nan.12677

54. Fanou EM, Coutinho JM, Shannon P, Kiehl TR, Levi MM, Wilcox ME, et al. Critical Illness-Associated Cerebral Microbleeds. *Stroke.* (2017) 48:1085–7. doi: 10.1161/STROKEAHA.116.016289

55. Nori P, Cowman K, Chen V, Bartash R, Szymczak W, Madaline T, et al. Bacterial and fungal coinfections in COVID-19 patients hospitalized during the New York City pandemic surge. *Infect Control Hosp Epidemiol.* (2021) 42:84–8. doi: 10.1017/ice.2020.368

56. Dudoignon E, Camelena F, Deniau B, Habay A, Coutrot M, Ressaire Q, et al. Bacterial pneumonia in COVID-19 critically ill patients: a case series. *Clin Infect Dis.* (2021) 72:905–6. doi: 10.1093/cid/ciaa762

57. Lansbury L, Lim B, Baskaran V, Lim WS. Co-infections in people with COVID-19: a systematic review and meta-analysis. *J Infect.* (2020) 81:266–75. doi: 10.1016/j.jinf.2020.05.046

58. El Bouzidi K, Howard M, Ali H, Khan M, Harris A, Zuckerman M. 'Test, test, test' even after death: persistence of SARS-CoV-2 RNA in postmortem nasopharyngeal swabs. *J Clin Pathol.* (2020). doi: 10.1136/jclinpath-2020-207091

59. Sawant OB, Singh S, Wright RE. 3rd, Jones KM, Titus MS, Dennis E, et al. Prevalence of SARS-CoV-2 in human post-mortem ocular tissues. *Ocul Surf.* (2021) 19:322–9. doi: 10.1016/j.jtos.2020.11.002

60. Servadei F, Mauriello S, Scimeca M, Caggiano B, Ciotti M, Anemona L, et al. Persistence of SARS-CoV-2 Viral RNA in nasopharyngeal swabs after death: an observational study. *Microorganisms.* (2021). 9. doi: 10.3390/microorganisms9040800

61. Beltempo P, Curti SM, Maserati R, Gherardi M, Castelli M. Persistence of SARS-CoV-2 RNA in post-mortem swab 35 days after death: A case report. *Forensic Sci Int.* (2021) 319:110653. doi: 10.1016/j.forsciint.2020.110653

62. Braunstein GD, Schwartz L, Hymel P, Fielding J. False positive results with SARS-CoV-2 RT-PCR tests and how to evaluate a RT-PCR-positive test for the possibility of a false positive result. *J Occup Environ Med.* (2021) 63:e159–e62. doi: 10.1097/JOM.0000000000002138

63. Skittrall JP, Wilson M, Smielewska AA, Parmar S, Fortune MD, Sparkes D, et al. Specificity and positive predictive value of SARS-CoV-2 nucleic acid amplification testing in a low-prevalence setting. *Clin Microbiol Infect.* (2021). 27:469 e9–e15. doi: 10.1016/j.cmi.2020.10.003

64. Hall JA, Harris RJ, Emmett HE, Lowe B, Singanayagam A, Twohig KA, et al. On the sensitivity and specificity of postmortem upper respiratory tract testing for SARS-CoV-2. *J Infect Dis.* (2021) 224:389–94. doi: 10.1093/infdis/jiab270

65. Jaafar R, Aherfi S, Wurtz N, Grimaldier C, Van Hoang T, Colson P, et al. Correlation between 3790 quantitative polymerase chain reaction-positives samples and positive cell cultures, including 1941. Severe acute respiratory syndrome coronavirus 2 isolates. *Clin Infect Dis.* (2021) 72:e921. doi: 10.1093/cid/ciab531

66. England JT, Abdulla A, Biggs CM, Lee AYY, Hay KA, Hoiland RL, et al. Weathering the COVID-19 storm: Lessons from hematologic cytokine syndromes. *Blood Rev.* (2021) 45:100707. doi: 10.1016/j.blre.2020.100707

67. Karki R, Sharma BR, Tuladhar S, Williams EP, Zalduondo L, Samir P, et al. Synergism of TNF-alpha and IFN-gamma triggers inflammatory cell death,

tissue damage, and mortality in SARS-CoV-2 infection and cytokine shock syndromes. *Cell.* (2021). 184:149–68 e17. doi: 10.1016/j.cell.2020.11.025

68. Nicosia RF, Ligresti G, Caporarello N, Akilesh S, Ribatti D. COVID-19 Vasculopathy: mounting evidence for an indirect mechanism of endothelial injury. *Am J Pathol.* (2021). doi: 10.1016/j.ajpath.2021.05.007

69. Ragab D, Salah Eldin H, Taeimah M, Khattab R, Salem R. The COVID-19 cytokine storm; what we know so far. *Front Immunol.* (2020) 11:1446. doi: 10.3389/fimmu.2020.01446

70. Zhang J, Wu H, Yao X, Zhang D, Zhou Y, Fu B, et al. Pyroptotic macrophages stimulate the SARS-CoV-2-associated cytokine storm. *Cell Mol Immunol.* (2021) 18:1305–7. doi: 10.1038/s41423-021-00665-0

7

Ferroptosis in Intrahepatic Cholangiocarcinoma: IDH1^{105GGT} Single Nucleotide Polymorphism is Associated with its Activation and Better Prognosis

Samantha Sarcognato[1]*, Diana Sacchi[1], Luca Fabris[2], Giacomo Zanus[3,4], Enrico Gringeri[4], Monia Niero[1], Giovanna Gallina[1] and Maria Guido[1,5]

[1] Department of Pathology, Azienda ULSS2 Marca Trevigiana, Treviso, Italy, [2] Department of Molecular Medicine – DMM, University of Padova, Padova, Italy, [3] 4th Surgery Unit, Azienda ULSS2 Marca Trevigiana, Treviso, Italy, [4] Department of Surgery, Oncology and Gastroenterology – DISCOG, University of Padova, Padova, Italy, [5] Department of Medicine – DIMED, University of Padova, Padova, Italy

*Correspondence:
Samantha Sarcognato
samantha.sarcognato@
aulss2.veneto.it

Objectives: Intrahepatic cholangiocarcinoma (ICC) has a dismal prognosis and often demonstrates an anti-apoptotic landscape, which is a key step to chemotherapy resistance. Isocitrate dehydrogenase 1 or 2 (*IDH1-2*)-mutated ICCs have been described and associated with better prognosis. Ferroptosis is a regulated iron-mediated cell death induced by glutathione peroxidase 4 (GPX4) inhibition, and may be triggered pharmacologically. GPX4 is overexpressed in aggressive cancers, while its expression is inhibited by *IDH1^{R132C}* mutation in cell lines. We investigated tissue expression of ferroptosis activation markers in ICC and its correlation with clinical-pathological features and *IDH1-2* status.

Materials and Methods: We enrolled 112 patients who underwent hepatic resection or diagnostic liver biopsy for ICC. Immunostaining for transferrin-receptor 1 and GPX4, and Pearls' stain for iron deposits were performed to evaluate ferroptosis activation. Immunostaining for STAT3 was performed to study pro-inflammatory and anti-apoptotic landscape. Main *IDH1-2* mutations were investigated in 90 cases by real-time polymerase chain reaction.

Results: GPX4 overexpression was seen in 79.5% of cases and related to poor histological prognostic factors (grading and perineural and vascular invasion; $p < 0.005$ for all) and worse prognosis (OS $p = 0.03$; DFS $p = 0.01$). STAT3 was expressed in 95.5% of cases, confirming the inflammation-related anti-apoptotic milieu in ICC, and directly related to GPX4 expression ($p < 0.0001$). A high STAT3 expression correlated to a worse prognosis (OS $p = 0.02$; DFS $p = 0.001$). Nearly 12% of cases showed *IDH1^{105GGT}* single nucleotide polymorphism, which was never described in ICC up to now, and was related to lower tumor grade ($p < 0.0001$), longer overall survival ($p = 0.04$), and lower GPX4 levels ($p = 0.001$).

Conclusion: Our study demonstrates for the first time that in most inflammatory ICCs ferroptosis is not active, and its triggering is related to *IDH1-2* status. This supports the possible therapeutic role of ferroptosis-inducer drugs in ICC patients, especially in drug-resistant cases.

Keywords: intrahepatic cholangiocarcinoma, ferroptosis, *IDH1*^{105GGT} single nucleotide polymorphism, STAT3, GPX4

INTRODUCTION

Intrahepatic cholangiocarcinoma (ICC) is the second most common primary liver tumor, whose incidence and mortality have increased worldwide over the last decades (1–6). Because of a frequent diagnosis at an advanced stage, ICC prognosis remains dismal. Surgical resection is the only potentially curative treatment option, but recurrence rates remain high. Patients with metastatic or unresectable disease undergo palliative non-curative systemic therapies, with only modest increases in overall survival and frequent development of chemoresistance, often due to an escape from drug-induced apoptosis by cancer cells (1, 3–5, 7, 8).

Advances have been made in the last decade regarding ICC molecular background. In particular, Sia et al. identified two molecular subclasses, named the proliferative and the inflammation-related classes (9). The latter is defined by the triggering of pro-inflammatory signaling pathways *via* different interleukins and the signal transducer and activator of transcription 3 (STAT3) protein (4, 9). STAT3 is involved in several cellular processes, inhibits apoptosis, and it is known to play a role in many cancer types, being associated with a worse prognosis (4, 10–13).

A subgroup of ICCs showing missense mutations in the isocitrate dehydrogenase 1 and 2 (*IDH1-2*) genes has also been described (14, 15). *IDH*-mutated ICCs exhibit high expression of mitochondrial genes and low expression of chromatin modifier genes and were demonstrated to have a better prognosis than cases with wild type *IDH1-2* (3, 4, 14–17).

Ferroptosis is a newly described form of regulated iron-mediated cell death type, whose activation requires high intracytoplasmic iron concentrations and the inhibition of the reduced glutathione (GSH)-dependent enzyme glutathione peroxidase 4 (GPX4) (18, 19). GPX4 overexpression has been described in many aggressive cancers, making it a potential therapeutic target able to promote death in drug-tolerant tumor cells. Many molecules currently exist that are able to trigger the ferroptotic cascade, known as ferroptosis inducers, either by decreasing GSH levels, such as erastin, or by directly inhibiting GPX4 activity, such as RSL3. Some of them are currently under investigation in clinical trials for cancer treatment (19, 20). So far, no data are reported in literature regarding the possible role of ferroptosis and ferroptosis inducers in ICC.

An *in vitro* study by Wang et al. (21) conducted on different cell lines firstly demonstrated that tumor-derived *IDH1*^{R132C} mutation sensitizes cells to ferroptosis, by reducing

GPX4 levels through the production of the oncometabolite 2-hydroxyglutarate (2-HG). In their work, mutated cells were able to undergo ferroptosis in response to erastin but not to RSL3, which acts in a concentration-dependent manner, implying that 2-HG acts directly on GPX4 expression (21).

Basing on this background, the aim of our study was to investigate tissue expression of ferroptosis activation markers in ICC cases, and to correlate it with clinical-pathological features, STAT3 expression, and *IDH1-2* status.

MATERIALS AND METHODS

Case Selection

We retrospectively collected a total of 112 consecutive patients with a diagnosis of ICC. Among them, 90 patients underwent laparoscopic hepatic resection with curative intent from January 2006 to May 2021. The remaining 22 patients were patients with liver mass who underwent diagnostic liver biopsy, eventually diagnosed as ICC, who subsequently underwent surgery in a different hospital. Thirty patients included in our cohort were already investigated before, as part of a previous study (22). Exclusion criteria were (i) the administration of any systemic or loco-regional therapy prior to surgery/biopsy, (ii) a survival of less than 3 months after surgery (for patients who underwent resection), to exclude deaths due to surgical complications, and (iii) the absence of available residual tumor tissue for immunohistochemical (IHC) stains and molecular tests. Only surgical specimens were considered for molecular analyzes. The study complies with the ethical guidelines of the 1975 Declaration of Helsinki and obtained the approval from the local Ethics Committee (Ethics Committee for Clinical Research—University Hospital of Padova, Italy; protocol #: 0038038/17). All of the patients gave their appropriate informed consent to any procedure.

Clinical Data

Patients' relevant clinical and laboratory data were retrieved from medical records, including sex, age, serum ferritin levels, the presence of any underlying chronic hepatic or biliary disease, the presence of cirrhosis, and the administration of adjuvant chemotherapy. We also reported whether lymphadenectomy was performed during surgery or not.

All patients who underwent surgery were clinically followed-up, and regularly subjected to ultrasonography and computed tomography to detect any recurrence of the disease. Overall and disease-free survival time was obtained from medical charts.

Histological Study

All of the cases were blindly and contemporarily reviewed by an experienced (MG) and two trainee (SS and DS) liver pathologists, and relevant histological features were recorded, including macroscopic tumor type, histotype, grade of differentiation, T stage (according to the revised 8th edition of the UICC staging system) (23), margin status (for surgical resections), and the presence of vascular and perineural invasion and lymph node metastasis.

Immunohistochemical Study

Tissue microarrays (TMAs) made of formalin-fixed paraffin-embedded ICC tissue cores (with a diameter of 2 mm) were obtained by selecting two or three representative tumor areas from each liver resection case, depending on tumor dimension. All of the samples were processed by using the TMA Master platform (3DHistech, Budapest, Hungary), a semi-automatic and computer-assisted TMA platform.

Immunostains were performed on TMA and liver biopsy sections by using the following antibodies: anti-STAT3 (clone F-2; Santa Cruz Biotechnology, Dallas, TX, United States; dilution 1:200; mouse monoclonal), anti-GPX4 (clone E-12; Santa Cruz Biotechnology, Dallas, TX, United States; dilution 1:400; mouse monoclonal), and anti-transferrin receptor 1 (TFR1; also known as CD71) (clone 10F11; Leica Biosystems, Newcastle upon Tyne, United Kingdom; dilution 1:100; mouse monoclonal). All IHC stains were conducted according to standard protocols by using the Dako Omnis autostainer (Dako, Glostrup, Denmark), and all of the slides were counterstained with hematoxylin. Appropriate positive and negative controls were used for each run. In evaluating the expression of all markers, only cytoplasmic staining was considered. STAT3 and GPX4 expression was semi-quantitatively scored from 0 to 2 +, as follows: 0 = negative; 1 + = expression in ≤ 50% of tumor cells (TCs); 2 + = expression in > 50% of TCs (**Figure 1**). Finally, TFR1 positivity was evaluated as follows: 0 = negative or positive in ≤ 10% of TCs; 1 + = expression in 11–50% of TCs; 2 + = expression in > 50% of TCs (**Figure 2**).

In every case, we also performed histochemical Perls' stain (Artisan Iron Stain Kit, Dako, Glostrup, Denmark) to detect intratumoral iron deposits, which were recorded as absent/present (**Figure 3**).

Molecular Study

As reported above, only surgical specimens (90 cases) were considered for molecular tests. For each case, DNA extraction was performed on selected representative areas of formalin-fixed paraffin-embedded ICC tissue, with Qiasymphony DSP DNA Mini Kit (Qiagen, Hilden, Germany). DNA quantity was measured spectrophotometrically by using NanoDrop ND 100 Spectrophotometer (Thermo Fisher Scientific, Waltham, MA, United States). Detection of the main *IDH1* (codons 105 and 132) and *IDH2* (codons 140 and 172) gene mutations was performed by real-time polymerase chain reaction (PCR) analysis (Easy PGX ready IDH1-2, Easy PGX platform, Diatech Pharmacogenetics, Jesi, Italy), according to the manufacturer's

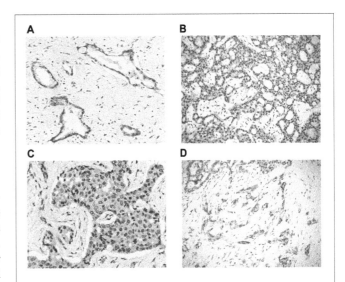

FIGURE 1 | STAT3 and GPX4 expression in ICC cases. Examples of 1 + and 2 + cytoplasmic positivity for STAT3 and GPX4 [(**A**) 1 + STAT3, original magnification 20x; (**B**) 2 + STAT3, original magnification 10x; (**C**) 1 + GPX4, original magnification 20x; (**D**) 2 + GPX4, original magnification 10x].

instructions. When necessary, the identified mutations were confirmed by PCR analysis and Sanger sequencing, by using the ABI PRISM 3500 Genetic Analyzer (Applied Biosystems, Waltham, MA, United States).

Statistical Analysis

Continuous variables were expressed as median (range) while categorical variables as frequency and percentage. For clinical-pathological correlations, appropriated tests were used, including Student's *t*-test, one-way ANOVA test, Spearman rank correlation test and Fisher exact probability test. The Kaplan–Meier method was used to create survival curves, which were compared by using both the log-rank and the Breslow (generalized Wilcoxon) tests. Multivariate Cox backward stepwise regression analyzes were performed including all of the variables identified as significant on univariate Cox regression analyzes. Hazard ratios (HRs) and their 95% confidence intervals (CIs) were calculated. *p* values < 0.05 were considered statistically significant. Data analyzes were performed by applying Statistical Package for the Social Science (SPSS, version 25, IBM SPSS Statistics, Chicago, IL, United States) and GraphPad (version 6, GraphPad Software, San Diego, CA, United States) statistical software.

RESULTS

Clinical Features

Overall, in our cohort of 112 patients there were 58 males (51.8%) and 54 females (48.2%), with a median age of 68 years (range 34–92 years). Seventeen patients (15.2%) had a cirrhotic liver, and 36 patients (32.1%) received adjuvant chemotherapy after resection/biopsy. Patients had a median follow-up of 1.7 years (range 0.3–8.8 years). Lymphadenectomy was performed in 33/90 patients who underwent surgery. Clinical and laboratory

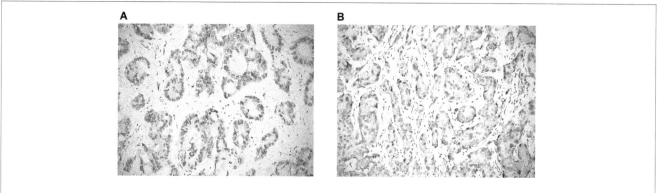

FIGURE 2 | TFR1 expression in ICC cases was semi-quantitatively evaluated as negative, 1 + [**(A)** original magnification 20x], and 2 + [**(B)** original magnification 20x].

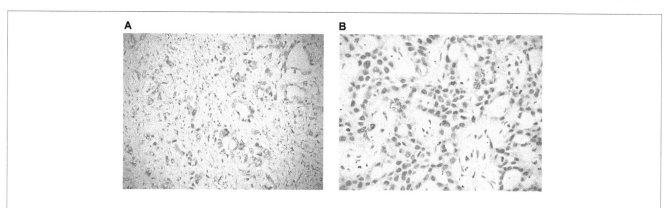

FIGURE 3 | Intratumoral iron deposits in ICC were evaluated as absent/present. Negative cases often showed iron deposition in peri-tumoral macrophages, but not in neoplastic cells [**(A)** original magnification 20x]; in positive cases, iron deposits appear as intracytoplasmic blue granules in tumor cells [**(B)** original magnification 40x].

features of all the patients are summarized in **Table 1**. Age, sex, the presence of underlying chronic liver diseases, and the administration of adjuvant chemotherapy were not related to patients' prognosis. Furthermore, overall and disease-free survivals were not different between patients with or without cirrhosis, probably because of the low number of cirrhotic patients in our cohort.

Histological Features and Clinical-Pathological Correlations

Macroscopically, all cases were mass forming, while, histologically, there were 82 cases (73.2%) of small duct type ICC and 30 cases (26.8%) of large duct type ICC. We observed vascular invasion in 78 out of 112 patients (69.6%), while perineural invasion was present in 50/112 cases (44.6%), as reported in **Table 2**. Among the 33 patients who underwent lymphadenectomy, 15 had lymph node metastases. Forty-seven patients out of the 90 who underwent surgery (52.2%) had a complete surgical excision of the tumor (R0 cases), while the remaining 43 patients (47.8%) showed a microscopic neoplastic infiltration of the resection margin (R1 cases).

As expected, grading and the presence of perineural and vascular neoplastic invasion were all related to worse overall

$(p = 0.009, p < 0.0001$, and $p = 0.004$, respectively) and disease-free survivals $(p = 0.01, p = 0.002$, and $p = 0.001$, respectively). An advanced T stage (i.e., T stage 3 and 4) was related to a reduced overall survival $(p = 0.06)$. We failed to find any correlation between patients' prognosis and histotype or resection margin status. We did not observe differences in survival times between cases with or without lymph node metastases.

Immunohistochemical Features and Clinical-Pathological Correlations

In our cohort, most of the cases showed GPX4 expression, either 1 + (43/112; 38.4%) or 2 + (46/112; 41.1%), while only 23 cases (20.5%) were completely negative. Twenty-two patients out of 112 (19.6%) showed 1 + TFR1 expression, while 7 cases showed a 2 + TFR1 positivity (6.3%). Intratumoral iron deposits were observed in only 2 cases (1.8%); among them, one showed a focal and one a diffuse deposition. Interestingly, the case that showed diffuse iron deposits had both a strong TFR1 expression and a completely negative GPX4 stain (**Supplementary Figure 1**). Taken together, these findings suggest an inhibition of the ferroptotic cascade in ICC. Most of our cases showed either a 1 + (56/112; 50%) or 2 + (51/112; 45.5%) STAT3 expression, with only 5 cases (4.5%) showing a completely negative reaction, suggesting an activation of the inflammatory pathway in our ICC

TABLE 1 | Clinical and laboratory features of the patients.

Feature	N = 112
Age [years]	
Median (range)	68 (34 − 92)
Sex N (%)	
Males	58 (51.8)
Females	54 (48.2)
Ferritin [ng/ml]	
Median (range)	260.5 (53 − 943.5)
Underlying diseases N (%)	
HBV hepatitis	6 (5.4)
HCV hepatitis	11 (9.8)
Alcoholic hepatitis	6 (5.4)
NAFLD/NASH	6 (5.4)
Cryptogenic cirrhosis	1 (0.9)
Cirrhosis N (%)	17 (15.2)
Adjuvant chemotherapy N (%)	36 (32.1)
Recurrence N (%)	60 (53.6)
Exitus N (%)	73 (65.2)

HBV, hepatitis B virus; HCV, hepatitis C virus; NAFLD, non-alcoholic fatty liver disease; NASH, non-alcoholic steatohepatitis.

TABLE 2 | Histological features of the patients.

Feature	N = 112
Histotype	
N (%)	
Small duct type	82 (73.2)
Large duct type	30 (26.8)
Grade	
N (%)	
G1	15 (13.4)
G2	49 (43.8)
G3	48 (42.8)
T stage [N = 90]	
N (%)	
T1a	13 (14.4)
T1b	11 (12.2)
T2	46 (51.1)
T3	13 (14.4)
T4	7 (7.9)
Vascular invasion N (%)	78 (69.6)
Perineural invasion N (%)	50 (44.6)
Lymph node metastasis [N = 33] N (%)	15 (45.5)
Resection margin status [N = 90]	
N (%)	
R0	47 (52.2)
R1	43 (47.8)

TABLE 3 | Histochemical and immunohistochemical expression of the different markers in ICC cases.

Marker	N = 112
GPX4	
N (%)	
0	23 (20.5)
1 +	43 (38.4)
2 +	46 (41.1)
TFR1	
N (%)	
0	83 (74.1)
1 +	22 (19.6)
2 +	7 (6.3)
Intratumoral iron deposits	
N (%)	
Absent	110 (98.2)
Present	2 (1.8)
STAT3	
N (%)	
0	5 (4.5)
1 +	56 (50)
2 +	51 (45.5)

association between the presence of the same unfavorable histological factors and STAT3 expression ($p = 0.001$, $p = 0.04$, and $p = 0.07$ for grading, perineural invasion, and vascular invasion, respectively), confirming what previously reported (4, 10). No associations were found between the same histological features and TFR1 expression, neither between them and the presence of iron deposits. No correlations were found between marker expression (and iron deposits) and tumor T stage. We observed a direct association between STAT3 and GPX4 expression ($p < 0.0001$) (**Supplementary Figure 2**), suggesting inhibition of ferroptosis in ICCs with an inflammatory background. Accordingly, we found an inverse correlation between STAT3 and TFR1 expression ($p = 0.04$). We failed to find any correlation between TFR1 and GPX4 expression, as well as between ferroptosis markers and STAT3 expression and the presence of intratumoral iron deposits.

Age, sex, the presence of any underlying chronic liver disease, the presence of cirrhosis, ferritin levels, tumor histotype, and the presence of nodal metastases were not related to the expression of any of the markers, neither to the presence of iron deposits.

As already reported in the literature, STAT3 expression was related to a worse overall ($p = 0.02$) and disease-free survival ($p = 0.001$) (**Figure 4**). We found significantly reduced overall ($p = 0.06$) and disease-free survivals ($p = 0.04$) in cases with a higher GPX4 expression, as shown by the Kaplan–Meyer curves (**Figure 5**). Considering GPX4 1 + and 2 + positive cases together, the association becomes even stronger for both overall and disease-free survival ($p = 0.03$ and $p = 0.01$, respectively) (**Figure 5**), suggesting that mild GPX4 presence is enough to inhibit ferroptosis and reduce survival times. TFR1 expression and the presence of iron deposits were not related to survival times.

cohort. Histochemical and immunohistochemical expressions of the different markers are summarized in **Table 3**.

Statistical analyzes showed a direct correlation between GPX4 expression and the presence of poor prognostic histological parameters, that is grading ($p < 0.0001$) and perineural ($p = 0.03$) and vascular invasion ($p < 0.0001$). We also found a direct

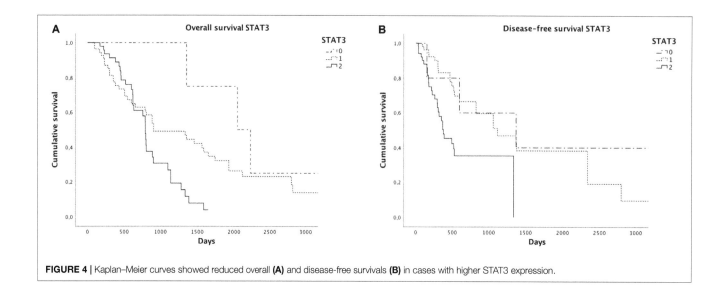

FIGURE 4 | Kaplan–Meier curves showed reduced overall **(A)** and disease-free survivals **(B)** in cases with higher STAT3 expression.

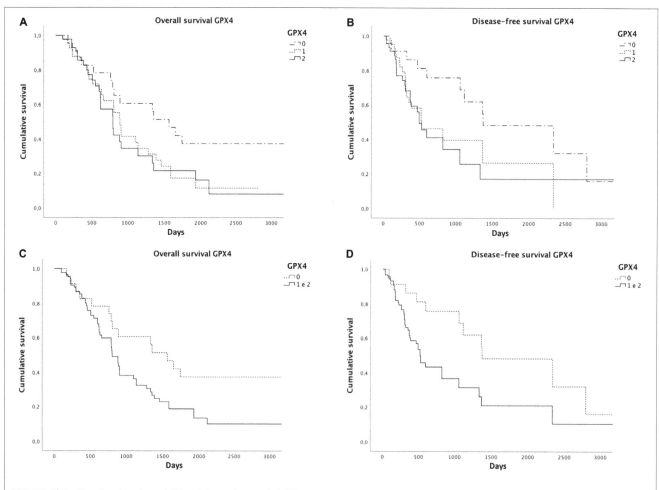

FIGURE 5 | Significantly reduced overall **(A)** and disease-free survivals **(B)** were observed in cases with higher GPX4 expression. Considering GPX4 1 + and 2 + positive cases together, the association becomes even stronger for both overall **(C)** and disease-free survivals **(D)**, as shown by the Kaplan–Meier curves.

Molecular Features and Clinical-Pathological Correlations

Molecular analysis results are reported in **Table 4**. As shown, they revealed *IDH1* point mutations in 15 out of 76 tested cases (19.7%), of which 14 involving codon 132 and one involving codon 105. Only one case showed a point mutation in *IDH2* codon 172 (1.3%). In 9 cases (11.8%) molecular tests described a single nucleotide polymorphism (SNP) in codon 105 of the *IDH1* gene, causing a change in the nucleotide sequence from GGC [Gly] to GGT [Gly] (C > T). Among them, two cases showed both a point mutation in *IDH1* (codon 132) and the $IDH1^{105GGT}$ SNP. No relationships were found between the presence of IDH1 point mutations and the presence of the $IDH1^{105GGT}$ SNP.

Statistical analyzes showed an inverse correlation between the presence of $IDH1^{105GGT}$ SNP and tumor grading ($p < 0.0001$). On the contrary, a direct relationship was found between tumor grading and the wild type status of *IDH1-2* genes ($p = 0.004$). No associations between tumor grading and the presence of point mutations in *IDH1-2* genes were observed. We also failed to find any correlation between *IDH1-2* status and age, sex, the presence of any underlying chronic liver disease, the presence of cirrhosis, ferritin levels, tumor histotype, the presence of perineural and vascular invasion, T stage and the presence of nodal metastases.

Furthermore, GPX4 expression was inversely correlated to the presence of $IDH1^{105GGT}$ SNP ($p = 0.001$) (**Supplementary Figure 3**), while it was directly related to the presence of an *IDH1-2* point mutation ($p = 0.06$) or wild type *IDH1-2* ($p = 0.04$). No associations were found between *IDH1-2* status and STAT3 and TFR1 expression, neither between *IDH1-2* status and intratumoral iron deposits.

Finally, cases with $IDH1^{105GGT}$ SNP showed a better overall survival than cases with wild type *IDH1-2* (1,648 days vs. 887 days; $p = 0.04$) and cases with *IDH1-2* point mutations (1,648 days vs. 1,333 days; $p = 0.09$) (**Figure 6**). We did not find any relationship between *IDH1-2* status and disease-free survival times. The multivariate Cox regression analysis, including

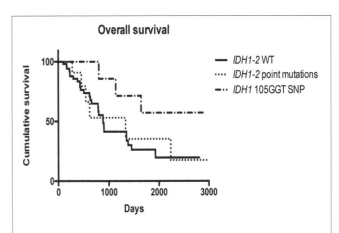

FIGURE 6 | Kaplan–Meier curves showed different overall survivals in cases bearing $IDH1^{105GGT}$ SNP, *IDH1-2* point mutations and wild type *IDH1-2*.

variables that were identified as significant on univariate survival analyzes (grading, perineural and vascular neoplastic invasion, T stage, STAT3 and GPX4 expression, and $IDH1^{105GGT}$ SNP) showed that only the presence of perineural invasion is an independent predictor of a worse overall survival [$p < 0.0001$, HR = 3.64 (95% CI: 1.86–7.11)], while the multivariate Cox regression analysis including grading, perineural and vascular neoplastic invasion, and STAT3 and GPX4 expression found that STAT3 expression and vascular invasion are independent predictors of a reduced disease-free survival [$p = 0.03$, HR = 1.81 (95% CI: 1.05–3.14), and $p = 0.05$, HR = 1.97 (95% CI: 1.02–3.84), respectively] (**Supplementary Table 1**).

DISCUSSION

In this study, we describe for the first time that in most inflammatory ICCs ferroptosis seems to be not active, and that its activation may depend on *IDH1-2* status. In our cohort, GPX4 was overexpressed in almost 80% of the cases, suggesting an inhibition of the ferroptotic cascade in most of our patients. GPX4 expression was found to be related to the presence of histological poor prognostic features, namely high grade and vascular and perineural invasion, and to reduced overall and disease-free survivals, implying that ferroptosis inhibition confers a worse prognosis, as expected.

We also observed that STAT3 was overexpressed in more than 90% of cases, indicating that they can be classified as inflammation-related ICC, according to the molecular classification proposed by Sia et al. (9). We confirm the poor prognostic role of STAT3 already reported in the literature (4, 10). In fact, we found a correlation between its expression and the presence of histological poor prognostic features, and worse overall and disease-free survivals in cases with higher STAT3 expression. Since this subclass of ICC is characterized by a pro-inflammatory and anti-apoptotic molecular milieu, and that pro-apoptotic drugs demonstrated only mild improvements in patients' prognosis and a frequent development of chemoresistance (4, 7, 11), the induction of other

TABLE 4 | *IDH1* and *IDH2* gene status in ICC cases.

Adequacy	N = 90
Inadequate samples	14/90 (15.6%)
Adequate samples	76/90 (84.4%)
Molecular alterations	**N = 76**
IDH1 point mutations*	15/76 (19.7%)
Arg132Cys	6/76 (7.9%)
Arg132His	2/76 (2.6%)
Arg132Val	1/76 (1.3%)
Arg132Ser	1/76 (1.3%)
Arg132X	4/76 (5.2%)
Gly105Asn	1/76 (1.3%)
IDH1^{105GGT} SNP*	9/76 (11.8%)
IDH2 Arg172X	1/76 (1.3%)
IDH1-2 WT	53/76 (69.7%)

*2 cases showed both an IDH1 point mutation in codon 132 (Arg132Cys and Arg132His) and IDH1^{105GGT} SNP. SNP, single nucleotide polymorphism; WT, wild type.

different cell death types, including ferroptosis, is a possible alternative way to kill resistant tumor cells. In line with this hypothesis, the high GPX4 levels found in our patients suggest that ferroptosis could be pharmacologically induced, by acting directly on GPX4 inhibition.

Molecular analyses on our cohort demonstrated *IDH1* (codon 132 or 105) or *IDH2* (codon 172) point mutations in nearly 20% of the cases, in line with the literature (3, 4, 14–17). Surprisingly, we found a SNP on codon 105 of the *IDH1* gene in 12% of our cases, which was never reported in ICC before. Patients bearing this molecular feature had a good histological profile, namely low histological tumor grade, and longer overall survival times. Synonymous SNPs are point mutations that cause a nucleotide change, which do not alter the amino acid sequence of the protein. However, sometimes they may lead to a protein defect and have functional consequences (24). The $IDH1^{105GGT}$ SNP we described in our cohort was previously reported in acute myeloid leukemia, gliomas, and thyroid tumors, and have a poorly understood role in tumorigenesis (24–27). Indeed, it was linked to an adverse prognosis in acute myeloid leukemia and glioblastomas, while it seemed to confer longer survivals in patients with grade II or III gliomas (28, 29), in line with our results. The explanation of this finding is not clear, since the biologic consequences of this SNP remain speculative. It has been hypothesized that $IDH1^{105GGT}$ SNP may alter *IDH1* mRNA stability or increase mRNA levels, leading to altered NADPH production (24, 28, 30), but further studies are needed to elucidate this issue. In line with previously reports (24, 28, 30), in two of our cases we described the concomitant presence of the $IDH1^{105GGT}$ SNP and a point mutation in *IDH1* (codon 132). It is known that, even if $IDH1^{105GGT}$ SNP is very close to codon 132, no correlation between the two molecular alterations exists (24, 30), as we confirm in our cohort.

The inverse correlation we observed between the presence of $IDH1^{105GGT}$ SNP and GPX4 levels may suggest an activation of the ferroptotic cascade in ICCs bearing this molecular feature, and eventually explains the longer overall survivals observed in these patients. On the other side, we failed to confirm the association between $IDH1^{R132C}$ mutation and reduced GPX4 levels reported by Wang et al. (21), but this might be explained by the different experimental conditions we worked under (cell lines versus ICC tissue and *in vitro* versus *in vivo*). Considering our survival data, it is possible that both $IDH1^{105GGT}$ SNP and $IDH1^{R132C}$ mutation act on GPX4 in different ways or with different intensity, since $IDH1^{R132C}$ mutation-bearing cases showed overall survival times shorter than those seen in $IDH1^{105GGT}$ SNP cases, but longer than those of patients with wild type *IDH1-2*. However, molecular mechanisms explaining how $IDH1^{105GGT}$ SNP act on GPX4 level reduction are unknown and impossible to infer basing on our data. So additional *in vitro* studies are indispensable to address this key issue. Moreover, the number of patients overall bearing the $IDH1^{105GGT}$ SNP in our cohort is low, and this limits the strength of our data, so additional studies based on larger cohorts may be of help to confirm our results. It is of interest to note that patients bearing $IDH1^{105GGT}$ SNP are not expected to respond to GPX4-inhibitor drugs, such as RSL3, since GPX4 levels are already

very low in these cases. However, as Wang et al. reported on $IDH1^{R132C}$-mutated cell lines (21), $IDH1^{105GGT}$ SNP-bearing ICCs may respond to ferroptosis-inducers acting on GSH levels, such as erastin. Therefore, knowing the molecular background in ICC patients is fundamental to choose the appropriate pharmacological therapy to induce tumor cell death, particularly in cases developing drug-resistance.

In conclusion, our study demonstrates for the first time that in most inflammatory ICCs ferroptosis seems to be not active, and that its triggering may be related to some molecular features of the tumor. *IDH1-2* status is essential to determine whether (and which type of) ferroptosis-inducer drugs might be useful in ICC patient treatment, especially in drug-resistant cases.

AUTHOR CONTRIBUTIONS

SS contributed to conception and design, acquisition of data, analysis and interpretation of data, writing and revision of the manuscript. DS contributed to conception and design, acquisition of data, analysis and interpretation of data, and revision of the manuscript. LF, GZ, and EG contributed to revision of the manuscript. MN contributed to development of methodology and technical and material support. GG contributed to development of methodology, analysis and interpretation of data, and technical and material support. MG contributed to conception and design, interpretation of data, revision of the manuscript, and study supervision. All authors contributed to the article and approved the submitted version.

ACKNOWLEDGMENTS

We thank Roberta Pozzobon, Irene Sarcinelli, and Ylenia Barbanera for the technical support.

REFERENCES

1. Mejia JC, Pasko J. Primary liver cancers: intrahepatic cholangiocarcinoma and hepatocellular carcinoma. *Surg Clin North Am.* (2020) 100:535–49. doi: 10.1016/j.suc.2020.02.013
2. Sarcognato S, Sacchi D, Fassan M, Fabris L, Cadamuro M, Guido M, et al. Cholangiocarcinoma. *Pathologica.* (2021) 113:158–69. doi: 10.32074/1591-951X-252
3. Sirica AE, Gores GJ, Groopman JD, Selaru FM, Strazzabosco M, Zhu AX, et al. Intrahepatic cholangiocarcinoma: continuing challenges and translational advances. *Hepatology.* (2019) 69:1803–15. doi: 10.1002/hep.30289
4. Acher AW, Paro A, Elfadaly A, Tsilimigras D, Pawlik TM. Intrahepatic cholangiocarcinoma: a summative review of biomarkers and targeted therapies. *Cancers (Basel).* (2021) 13:5169. doi: 10.3390/cancers13205169
5. El-Diwany R, Pawlik TM, Ejaz A. Intrahepatic cholangiocarcinoma. *Surg Oncol Clin N Am.* (2019) 28:587–99. doi: 10.1016/j.soc.2019.06.002
6. Sung H, Ferlay J, Siegel RL, Laversanne M, Soerjomataram I, Freddie Bray F, et al. Global cancer statistics 2020: GLOBOCAN estimates of incidence and mortality worldwide for 36 cancers in 185 countries. *CA Cancer J Clin.* (2021) 71:209–49. doi: 10.3322/caac.21660
7. Cadamuro M, Brivio S, Spirli C, Joplin RE, Strazzabosco M, Fabris L. Autocrine and paracrine mechanisms promoting chemoresistance in cholangiocarcinoma. *Int J Mol Sci.* (2017) 18:149. doi: 10.3390/ijms18010149
8. Morton SD, Cadamuro M, Brivio S, Vismara M, Stecca T, Strazzabosco M, et al. Leukemia inhibitory factor protects cholangiocarcinoma cells from drug-induced apoptosis via a PI3K/AKT-dependent Mcl-1 activation. *Oncotarget.* (2015) 6:26052–64. doi: 10.18632/oncotarget.4482

9. Sia D, Hoshida Y, Villanueva A, Roayaie S, Ferrer J, Llovet JM, et al. Integrative molecular analysis of intrahepatic cholangiocarcinoma reveals 2 classes that have different outcomes. *Gastroenterology.* (2013) 144:829–40. doi: 10.1053/j.gastro.2013.01.001

10. Johnston P, Grandis JR. STAT3 SIGNALING: anticancer strategies and challenges. *Mol Interv.* (2011) 11:18–26. doi: 10.1124/mi.11.1.4

11. Jin K, Li T, Sánchez-Duffhues G, Zhou F, Zhang L. Involvement of inflammation and its related microRNAs in hepatocellular carcinoma. *Oncotarget.* (2017) 8:22145–65. doi: 10.18632/oncotarget.13530

12. Yu H, Lee H, Herrmann A, Buettner R, Jove R. Revisiting STAT3 signalling in cancer: new and unexpected biological functions. *Nat Rev Cancer.* (2014) 14:736–46. doi: 10.1038/nrc3818

13. Darnell J, Kerr I, Stark G. Jak-STAT pathways and transcriptional activation in response to IFNs and other extracellular signaling proteins. *Science.* (1994) 264:1415–21. doi: 10.1126/science.8197455

14. Farshidfar F, Zheng S, Gingras M, Newton Y, Shih J, Kleiner DE, et al. Integrative genomic analysis of cholangiocarcinoma identifies distinct IDH-mutant molecular profiles. *Cell Rep.* (2017) 19:2878–80. doi: 10.1016/j.celrep.2017.06.008

15. Borger DR, Tanabe KK, Fan KC, Lopez HU, Fantin VR, Iafrate AJ, et al. Frequent mutation of isocitrate dehydrogenase (IDH)1 and IDH2 in cholangiocarcinoma identified through broad-based tumor genotyping. *Oncologist.* (2012) 17:72–9. doi: 10.1634/theoncologist.2011-0386

16. Haber PK, Sia D. Translating cancer genomics for precision oncology in biliary tract cancers. *Discov Med.* (2019) 28:255–65.

17. Moeini A, Sia D, Bardeesy N, Mazzaferro V, Llovet JM. Molecular pathogenesis and targeted therapies for intrahepatic cholangiocarcinoma. *Clin Cancer Res.* (2016) 22:291–300. doi: 10.1158/1078-0432.CCR-14-3296

18. Galluzzi L, Vitale I, Aaronson SA, Abrams JM, Adam D, Agostinis P, et al. Molecular mechanisms of cell death: recommendations of the nomenclature committee on cell death 2018. *Cell Death Differ.* (2018) 25:486–541. doi: 10.1038/s41418-017-0012-4

19. Xu T, Ding W, Ji X, Ao X, Liu Y, Yu W, et al. Molecular mechanisms of ferroptosis and its role in cancer therapy. *J Cell Mol Med.* (2019) 23:4900–12. doi: 10.1111/jcmm.14511

20. Wang H, Lin D, Yu Q, Li Z, Lenahan C, Shao A, et al. A promising future of ferroptosis in tumor therapy. *Front Cell Dev Biol.* (2021) 9:629150. doi: 10.3389/fcell.2021.629150

21. Wang T, Liang J, Zhang C, Xiong Y, Guan K, Yuan H. The oncometabolite 2-hydroxyglutarate produced by mutant IDH1 sensitizes cells to ferroptosis. *Cell Death Dis.* (2019) 10:755. doi: 10.1038/s41419-019-1984-4

22. Sarcognato S, Gringeri E, Fassan M, Di Giunta M, Cillo U, Guido M, et al. Prognostic role of BAP-1 and PBRM-1 expression in intrahepatic cholangiocarcinoma. *Virchows Arch.* (2019) 474:29–37. doi: 10.1007/s00428-018-2478-y

23. Brierley J, Gospodarowicz MK, Wittekind C. *TNM Classification of Malignant Tumours.* Eighth ed. Hoboken, NJ: John Wiley & Sons, Inc (2017).

24. Acquaviva G, Visani M, de Biase D, Marucci G, Franceschi E, Tallini G, et al. Prevalence of the single-nucleotide polymorphism rs11554137 (IDH1 105GGT) in brain tumors of a cohort of Italian patients. *Sci Rep.* (2018) 8:4459. doi: 10.1038/s41598-018-22222-y

25. Ho PA, Kopecky KJ, Alonzo TA, Gerbing RB, Miller KL, Kuhn J, et al. Prognostic implications of the IDH1 synonymous SNP rs11554137 in pediatric and adult AML: a report from the Children's Oncology Group and SWOG. *Blood.* (2011) 118:4561–6. doi: 10.1182/blood-2011-04-348888

26. Hemerly JP, Bastos AU, Cerutti JM. Identification of several novel non-p.R132 IDH1 variants in thyroid carcinomas. *Eur J Endocrinol.* (2010) 163:747–55. doi: 10.1530/EJE-10-0473

27. Murugan AK, Bojdani E, Xing M. Identification and functional characterization of isocitrate dehydrogenase 1 (IDH1) mutations in thyroid cancer. *Biochem Biophys Res Commun.* (2010) 393:555–9. doi: 10.1016/j.bbrc.2010.02.095

28. Wang X, Boisselier B, Rossetto M, Marie Y, Idbaih A, Sanson M, et al. Prognostic impact of the isocitrate dehydrogenase 1 single-nucleotide polymorphism rs11554137 in malignant gliomas. *Cancer.* (2013) 119:806–13. doi: 10.1002/cncr.27798

29. Franceschi E, De Biase D, Di Nunno V, Pession A, Tosoni A, Brandes AA, et al. IDH1 105GGT single nucleotide polymorphism improves progression free survival in patients with IDH mutated grade II and III gliomas. *Pathol Res Pract.* (2021) 221:153445. doi: 10.1016/j.prp.2021.153445

30. Wagner K, Damm F, Göhring G, Görlich K, Heuser M, Schäfer I, et al. Impact of IDH1 R132 mutations and an IDH1 single nucleotide polymorphism in cytogenetically normal acute myeloid leukemia: SNP rs11554137 is an adverse prognostic factor. *J Clin Oncol.* (2010) 28:2356–64. doi: 10.1200/JCO.2009.27.6899

8

Resection of Thymic Neuroendocrine Carcinoma Guided by Three-Dimensional Reconstruction

Fang Liu[1], Hengxiao Lu[2], Liqian Chen[3], Junfeng Geng[4] and Tongzhen Xu[2]*

[1] Department of Respiratory Medicine, Weifang People's Hospital, The First Affiliated Hospital of Weifang Medical University, Weifang, China, [2] Department of Thoracic Surgery, Weifang People's Hospital, The First Affiliated Hospital of Weifang Medical University, Weifang, China, [3] Department of Pathology, Weifang People's Hospital, The First Affiliated Hospital of Weifang Medical University, Weifang, China, [4] Department of Thoracic Surgery, Shanghai Chest Hospital, Shanghai Jiao Tong University, Shanghai, China

Correspondence:
Tongzhen Xu
xtz521@126.com

Primary thymic small cell neuroendocrine carcinoma (SCNEC), which possesses a more aggressive biological behaviour, including invasion of proximal structures, local recurrence, and distant metastasis, is extremely rare. According to a previous literature report, only a few patients with this disease have been reported, compared to patients with distant metastasis of bones, lungs, spleen, liver, and adrenal glands (1, 2). The report data suggest that SCNEC is a highly malignant tumour compared to most other tumours of the human body. In this study, we presented the case of a patient who underwent surgery guided by three-dimensional reconstruction modelling before the operation. We were fully prepared for the resection of this tumour using three-dimensional reconstruction modelling, even after reading the computed tomography (CT) images that showed a closed relationship with the pericardium, the vein of the right middle lung lobe, and the phrenic nerve. All these features demonstrate that SCNEC is highly malignant. To date, there are no procedural reports for three-dimensional reconstruction modelling in malignant thymus tumours.

Keywords: thymic small cell neuroendocrine carcinoma, three-dimensional reconstruction, surgical planning, uniport video-assisted thoracoscopy, prognosis, video-assisted thoracoscopy

INTRODUCTION

Thymic neuroendocrine carcinoma (NEC) is a malignant tumour originating from thymic tissue with neuroendocrine cells. It is rare in the clinic and accounts for 2–4% of mediastinal tumours (3). There were no specific symptoms or signs except for the invasion of surrounding tissues. The computed tomography (CT) displayed a large soft tissue mass with uniform density and local necrosis located in the anterior mediastinum. The enhanced CT scan also showed mild to moderate tumour enhancement. Thymic NEC possesses a more aggressive biological behaviour, including invasion of proximal structures, local recurrence, and distant haematogenous metastasis. Distant metastasis is often observed in the bones, lungs, spleen, liver, and adrenal glands. However, a study reported a patient with pancreatic metastasis resulting from thymic NEC.

CASE REPORT

A 71-year-old male patient was admitted to Weifang Peoples Hospital (The First Affiliated Hospital of Weifang Medical University, Weifang, China) in April 2021 with a 3.5 × 2.7 cm anterior mediastinal mass, which was observed on routine chest-enhanced CT. The patient had no symptoms, signs, or discomforts. The medical history of the patient revealed no special case earlier and no basic illness, including hypertension, diabetes, or coronary heart disease. A general physical examination was unremarkable. We completed various tests and inspections after hospitalisation. The enhanced CT scan showed that the soft tissue mass enclosed proximal structures, including lung tissue, pulmonary vein, pericardium, and phrenic nerve (**Figure 1**). We could tell that the operation would be very difficult and high risk. As a result, we performed three-dimensional reconstruction modelling of this mass as well as proximal structures to develop a safe surgical plan. Literature reports on three-dimensional reconstruction modelling applications in this area are rare. We could clearly see the relative positional relationship between the mass and the surrounding tissues, which provided us with a clear understanding of this mass. The mass clearly invaded the pericardium and right middle lobe (RML) tissue, with an extremely closed relationship between the pulmonary vein as well as the phrenic nerve (**Figure 2**). The patient underwent surgery to resect the mass through UniProt video-assisted thoracoscopy (VATS) (**Figure 3**). We performed a left lateral decubitus position surgery similar to the right lung lobectomy after communicating with Professor Junfeng Geng in the Department of Thoracic Surgery, Shanghai Chest Hospital, which is the most authoritative hospital on the chest in China. During the surgery, the tumour was observed to be located in the anterior mediastinum with an invasion of the adjacent structures, including the pericardium, RML and vein, superior vena cava, and phrenic nerve. The tumour invaded the pericardium and phrenic nerve, which did not remain intact. As a result, we resected part of the pericardium, RML, and phrenic nerve. We also performed sidewall moulding on the pulmonary vein, which was the main return path of the RML, instead of cutting it off. Eventually, the tumour was completely resected using three-dimensional reconstruction modelling preoperative planning that ensured the operation went smoothly. The postoperative pathological results were small cell neuroendocrine carcinoma (SCNEC) with a volume of 3.5 cm × 2.7 cm × 1.2 cm, accompanied by massive haemorrhage and local necrosis. Tumour thrombus was seen in the vessel and invaded the nerve. The staining results of immunohistochemistry were as follows: CK (+), CD117 (+), CD56 (+), Syn (+), CgA (+), CK7 (–), CK19 (–), CK20 (–), CK5/6 (–), P40 (–), TTF-1 (–), CD3 (–), CD20 (–), TdT (–), CD5 (–), and Ki-67 (30%).

DISCUSSION

Thymic neuroendocrine tumours are rare, with a variety of variations in their form, and are easily confused with other

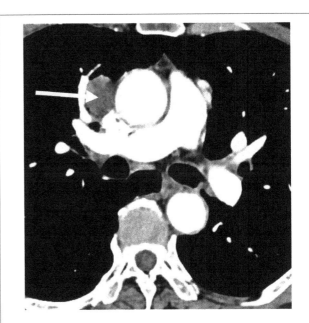

FIGURE 1 | CT scans of the patient showing thymic neuroendocrine carcinoma with a closed relationship of proximal structures.

tumours. In 2004, the WHO carried out a new classification of thymic neuroendocrine tumours and put forward diagnostic criteria, which are of great significance to clinicopathological diagnosis (4). We first learn more about this rare disease from the following aspects:

Definition

Thymic neuroendocrine tumours are epithelial tumours consisting mainly or entirely of neuroendocrine cells. It must be identified with thymus cancers and non-neuroepithelial tumours, especially paraneurotransplants, which contain scattered and congenital neuroendocrine cells. The origin of tissue in thymic neuroendocrine tumours is unknown. Neuroendocrine cancer is often associated with thymic scale cancer and, in occasional cases, can be mixed with thymus tumours, which supports the idea that common thymic epithelial precursor cells were the ancestors of thymic neuroendocrine cancer (5).

Pathological Type

The WHO has carried out a new classification of neuroendocrine tumours in the thymus and proposed diagnostic criteria, which are of great significance for clinicopathological diagnosis. According to the recent WHO classification criteria, thymic neuroendocrine tumours are divided into the following 2 categories: well-differentiated neuroendocrine carcinoma, containing typical classic carcinoid and atypical carcinoid, and poorly differentiated neuroendocrine carcinoma, containing small cell carcinoma (SCC) and large cell neuroendocrine carcinoma (LCNEC). Thymic SCC is an advanced tumour composed of small cells with unclear

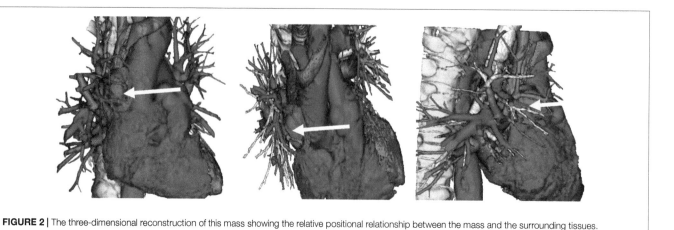

FIGURE 2 | The three-dimensional reconstruction of this mass showing the relative positional relationship between the mass and the surrounding tissues.

boundaries. Tumour cells are egg-shaped and shuttle-shaped, and nuclear division is common. Its cellular morphology is indicative of small cell lung cancer (SCLC). The variant type is complex SCC, which combines non-SCC components, such as squamous cell carcinoma and adenocarcinoma (6).

Aetiology

Approximately 25% of patients with thymus cancer have a MEN-1-positive family history, whereas 8% have thymus cancer in MENen-1 patients. As cases of thymic neuroendocrine cancer are concentrated in a small number of MEN-1 families and can manifest with various types of mutations other than 11q13 (MEN-1) site heterocyclic deficiency (LOH), mutations in genes and MEN-1 abnormalities (which may affect chromosome 1p tumour suppressor genes) lead to the occurrence of thymus cancer (7).

Clinical Characteristics

Thymic neuroendocrine cancer often occurs in the anterior mediastinum, and cases have been reported to occur in

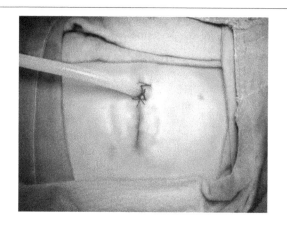

FIGURE 3 | The patient underwent surgery through uniport video-assisted thoracoscopy (VATS).

ectopic thymus tissue next to the thyroid gland. Most poorly differentiated thymic neuroendocrine cancers and approximately 50% of differentiated neuroendocrine cancers can have local symptoms such as chest pain, cough, dyspnoea, or upper cavity vein syndrome. It is very rare for patients to have cancer-like syndrome (<1%). Notably, 17–30% of adults and more than 50% of children with thymus cancer were accompanied by Cushing syndrome due to the tumour cell secretion of adrenocorticotropic hormone (ACTH). It is noted that 10% of all ectopic ACTH syndromes are caused by thymus cancer. In fact, thymic SCC rarely causes Cushing syndrome (8).

This 71-year-old male patient was asymptomatic, and the tumours were incidentally observed on routine chest CT without any positive signs by physical examination. Similar to the case presented in this study, over one-third of patients are asymptomatic, which reduces the early detection rate to a certain extent.

Treatments for thymic neuroendocrine cancer are very limited thus far. Surgery is the most effective treatment for thymic neuroendocrine cancer, and radical excision is the most critical factor for predicting the long-term survival of patients. Similar to the operation performed on this patient, radical excision often consists of en bloc resection of the tumour as well as the involved structures (9). The role of radiotherapy and chemotherapy in the treatment of thymic NEC is controversial. Radiotherapy and chemotherapy usually play secondary roles, while patients still have the possibility of surgical resection. Radiotherapy is recommended to prevent local recurrence of invasive tumours, and chemotherapy is usually used as an adjuvant treatment after surgery (10). Radiotherapy combined with chemotherapy in patients who do not qualify for surgery remains controversial because the effectiveness is difficult to evaluate. Fortunately, this patient was discovered in a timely manner and underwent surgical resection in time. Testing during the operation indicated that the tumour was highly malignant, and pathology results confirmed this after surgery. The tumour cells were small, with fewer than 3 quiescent lymphocytes, with few cytoplasmic cells that were densely crowded and arranged in nests and sheets. Abundant apoptotic debris and mitotic figures were found, and

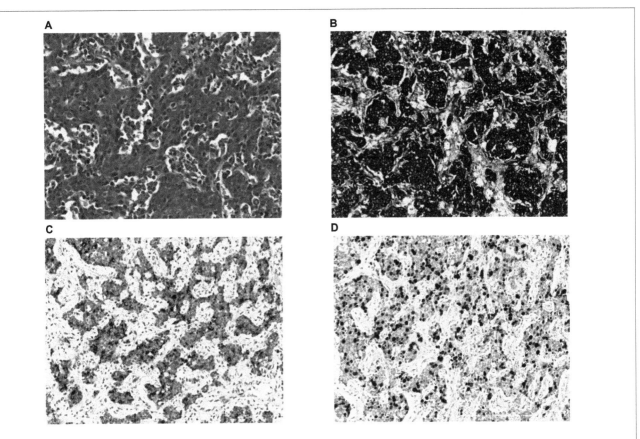

FIGURE 4 | (A) A high-power view of the tumour biopsy under a light microscope. Hematoxylin and eosin staining (magnification, 40×); **(B)** synaptophysin staining (magnification, 20×); **(C)** chromogranin A staining (magnification, 20×); **(D)** Ki-67 staining. In total, ~30% of the tumour cells are positive (magnification, 20×).

immunohistochemical stains were strongly positive for CK, Syn, CgA, and CD56 (**Figure 4**). Adenocarcinoma synaptophysin (Syn) and chromogranin (CgA) are currently recognised as neuroendocrine markers (7), and combined detection can improve the diagnosis rate. At the same time, electron microscope observation found that neuroendocrine granules (NSGs), tension fibrils, and desmosomes were of decisive significance in confirming neuroendocrine cancer. Depending on the four main types, typical carcinoid, atypical carcinoid, LCNEC, and SCC, and according to the immunohistochemical and morphological diagnostic criteria, the patient in this study was diagnosed with thymic SCNEC.

Morphologically, thymic SCNEC and small cell lung neuroendocrine carcinoma cannot be distinguished, and some immunological markers must be used to distinguish these two. TTF-1 may help to differentiate lung and thymic SCC. Most thymic carcinoids and neuroendocrine carcinomas do not express TTF-1, while 50–75% of lung neuroendocrine carcinomas express TTF-1. Carcinoids located in the mediastinum do not express TTF-1, which cannot be excluded from carcinoids metastasised from the gastrointestinal tract and pancreas because carcinoids of the gastrointestinal tract and pancreas often do not express TTF-1. The patient underwent a colour Doppler ultrasound examination of the abdomen as well as brain CT, and the

inspection results showed no obvious abnormalities. In addition, the immunohistochemistry results showed TTF-1 (–) in this patient. According to related literature reports, Syn and CgA are not expressed in adenocarcinoma but are in thymic carcinoids and neuroendocrine carcinomas. Syn and CgA were all positively expressed according to the pathological results. These results all support that this tumour is of thymic origin, which is rare in the clinic. The patient was discharged smoothly, and the follow-up treatment was radiotherapy combined with chemotherapy, according to the advice from Shanghai Chest Hospital. We will continue to pay close attention to the patient's condition.

In general, thymic SCNEC is a type of highly malignant tumour, is poorly differentiated, is easy to metastasise, and has a poor prognosis. The diagnosis relies on pathology and immunohistochemistry. The treatment is mainly combined with surgery, radiotherapy, and chemotherapy combined with biological therapy, but the effect is low. Therefore, early detection, diagnosis, and early treatment are the keys to improve prognosis. For malignant tumours that easily invade proximal structures, surgical planning under the guidance of three-dimensional reconstruction modelling before surgery will greatly reduce the risk of surgery and increase the complete resection rate, thereby improving the prognosis of patients. The three-dimensional reconstruction modelling technology is rarely used in clinical practice for mediastinal tumours and can provide surgeons with a safer and more intuitive operation plan.

AUTHOR CONTRIBUTIONS

TX, HL, and JG made contributions to the surgery. FL made contributions to the three-dimensional reconstruction which played an important role during the surgical planning. LC contributed prominently to the pathology discussion section of the article. All authors contributed to the article and approved the submitted version.

REFERENCES

1. Filosso PL, Yao X, Ahmad U, Zhan Y, Huang J, Ruffini E, et al. Outcome of primary neuroendocrine tumors of the thymus: a joint analysis of the international thymic malignancy interest group and the European society of thoracic surgeons databases. *J Thorac Cardiovasc Surg.* (2015) 149:103–9.e2. doi: 10.1016/j.jtcvs.2014.08.061

2. Song Z, Zhang Y. Primary neuroendocrine tumors of the thymus: clinical review of 22 cases. *Oncol Lett.* (2014) 8:2125–9. doi: 10.3892/ol.2014. 2490

3. Goto K, Kodama T, Matsuno Y, Yokose T, Asamura H, Kamiya N, et al. Clinicopathologic and DNA cytometric analysis of carcinoid tumors of the thymus. *Mod Pathol.* (2001) 14:985–94. doi: 10.1038/modpathol.3880423

4. Park MS, Chung KY, Kim KD, Yang WI, Chung JH, Kim YS, et al. Prognosis of thymic epithelial tumors according to the new World Health Organization histologic classification. *Ann Thorac Surg.* (2004) 78:992–7. doi: 10.1016/j. athoracsur.2004.03.097

5. Cardillo G, Rea F, Lucchi M, Paul MA, Margaritora S, Carleo F, et al. Primary neuroendocrine tumors of the thymus: a multicenter experience of 35 patients.

Ann Thorac Surg. (2012) 94:241–5. doi: 10.1016/j.athoracsur.2012.03.062

6. Moran CA, Suster S. Neuroendocrine carcinomas (carcinoid tumor) of the thymus. A clinicopathologic analysis of 80 cases. *Am J Clin Pathol.* (2000) 114:100–10. doi: 10.1309/3PDN-PMT5-EQTM-H0CD

7. Teh BT, McArdle J, Chan SP, Menon J, Hartley L, Pullan P, et al. Clinicopathologic studies of thymic carcinoids in multiple endocrine neoplasia type 1. *Medicine.* (1997) 76:21–9. doi: 10.1097/00005792-199701000-00002

8. Kondo K, Monden Y. Therapy for thymic epithelial tumors: a clinical study of 1,320 patients from Japan. *Ann Thorac Surg.* (2003) 76:878–84. doi: 10.1016/ s0003-4975(03)00555-1

9. Spaggiari L, Pastorino U. Double transmanubrial approach and sternotomy for resection of a giant thymic carcinoid tumor. *Ann Thorac Surg.* (2001) 72:629–31. doi: 10.1016/s0003-4975(01)02710-2

10. Filosso PL, Actis Dato GM, Ruffini E, Bretti S, Ozzello F, Mancuso M. Multidisciplinary treatment of advanced thymic neuroendocrine carcinoma (carcinoid): report of a successful case and review of the literature. *J Thorac Cardiovasc Surg.* (2004) 127:1215–9. doi: 10.1016/j.jtcvs.2003.09.058

9

StainNet: A Fast and Robust Stain Normalization Network

Hongtao Kang [1,2], Die Luo [1,2], Weihua Feng [1,2], Shaoqun Zeng [1,2], Tingwei Quan [1,2], Junbo Hu [3] and Xiuli Liu [1,2*]*

[1] *Britton Chance Center for Biomedical Photonics, Wuhan National Laboratory for Optoelectronics, Huazhong University of Science and Technology, Wuhan, China,* [2] *Ministry of Education (MOE) Key Laboratory for Biomedical Photonics, School of Engineering Sciences, Huazhong University of Science and Technology, Wuhan, China,* [3] *Department of Pathology, Hubei Maternal and Child Health Hospital, Wuhan, China*

*Correspondence:
Junbo Hu
cqjbhu@163.com
Xiuli Liu
xlliu@mail.hust.edu.cn

Stain normalization often refers to transferring the color distribution to the target image and has been widely used in biomedical image analysis. The conventional stain normalization usually achieves through a pixel-by-pixel color mapping model, which depends on one reference image, and it is hard to achieve accurately the style transformation between image datasets. In principle, this difficulty can be well-solved by deep learning-based methods, whereas, its complicated structure results in low computational efficiency and artifacts in the style transformation, which has restricted the practical application. Here, we use distillation learning to reduce the complexity of deep learning methods and a fast and robust network called StainNet to learn the color mapping between the source image and the target image. StainNet can learn the color mapping relationship from a whole dataset and adjust the color value in a pixel-to-pixel manner. The pixel-to-pixel manner restricts the network size and avoids artifacts in the style transformation. The results on the cytopathology and histopathology datasets show that StainNet can achieve comparable performance to the deep learning-based methods. Computation results demonstrate StainNet is more than 40 times faster than StainGAN and can normalize a 100,000 × 100,000 whole slide image in 40 s.

Keywords: stain normalization, cytopathology, histopathology, convolutional neural network (CNN), generative adversarial network (GANs)

INTRODUCTION

Tissues or cells are usually transparent and need to be stained before observation under a microscope. However, the potential factor in the staining reagent, staining process, and slide scanner specifications often result in inconsistency of pathological images (1). These variations not only affect the judgment of pathologists but also weaken the performance of CAD systems and hamper their applications in pathology (2–4). So, stain normalization is a routine pre-processing operation for pathological images, especially for CAD systems, and it is reported to help increase the prediction accuracy, such as tumor classification (5). Stain normalization algorithms usually transfer the color style of the source image to that of a target image (6) while preserving the other information in the processed image (7), which can be broadly classified into two classes: conventional methods and deep learning-based methods.

Conventional methods are mainly realized by analyzing, converting, and matching color components, which can be divided into color matching and stain-separation methods. Color matching methods calculated the mean and SD of source images and matched them to a reference image in the Lab color space (8, 9). Stain-separation methods try to separate and normalize each staining channel independently (10–12). For instance, Ruifrok and Johnston (10) proposed to measure the relative proportion for three channels (R, G, and B) with the slides stained by only a single stain reagent (Hematoxylin or Eosin) to estimate stain vectors. And different mathematical methods were applied to compute stain vectors, such as singular value decomposition (SVD) in Optical Density (OD) space (11), sparse non-negative matrix factorization (SNMF) (12), or a pertained classifier (6). However, Pap stain used in cervical cytopathology involves not only Hematoxylin and Eosin but also Orange, Light Green, and Bismarck Brown (13), which makes it more difficult to distill the various dye vectors on cervical cytopathology. Nevertheless, most of these methods rely on a reference image to estimate stain parameters, but it is hard for one reference image to cover all staining phenomena or represent all input images, which usually causes misestimation of stain parameters and thus delivers inaccurate normalization results (14, 15).

Deep learning-based methods mostly apply generative adversarial networks (GANs) to achieve stain normalization (3, 7, 8, 16–18). Shaban et al. (8) proposed an unsupervised stain normalization method named StainGAN based on CycleGAN (16) to transfer the stain style. Cai et al. (3) proposed a new generator to improve the image quality and accelerate the networks. On the other hand, Cho et al. (18), Salehi et al. (7), and Tellez et al. (17) reconstructed original images from the images with color augmentations, e.g., grayscale and Hue-Saturation-Value (HSV) transformation, and tried to normalize other color styles to the original. However, due to the complexity of deep neural networks and the instability of GANs, it is hard to preserve all source information; sometimes, it has a risk of introducing some artifacts, which has some adverse effects on subsequent analysis (19). At the same time, the network of deep learning-based methods usually contains millions of parameters, so it generally requires high-computing resources and the computing efficiency is generally low (14).

Deep learning-based methods perform well in stain normalization, but they are not satisfactory in the robustness and computational efficiency. In this paper, we propose a stain normalization network named StainNet, which employs a fully 1×1 convolution network to adjust the color value in a pixel-by-pixel manner. In the method, StainGAN was used as the teacher network and StainNet as the student network to learn the color mapping by distillation learning. Results show that StainNet can achieve comparable normalization performance with StainGAN but retains the source information better. The results also demonstrate that StainNet was more than 40 times faster than StainGAN in computational efficiency, which allows StainNet to normalize a $100,000 \times 100,000$ whole slide image in 40 s.

MATERIALS AND METHODS

Dataset

Five datasets were used to evaluate the performance of different methods. Among them, the aligned cytopathology dataset and

the aligned histopathology dataset are used to evaluate the similarity between the normalized image and the target image. The cytopathology classification dataset and the histopathology classification dataset are used to verify normalization algorithms in the classification task. Twenty metastases whole slide images (WSIs) from the University Medical Center Utrecht in Camelyon16 testing part was used to test the effects of the StainNet normalization on the clinical diagnostics. This study was approved by the Ethics Committee of Tongji Medical College, Huazhong University of Science and Technology.

The Aligned Cytopathology Dataset for Evaluating the Similarity

These cytopathology datasets are taken from the same slides (Thinprep cytologic test slides from the Maternal and Child Hospital of Hubei Province) with two slide scanners. One scanner is custom constructed, called Scanner O, equipped with a 20x objective lens with a pixel size of $0.2930 \, \mu m$. The other from Shenzhen Shengqiang Technology Co., Ltd., called scanner T, has a 40x objective lens and a pixel size of $0.1803 \, \mu m$. We resampled the images from scanner T to reduce the pixel size to $0.2930 \, \mu m$, and then performed rigid and no-rigid registration to align the resampled images to these from scanner O. Finally, 3,223 aligned image pairs with the size of 512×512 pixels were collected. Among these images, 2,257 pairs of images were randomly selected as the training set, and the remaining 966 pairs of images were used as the test set. The images from the scanner O and T are seen as source images and target images, respectively.

The Cytopathology Classification Dataset for Verifying Normalization Algorithms

This dataset used the same data source as that in section The Aligned Cytopathology Dataset for Evaluating the Similarity. The patches from scanner T are used as the training set to train the classifier, and these from scanner O are used as the test set to evaluate the classifier. In this dataset, the patches with abnormal cells were labeled by cytopathologists as abnormal patches and the patches without abnormal cells as normal patches. There are 6,589 abnormal patches, 6,589 normal patches in the training dataset, 3,343 abnormal patches, and 3,192 normal patches in the test dataset. The resolution of patches was resampled to 256×256 with $0.4862 \, \mu m$ per pixel. We used StainGAN and StainNet trained on the aligned cytopathology dataset in section The Aligned Cytopathology Dataset for Evaluating the Similarity to normalize the patches in the test set to the style of the training set. Then, we used the original test set and the normalized test set to verify the necessity of stain normalization and evaluate the performance of StainGAN and StainNet.

The Aligned Histopathology Dataset for Evaluating the Similarity

The histopathology dataset is from the publicly available part of the MITOS-ATYPIA ICPR'14 challenge (20). In the MITOS-ATYPIA dataset (20), there are 16 slides with standard hematoxylin and eosin (H&E) staining, 11 slides as the training set, and 5 slides as the test set. And all the aligned images are taken from the same slide but using two slide scanners: Aperio

Scanscope XT called scanner A and Hamamatsu Nanozoomer 2.0-HT called scanner H. The number of image frames is variable from slide to slide. The training data set contains 1,200 frames, and the test data set contains 496 frames at 40x magnification. The resolution of the frames from scanner H was resampled to that of frames from scanner A, and then performed rigid and no-rigid registration to align the resampled frames to these from scanner A. We cropped 16 patches with the size of 256 × 256 from every frame without overlap, so there are 19,200 patch pairs in our training set and 7,936 patch pairs in our testing set. In this dataset, the images from the scanners A and H are seen as source images and target images, respectively.

The Histopathology Classification Dataset for Verifying Normalization Algorithms

The publicly available Camelyon16 dataset (21) is used, which contains 399 WSIs from two centers. In our experiments, 170 WSIs from Radboud University Medical Center in Camelyon16 training part were used to extract the training patches, and 50 WSIs from University Medical Center Utrecht in Camelyon16 testing part were used to extract the test patches. We labeled the patches containing tumor cells as abnormal and the patches not containing any tumor cells as normal. For abnormal patches, we extracted patches of size 256 × 256 from the tumor area in tumor slides. For normal patches, we randomly extracted patches of size 256 × 256 from the normal area in tumor slides and normal slides until the number of normal patches was equal to the number of abnormal patches. In this way, there are 40,000 patches in our training set and 10,000 patches in the testing set. In addition, we also randomly extracted 6,000 patches from the training set and test set to train StainGAN and StainNet, where the patches from the test set were used as the source image, and the patches from the training set were used as the target image. For the classifier trained on the training set, we used the original test set and the normalized test set to evaluate the classifier and the performance of StainGAN and StainNet.

StainNet for Stain Normalization

The framework is shown in **Figure 1**, which mainly consists of two steps: one step is StainGAN training, a generative confrontation network with two generators and two discriminators, and the other step is StainNet generation, which is composed of a fully convolutional neural network. StainNet needs paired source and target images to learn the transformation from the source color space to the target color space. In practice, it is hard to get the paired images and align the images perfectly; we used StainGAN as the teacher network and StainNet as the student network. That is, StainNet uses the L1 loss to learn the output of StainGAN.

There are two generators (G_A and G_B) and a discriminator (D_A and D_B) in StainGAN. G_A is used to transfer the image from the source domain to the target domain, and G_B is used to transfer from the target domain to the source domain. D_A is used to distinguish the image generated by G_A and a real target image, D_B is used to distinguish the image generated by G_B or a real source image. There are two losses in StainGAN,

namely cycle-consistency loss and adversarial loss. The cycle-consistency loss (16) ensures that the generated images by G_A can be reconstructed to source image by G_B, and the generated images by G_B can be reconstructed to target image by G_A. The adversarial loss tries to ensure the stain distribution of the generated images is consistent with the real distribution.

In the current convolutional neural network, convolution operations employ a kernel size of 3 × 3 or larger. However, a 3 × 3 or larger convolution performs a weighted summation in the local neighborhood of the input image. Therefore, the pixel value in the output image is inevitably affected by the local neighborhood of the input image. Unlike the 3 × 3 convolutions, the 1 × 1 convolution only maps a single pixel and has nothing to do with the local neighborhood values. That is, it will not be affected by the texture and can keep the source information of inputs. Following this, a fully 1 × 1 convolutional neural network named StainNet is used to extract the mapping relationship from StainGAN. Except for the last convolutional layer, ReLU is used as a convolutional layer to enhance the non-linear mapping ability. Considering the balance of performance and computational efficiency, we used three convolutional layers with 32 channels by default. Therefore, our network only contains about 1,000 parameters, whereas the generator in StainGAN contains millions of parameters.

The training process mainly consists of three steps. Firstly, we trained StainGAN using an unpaired source and target images. Then, the generator of StainGAN was used to normalize the source images. At last, the normalized images were taken as the Ground Truths to train StainNet with L1 Loss and SGD optimizer. The mapping relationship of StainGAN is based on the image content, that is, the mapping relationship will change accordingly with the different image contents. By learning the normalized images by StainGAN, StainNet can transfer the mapping relationship of StainGAN based on image content into a mapping relationship based on pixel values.

EXPERIMENTS AND RESULTS

In this section, StainNet is compared with the state-of-the-art methods of Reinhard (9), Macenko (11), Vahadane (12), and StainGAN on the cytopathology and histopathology dataset. We report: (1) Quantitative comparison of different methods in the visual appearance, (2) Application results on the cytopathology and histopathology classification task, (3) Quantitative comparison between the whole slide images normalization results and the whole slide images metastasis detection results.

Evaluation Metrics

In order to evaluate the performance of different methods, we measured the similarity between the normalized image and the target image, and the consistency between the normalized image and the source image.

Two similarity metrics—Structural Similarity index (SSIM) (21) and Peak Signal-to-Noise Ratio (PSNR)—are used to evaluate the performance. The SSIM and PSNR of the target image (SSIM Target and PSNR Target) are used to evaluate the

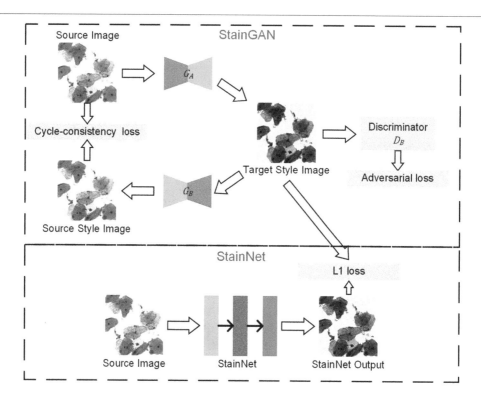

FIGURE 1 | The framework of StainNet. First, StainGAN normalizes the images from the source domain to the target domain. Then, the normalized images by StainGAN are set as Ground Truth to train StainNet. The images from the source domain are mapped to the source domain and then back to the target domain by StainGAN. The same reverse process is also performed for images from the target domain. StainNet is a fully 1 × 1 convolutional neural network, which can directly map the images from the source domain to the target domain.

TABLE 1 | Evaluation metrics of various stain normalization methods on the cytopathology dataset.

Methods	SSIM target	PSNR target	SSIM source	FPS
Reinhard	0.739 ± 0.046	19.8 ± 3.3	0.885 ± 0.042	54.8
Macenko	0.731 ± 0.054	22.5 ± 3.1	0.853 ± 0.054	4.0
Vahadane	0.739 ± 0.050	22.6 ± 3.0	0.867 ± 0.050	0.5
StainGAN	0.764 ± 0.030	29.7 ± 1.6	0.905 ± 0.021	19.6
StainNet	0.809 ± 0.027	29.8 ± 1.7	0.945 ± 0.025	881.8

TABLE 2 | Evaluation metrics of various stain normalization methods on the histopathology dataset.

Methods	SSIM target	PSNR target	SSIM source
Reinhard	0.617 ± 0.106	19.9 ± 2.1	0.964 ± 0.031
Macenko	0.656 ± 0.115	20.7 ± 2.7	0.966 ± 0.049
Vahadane	0.664 ± 0.116	21.1 ± 2.8	0.967 ± 0.046
StainGAN	0.706 ± 0.099	22.7 ± 2.6	0.912 ± 0.025
StainNet	0.691 ± 0.107	22.5 ± 3.3	0.957 ± 0.007

similarity between the normalized image and the target image. The extent of source information preservation is weighed by the SSIM of the source image (SSIM Source), which also was used to measure the similarity between the normalized image and the source image. SSIM Target and PSNR Target are calculated using the original RGB values. SSIM Source is used to measure the preservation of the source image texture information, similar to (22), we used grayscale images to calculate SSIM Source. And the statistic results of SSIM Target, PSNR Target, and SSIM Source on the testing set in the aligned cytopathology dataset and the aligned histopathology dataset are shown in **Tables 1**, **2**, which contain 966 and 7,936 patch pairs, respectively.

The Area Under the Curve (AUC) of the Receiver Operating Characteristics (ROC) is used to evaluate the

classifier performance. The statistic results of AUC on the cytopathology and histopathology datasets are shown in **Table 3**, as Mean ± standard deviation, which contain 6,535 and 10,000 patches, respectively.

Implementation

For conventional methods, Reinhard (9), Macenko (11), and Vahadane (12), a carefully picked image was used as the reference image. For the StainGAN, the model was trained using Adam optimizer, and training was stopped at the 100th epoch, which was chosen experimentally. For StainNet, the trained StainGAN was used to normalize the source images in both the training dataset and the test dataset. Then, the normalized images were used as the ground truths during training. StainNet was trained with stochastic gradient descent (SGD) optimizer, an initial learning rate of .01, and a batch size of 10. The L1 loss was used to minimize the difference between the output of the network and the normalized image by the trained StainGAN. A cosine annealing scheduler was adopted to decay the learning rate from 0.01 to 0 during 300 epochs. The weights corresponding to the model with the lowest test loss were selected during the training.

TABLE 3 | The AUC for various stain normalization methods on the cytopathology and the histopathology classification dataset.

AUC	The cytopathology classification dataset	The histopathology classification dataset
Original	0.832 ± 0.016	0.685 ± 0.033
Reinhard	0.738 ± 0.014	0.821 ± 0.005
Macenko	0.872 ± 0.006	0.843 ± 0.007
Vahadane	0.832 ± 0.011	0.847 ± 0.005
StainGAN	0.896 ± 0.002	0.905 ± 0.006
StainNet	0.901 ± 0.002	0.895 ± 0.009

On the application task, stain normalization was used as a pre-processing step to increase the performance of the CAD system. A classifier was trained on the cytopathology classification dataset and histopathology classification dataset to prove this. We used a pre-trained SqueezeNet (23) on ImageNet (24) as the classifier and fine-tuned it on the images of the training dataset. The classifier was trained with Adam optimizer, an initial learning rate of 2e-4, and a batch size of 64. Cross-entropy loss was used as our loss function. A cosine annealing scheduler was adopted to decay the learning rate from 2e-3 to 0 in 60 epochs. The training was stopped at the 60th epoch, which was chosen experimentally. The experiment was repeated 20 times in order to enhance reliability.

Results

Stain Transfer Results

Firstly, we evaluated the effectiveness of our method. The normalized images by StainNet are evaluated with the target images through vision and the gray value profiles around the cell nucleus shown in **Figures 2**, **3**. The results on the aligned cytopathology dataset are shown in **Figure 2**, the source images

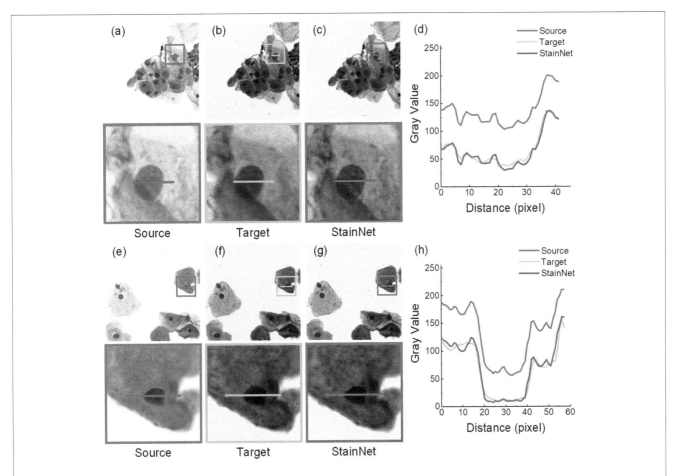

FIGURE 2 | StainNet normalization effects on the cytopathology image. The source images, the target images, and the normalized images by StainNet are shown in **(a,e)**, **(b,f)**, and **(c,g)**, respectively. The image in the box is enlarged below. Gray value profiles of the lines on **(a–c)** are shown in the line chart **(d)**, and the lines in **(e–g)** are shown in the line chart **(h)**.

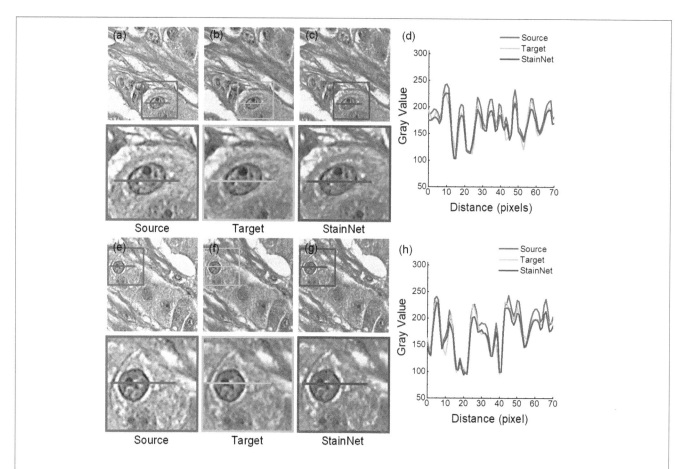

FIGURE 3 | StainNet normalization effects on the histopathology image. The source images, the target images, and the normalized images by StainNet are shown in **(a,e) (b,f)**, and **(c,g)**, respectively. The image in the box is enlarged below. Gray value profiles of the lines on **(a–c)** are shown in the line chart **(d)**, and the lines in **(e–g)** are shown in the line chart **(h)**.

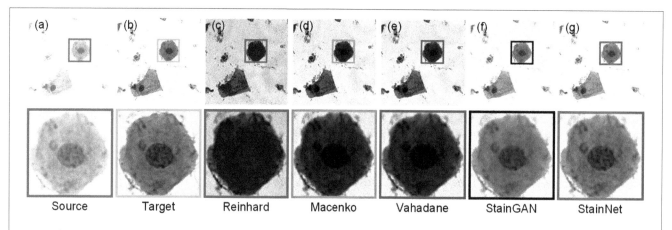

FIGURE 4 | Visual comparison of different normalization methods on the aligned cytopathology dataset. Source image **(a)**, target image **(b)**, and normalized image by Reinhard **(c)**, Macenko **(d)**, Vahadane **(e)**, StainGAN **(f)**, and StainNet **(g)** are listed.

are from scanner O, and the target images are from scanner T. From the figure, the normalized images in **Figures 2c,g** are similar to the target images in **Figures 2b,f**. The gray value profiles at the nucleus of the source images, target images,

and normalized images are shown in **Figures 3d,h**. The gray value profiles of the normalized images by StainNet and the target images coincide on the whole indicating that, after being normalized by StainNet, the normalized images have similar

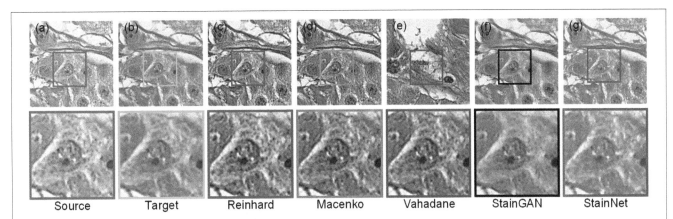

FIGURE 5 | Visual comparison of different normalization methods on the aligned histopathology dataset. Source image **(a)**, target image **(b)**, and normalized image by Reinhard **(c)**, Macenko **(d)**, Vahadane **(e)**, StainGAN **(f)**, and StainNet **(g)** are listed.

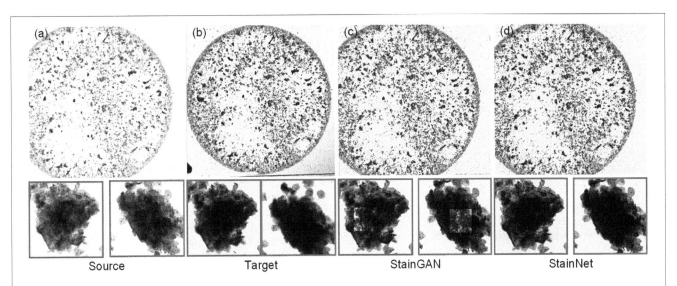

FIGURE 6 | The whole slide image normalization result on the cytopathology dataset. The source slide **(a)**, the target slide **(b)**, the normalized slide by StainGAN **(c)**, and the normalized slide by StainNet **(d)** are listed.

color distribution with the target images. In terms of local gray value profiles, the changing trend of the normalized images by StainNet is the same as that of the source images, which shows that StainNet can fully retain the information of the source images.

The results on the aligned histopathology dataset are shown in **Figure 3**. The histopathology dataset was from the publicly available part of the MITOS-ATYPIA ICPR'14 challenge (20). The aligned images are taken from the same slide but using two slide scanners: Aperio Scanscope XT called scanner A and Hamamatsu Nanozoomer 2.0-HT called scanner H. From the figure, we can see, after normalization, the images have a similar vision and the gray value profiles with the target images.

Furthermore, we compare the normalization effect of StainNet with the other four classic methods, Reinhard, Macenko, Vahadane, and StainGAN. Results are shown in **Figure 4**. From the figure, we can see the Reinhard method performs badly

because it is hard to choose an image to represent the entire dataset due to the discreteness of cytopathological images. Macenko and Vahadane, based on stain separation, perform poorly on cytopathological images. Both StainGAN and StainNet perform well.

The quantitative results on the aligned cytopathology dataset are shown in **Table 1**. From **Table 1**, parameters PSNR Target of the conventional methods is lower than that of StainGAN and StainNet. StainNet outperforms other methods in all indicators. Among them, SSIM Target and SSIM Source are 0.809 and 0.945 higher than 0.764 and 0.905 of StainGAN, which shows that StainNet is not only more similar to the target image but also better to retain the source image information.

The visual comparison of the aligned histopathology dataset is shown in **Figure 5**. From it, the normalized images by the conventional methods are still visually different from the target image due to the dependence on the reference image and the

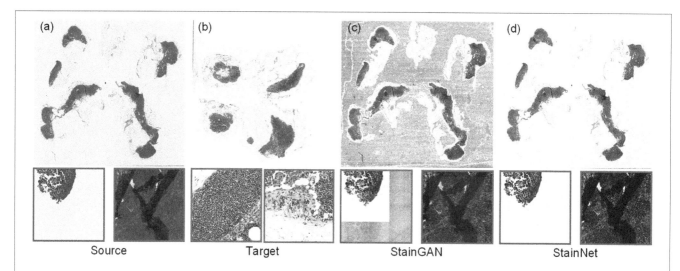

(a) (b) (c) (d)

Source   Target   StainGAN   StainNet

FIGURE 7 | The whole slide image normalization result on the Camelyon16 dataset. The source slide **(a)**, the target slide **(b)**, the normalized slide by StainGAN **(c)**, and the normalized slide by StainNet **(d)** are listed.

TABLE 4 | The SSIM source of the normalized whole slide image by StainGAN and StainNet.

	StainGAN	StainNet
The cytopathology WSIs	0.905 ± 0.093	0.954 ± 0.050
The histopathology WSIs	0.762 ± 0.182	0.980 ± 0.013

difficulty of image selection of the conventional methods. The normalized images by StainGAN and StainNet are consistent with the style of the target image. In addition, the normalized image by StainNet not only has a similar color to the target image but also retains more source information.

The quantitative comparison of the aligned histopathology dataset is shown in **Table 2**. The test data and training data are completely separated at the slide level and divided in the same way as in the MITOS-ATYPIA ICPR'14 challenge (20), so there is no deviation caused by personal factors. Due to the rigid and non-rigid registration, the source image and the target image can be precisely matched. The dataset division and image registration make our results more reliable. StainGAN and StainNet are higher than conventional methods in the similarity of SSIM Target and PSNR Target with the target images. The SSIM Target and PSNR Target of StainNet are 0.691 and 22.5, respectively, which are slightly lower than 0.706 and 22.7 of StainGAN, 0.957 of StainNet is higher than 0.912 of StainGAN in the SSIM Source. Therefore, StainNet can obtain normalized results comparable to StainGAN but retain the source image information better, which is important in real CAD systems.

Next, we compared the normalization effects StainNet and StainGAN on image classification. SqueezeNet (22) pre-trained on ImageNet (23) was chosen as the classifier because of its small size and relatively high accuracy. On the cytopathology classification dataset, we used 13,178 image patches from scanner T to train the classifier and use 6,535 image patches from scanner

O to evaluate the classifier. On the histopathology classification dataset, the classifier was trained with 40,000 image patches from Radboud University Medical Center, and the classifier was evaluated with 10,000 image patches from University Medical Center Utrecht. **Table 3** shows the performance of the classifier with normalization and not with normalization. For the original images in the test set, there is only an AUC of 0.832 on the cytopathology classification dataset, and only 0.685 on the histopathology classification dataset. It shows that the classifier has a strong color bias and cannot be directly applied to the test data with different color styles from the training data. The AUC was increased to 0.896 and 0.905 by using StainGAN and 0.901 and 0.895 by using StainNet on the cytopathology classification dataset and histopathology classification dataset. The conventional stain normalization methods hardly achieve a better AUC, especially in the histopathology classification dataset, and the performance of the conventional method is lower than StainGAN and StainNet. The above results show that both StainGAN and StainNet can effectively improve the accuracy of the classifier, and the performance of the StainNet method and the StainGAN method is comparable.

Whole Slide Images Results

For a whole slide image (WSI), there are two main challenges in stain normalization: One is that WSIs are very large: a typical WSI may contain 100,000 × 100,000 pixels. So, computational efficiency is very important. The other is that WSIs may contain many naturally occurring and human-induced artifacts, e.g., air bubbles, dust, and out-of-focus. So, the methods must be robust to these phenomena when they are applied in a real-world system. Since StainNet has a very concise structure and only maps based on color values, it is less affected by the distribution of the training data and has better robustness.

In this experiment, we randomly selected 20 cytopathology WSIs from the same data source in section The Aligned

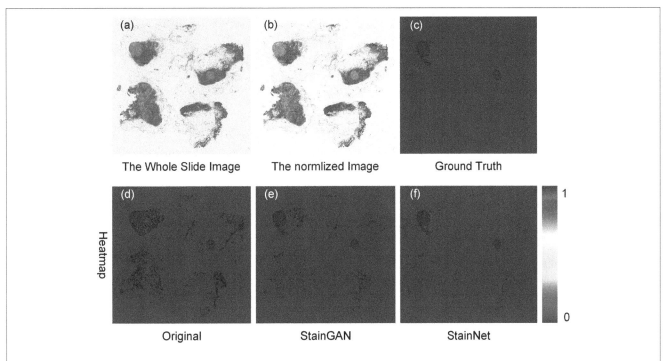

FIGURE 8 | Effects of color normalization on metastasis cancer tissue detection. The original whole slide image **(a)**, the normalized image by StainNet **(b)**, the ground truth **(c)** of the metastasis cancer, and the detection heat maps from the original image **(d)**, from the image by normalized StainGAN **(e)**, and from the image by normalized StainNet **(f)**.

Cytopathology Dataset for Evaluating the Similarity and 20 histopathology WSIs from the Camelyon16 dataset. StainGAN and StainNet are used to normalize these WSIs to the target style. Results show the computational efficiency of StainNet is more than 40 times that of StainGAN and can normalize a 100,000 × 100,000 whole slide image in 40 s, which is very important for real-time application.

For the cytopathology WSIs, StainGAN and StainNet trained on the aligned cytopathology dataset were used to perform normalization, as shown in **Figure 6**. From **Figure 6**, the normalized WSI by StainGAN has artifacts in the center of crowded cell clusters. Our proposed StainNet achieves better results maybe because of its robustness and less reliance on the distribution of the training set.

For the histopathology WSIs, StainGAN and StainNet trained on the histopathology classification dataset were used to perform normalization, as shown in **Figure 7**. StainGAN has artifacts in the blank background area and the out-of-focus area. Similar to the cytopathology WSIs, StainNet achieves a better performance.

SSIM Source was used to quantitatively evaluate the normalized performance by StainGAN and StainNet in this experiment. In **Table 4**, StainNet has a higher mean value and a lower standard deviation, which shows that StainNet not only can obtain better image quality but also has consistent and robust performance on the WSIs. The standard deviation of StainGAN is increased, which shows that the performance of StainGAN is not stable enough on the WSIs.

Furthermore, we tested the effects of the StainNet normalization on clinical diagnostics. Here, we chose the

TABLE 5 | The recall, precision, and accuracy of the metastasis detection at the WSI level.

	Recall	Precision	Accuracy
The original WSIs	0.781	0.368	0.940
The normalized WSIs by StainGAN	0.686	0.708	0.977
The normalized WSIs by StainNet	0.629	0.781	0.979

metastasis cancer slides and demonstrated the detection results on the WSI level. Twenty metastases WSIs from the University Medical Center Utrecht in Camelyon16 testing part were used, and the whole slide image was divided into several 256 × 256 image blocks with a 64 × 64 stride by a sliding window way. SqueezeNet was trained on the histopathology classification dataset, and then to detect the original WSIs and the normalized WSIs by StainGAN and StainNet, shown in **Figure 8**. From the picture, we can see, compared with the grand truth, there are a large number of normal areas that are misidentified as metastasis areas. After being normalized with StainGAN and StainNet, the misidentification area is reduced. The statistic results are shown in **Table 5**; the parameters of recall, precision, and accuracy are used to quantitatively evaluate the metastasis detection results on the WSIs. It can be seen that the precision of the original WSIs is only 0.368, and StainGAN and StainNet can improve the precision of recognition, which are 0.708 and 0.781, respectively. For the accuracy of recognition of all image blocks on the whole slide image, the accuracy of the original image without normalization is 0.940, and the accuracy of StainGAN and

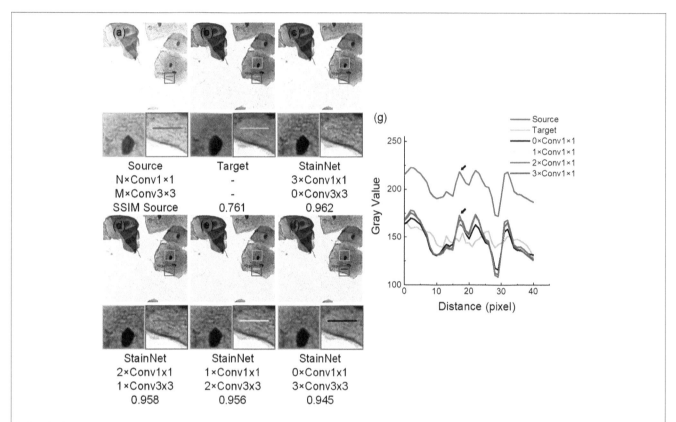

FIGURE 9 | Effects of 1 × 1 and 3 × 3 convolutions. NxConv1x1 and MxConv3x3 refer to the number of 1 × 1 convolution and 3 × 3 convolutions. StainNet contains only three convolution layers, so the total number of 1 × 1 convolution and 3 × 3 convolutions is three, that is, M + N = 3. The image in the dashed box is enlarged below. Gray value profiles of the straight lines in **(a–f)** are shown in the line chart **(g)**.

StainNet is 0.977 and 0.979, respectively. The preliminary results show that our method is better than StainGAN in accuracy and precision in the application of WSI metastasis detection.

The effectiveness of 1 × 1 convolution is verified by replacing the three 1 × 1 convolutions in StainNet with 3 × 3 convolutions in turn. The source image, target image, and normalized image by different structures of StainNet are shown in **Figures 9a–f**, and the gray value profiles of the straight lines in **Figures 9a–f** are shown in **Figure 9g**. It is clear that, with the increase of 3 × 3 convolutions, the normalized image becomes more blurred, and the ability to preserve the source information is getting worse. The best image quality can be obtained fully using 1 × 1 convolution in **Figure 9c**. In particular, at the place pointed by the black arrow in **Figure 9g**, only a fully 1 × 1 convolutional network can best preserve the grayscale changes of the source image.

The different evaluation metrics, SSIM Target, PSNR Target, and SSIM Source for different structures of StainNet are reported in **Table 6**. Although the 3 × 3 convolutions may help improve the similarity with the target images, they affect the ability to preserve the source information. Not changing the information of the source image is a basic requirement for stain normalization, so a fully 1 × 1 convolutional network is chosen.

TABLE 6 | Evaluation metrics of different StainNet structures.

Number of Conv 1 x 1	Number of Conv 3 x 3	SSIM target	PSNR target	SSIM source
3	0	0.808	29.8	0.960
2	1	0.814	30.0	0.958
1	2	0.814	30.0	0.956
0	3	0.804	29.8	0.950

DISCUSSION AND CONCLUSION

In this paper, we achieved stain normalization by using a fully 1 × 1 convolutional network in a pixel-to-pixel manner, which not only avoids the low computational efficiency and possible artifacts of deep learning-based methods but also preserves well the information of the source image. Compared with conventional methods, StainNet learns the mapping relationship from the whole dataset instead of relying on one single reference image, so it can obtain the normalized image with high similarity. Furthermore, StainNet has been validated on four datasets, including two public datasets, and the results show that StainNet has better performance, especially in computational efficiency and robustness.

Compared with the traditional methods, StainNet avoids the difficulty of choosing reference images. For the cytopathy image, the proportion of blank backgrounds is various, so the standard deviation and mean of the different images also are different, and we cannot find an image to represent the entire dataset. This is the reason that the Reinhard method does not perform well in **Figure 4c**. For Macenko and Vahadane, the color normalization method is based on stain separation, it is difficult to perform stain separation correctly due to the use of multiple stains for cytopathological images instead of only eosin and hematoxylin in histopathology.

Compared with StainGAN, StainNet achieves comparable normalization performance. At the same time, StainNet is more than 40 times that of StainGAN in the computational efficiency and can normalize a giga-pixel WSI in 40 s. And, more importantly, StainNet retains the source information better and would not produce some artifacts. StainNet retains the advantages of better color normalization of StainGAN, while a fully 1×1 convolutional network overcomes the determination of slow speed and instability.

In short, StainNet, a fast and robust stain normalization network, has the potential to perform normalization in real-time in a real-world CAD system.

AUTHOR CONTRIBUTIONS

HK contributed to the conception, implemented the experiments, and wrote the first draft of the manuscript. JH provided a cytopathology dataset and annotated the cytopathology images. HK, DL, WF, JH, SZ, TQ, and XL designed the study and contributed to the result analysis and manuscript revision. All authors approved the manuscript.

REFERENCES

1. Salvi M, Michielli N, Molinari F. Stain Color Adaptive Normalization (SCAN) algorithm: separation and standardization of histological stains in digital pathology. *Comput Methods Programs Biomed.* (2020) 193:105506. doi: 10.1016/j.cmpb.2020.105506

2. Ciompi F, Geessink O, Bejnordi BE, De Souza GS, Baidoshvili A, Litjens G, et al. The importance of stain normalization in colorectal tissue classification with convolutional networks. In: *Proceedings - International Symposium on Biomedical Imaging.* Melbourne, VIC: IEEE (2017). p. 160–3. doi: 10.1109/ISBI.2017.7950492

3. Cai S, Xue Y, Gao Q, Du M, Chen G, Zhang H, et al. Stain style transfer using transitive adversarial networks. In: Knoll F, Maier A, Rueckert D, Ye JC, editors. *Machine Learning for Medical Image Reconstruction.* Cham: Springer International Publishing (2020). p. 163–72.

4. Ismail SM, Colclough AB, Dinnen JS, Eakins D, Evans DM, Gradwell E, et al. Observer variation in histopathological diagnosis and grading of cervical intraepithelial neoplasia. *BMJ.* (1989) 298:707–10. doi: 10.1136/bmj.298.6675.707

5. Anghel A, Stanisavljevic M, Andani S, Papandreou N, Rüschoff JH, Wild P, et al. High-performance system for robust stain normalization of whole-slide images in histopathology. *Front Med.* (2019) 6:193. doi: 10.3389/fmed.2019.00193

6. Khan AM, Rajpoot N, Treanor D, Magee D, A. nonlinear mapping approach to stain normalization in digital histopathology images using image-specific color deconvolution. *IEEE Trans Biomed Eng.* (2014) 61:1729–38. doi: 10.1109/TBME.2014.2303294

7. Salehi P, Chalechale A. Pix2Pix-based stain-to-stain translation: a solution for robust stain normalization in histopathology images analysis. In: *2020 International Conference on Machine Vision and Image Processing (MVIP 2020).* Qom (2020). p. 1–7. doi: 10.1109/MVIP49855.2020.9116895

8. Shaban MT, Baur C, Navab N, Albarqouni S. Staingan: stain style transfer for digital histological images. In: *2019 IEEE 16th International Symposium on Biomedical Imaging (ISBI).* Venice: IEEE (2019). p. 953–6. doi: 10.1109/ISBI.2019.8759152

9. Reinhard E, Adhikhmin M, Gooch B, Shirley P. Color transfer between images. *IEEE Comput Graph Appl.* (2001) 21:34–41. doi: 10.1109/38.946629

10. Ruifrok AC, Johnston DA. Quantification of histochemical staining by color deconvolution. *Anal Quant CytolHistol.* (2001) 23:291–9.

11. Macenko M, Niethammer M, Marron JS, Borland D, Woosley JT, Xiaojun Guan, et al. A method for normalizing histology slides for quantitative analysis. In: *2009 IEEE International Symposium on Biomedical Imaging: From Nano to Macro.* (2009). p. 1107–10. doi: 10.1109/ISBI.2009.5193250

12. Vahadane A, Peng T, Sethi A, Albarqouni S, Wang L, Baust M, et al. Structure-preserving color normalization and sparse stain separation for histological images. *IEEE Trans Med Imaging.* (2016) 35:1962–71. doi: 10.1109/TMI.2016.2529665

13. Gill GW. Papanicolaou stain. In: *Cytopreparation: Principles & Practice.* New York, NY: Springer New York (2012). p. 143–89. doi: 10.1007/978-1-4614-4933-1_10

14. Zheng Y, Jiang Z, Zhang H, Xie F, Hu D, Sun S, et al. Stain standardization capsule for application-driven histopathological image normalization. *IEEE J Biomed Heal Informatics.* (2020) 25:337–47. doi: 10.1109/JBHI.2020.2983206

15. Zhou N, Cai D, Han X, Yao J. Enhanced cycle-consistent generative adversarial network for color normalization of H&E stained images. In: Shen D, Liu T, Peters TM, Staib LH, Essert C, Zhou S, Yap PT, Khan A, editors. *Medical Image Computing and Computer Assisted Intervention – MICCAI 2019.* Cham: Springer International Publishing (2019). p. 694–702.

16. Zhu JY, Park T, Isola P, Efros AA. Unpaired image-to-image translation using cycle-consistent adversarial networks. *Proc IEEE Int Conf Comput Vis.* (2017). p. 2242–51. doi: 10.1109/ICCV.2017.244

17. Tellez D, Litjens G, Bándi P, Bulten W, Bokhorst J-M, Ciompi F, et al. Quantifying the effects of data augmentation and stain color normalization in convolutional neural networks for computational pathology. *Med Image Anal.* (2019) 58:101544. doi: 10.1016/j.media.2019.101544

18. Cho H, Lim S, Choi G, Min H. Neural stain-style transfer learning using gan for histopathological images. *arXiv* [Preprint]. (2017) 1710:08543. Available online at: https://arxiv.org/abs/1710.08543

19. Lei G, Xia Y, Zhai DH, Zhang W, Chen D, Wang D. StainCNNs: an efficient stain feature learning method. *Neurocomputing.* (2020) 406:267–73. doi: 10.1016/j.neucom.2020.04.008

20. Roux L. Detection of mitosis and evaluation of nuclear atypia score in breast cancer histological images. In: *22nd International Conference on Pattern Recognition (ICPR 2014).* Stockholm: MITOS-ATYPIA Contest (2014). Available online at: http://ludo17.free.fr/mitos_atypia_2014/icpr2014_MitosAtypia_DataDescription.pdf

21. Bejnordi BE, Veta M, Van Diest PJ, Van Ginneken B, Karssemeijer N,

Litjens G, et al. Diagnostic assessment of deep learning algorithms for detection of lymph node metastases in women with breast cancer. *JAMA.* (2017) 318:2199–210. doi: 10.1001/jama.2017.14585

22. Shrivastava A, Adorno W, Sharma Y, Ehsan L, Ali SA, Moore SR, et al. Self-attentive adversarial stain normalization. In: Del Bimbo A, Cucchiara R, Sclaroff S, Farinella GM, Mei T, Bertini M, Escalante HJ, Vezzani R, editors. *Pattern Recognition. ICPR International Workshops and Challenges. ICPR 2021.* Cham: Springer International Publishing (2021). p. 120–40. doi: 10.1007/978-3-030-68763-2_10

23. Iandola FN, Han S, Moskewicz MW, Ashraf K, Dally WJ, Keutzer K. SqueezeNet: AlexNet-level accuracy with 50x fewer parameters and < 0.5 MB model size. *arXiv [Preprint].* (2016) 1602:07360. Available online at: https://arxiv.org/abs/1602.07360

24. Deng J, Dong W, Socher R, Li L, Li K, Li FF. ImageNet: a large-scale hierarchical image database. In: *2009 IEEE Conference on Computer Vision and Pattern Recognition.* (2009). p. 248–55. doi: 10.1109/CVPR.2009.5206848

10

Code-Free Development and Deployment of Deep Segmentation Models for Digital Pathology

Henrik Sahlin Pettersen [1,2,3*], *Ilya Belevich* [4], *Elin Synnøve Røyset* [1,2,3], *Erik Smistad* [5,6], *Melanie Rae Simpson* [7,8], *Eija Jokitalo* [4], *Ingerid Reinertsen* [5,6], *Ingunn Bakke* [2,3] *and André Pedersen* [2,5,9]

[1] Department of Pathology, St. Olavs Hospital, Trondheim University Hospital, Trondheim, Norway, [2] Department of Clinical and Molecular Medicine, Faculty of Medicine and Health Sciences, NTNU - Norwegian University of Science and Technology, Trondheim, Norway, [3] Clinic of Laboratory Medicine, St. Olavs Hospital, Trondheim University Hospital, Trondheim, Norway, [4] Electron Microscopy Unit, Institute of Biotechnology, Helsinki Institute of Life Science, University of Helsinki, Helsinki, Finland, [5] Department of Health Research, SINTEF Digital, Trondheim, Norway, [6] Department of Circulation and Medical Imaging, Faculty of Medicine and Health Sciences, NTNU - Norwegian University of Science and Technology, Trondheim, Norway, [7] Department of Public Health and Nursing, Faculty of Medicine and Health Sciences, NTNU - Norwegian University of Science and Technology, Trondheim, Norway, [8] The Clinical Research Unit for Central Norway, Trondheim, Norway, [9] The Cancer Foundation, St. Olavs Hospital, Trondheim University Hospital, Trondheim, Norway

Correspondence:
Henrik Sahlin Pettersen
henrik.s.pettersen@ntnu.no

Application of deep learning on histopathological whole slide images (WSIs) holds promise of improving diagnostic efficiency and reproducibility but is largely dependent on the ability to write computer code or purchase commercial solutions. We present a code-free pipeline utilizing free-to-use, open-source software (QuPath, DeepMIB, and FastPathology) for creating and deploying deep learning-based segmentation models for computational pathology. We demonstrate the pipeline on a use case of separating epithelium from stroma in colonic mucosa. A dataset of 251 annotated WSIs, comprising 140 hematoxylin-eosin (HE)-stained and 111 CD3 immunostained colon biopsy WSIs, were developed through active learning using the pipeline. On a hold-out test set of 36 HE and 21 CD3-stained WSIs a mean intersection over union score of 95.5 and 95.3% was achieved on epithelium segmentation. We demonstrate pathologist-level segmentation accuracy and clinical acceptable runtime performance and show that pathologists without programming experience can create near state-of-the-art segmentation solutions for histopathological WSIs using only free-to-use software. The study further demonstrates the strength of open-source solutions in its ability to create generalizable, open pipelines, of which trained models and predictions can seamlessly be exported in open formats and thereby used in external solutions. All scripts, trained models, a video tutorial, and the full dataset of 251 WSIs with ~31 k epithelium annotations are made openly available at https://github.com/andreped/NoCodeSeg to accelerate research in the field.

Keywords: computational pathology, deep learning, code-free, semantic segmentation, U-Net, open datasets, inflammatory bowel disease, colon

INTRODUCTION

Visual evaluation of histopathological whole slide images (WSIs) is the gold standard for diagnosing an array of medical conditions ranging from cancer subtyping and staging to inflammatory and infectious diseases. The increasing shortage of pathologists, in combination with continually increasing biopsy load and lack of reproducibility for several common diagnoses between pathologists, calls for the application of novel methods to improve both diagnostic efficiency and reproducibility (1–5). Application of deep learning-based methods to histopathological WSIs holds promise of improving diagnostic efficiency and reproducibility, but is largely dependent on the ability to write computer code or buy commercial solutions. The introduction of large-scale digitization of histopathological WSIs has moved several pathology departments away from manual microscopy diagnostics to diagnosing digitized WSIs on computer screens (6). The successful application of deep learning-based classification and segmentation of WSIs holds great promise for a continually increasing introduction of computer assisted diagnostics for pathologists, possibly alleviating both pathologist workload and increasing reproducibility (7, 8). Many current solutions are either commercial software with limited transparency of the applied algorithms, limited export/import capability for other software, and limited availability for diagnostic departments with strained budgets. Existing commercial solutions include software such as Visiopharm,[1] Halo AI,[2] and Aiforia,[3] but also, open-source alternatives such as MONAI-Label,[4] H-AI-L, QuickAnnotator (9–12), and ZeroCostDL4Mic (12). These open-source solutions, however, either lack a full annotation, training and visualization pipeline, require some degree of programming experience, or use commercial servers. This calls for the development and use of open-source solutions that enable transparency of the image analysis pipelines, the possibility of exporting and importing results and data between applications and use of local data without the requirement of uploading restricted images to commercial serves.

The open-source software QuPath is a user-friendly solution for WSI analysis (13). Its tools offer means for tumor identification and biomarker evaluation using conventional non-deep learning-based machine learning methods with possibilities of batch-processing and scripting, as well as communication with auxiliary image analysis applications such as ImageJ. However, no deep learning-based image segmentation functionality exists for QuPath to date, except for the possibility of calling the StarDist nucleus segmentation method (14) from a customizable script in the latest 0.3.x release.

Application of deep learning approaches to biological imaging during recent years has significantly boosted our capabilities to segment structures of interest from collected images and make them ready for visualization and quantitative analysis (15). Despite the potential quality of generated results, use of deep learning in routine research projects is still quite limited. This limitation is mostly due to a relatively high threshold barrier that is hard to overcome by researchers without extensive knowledge of computer science and programming experience. The typical deep learning workflows require knowledge of deep learning architectures, Python programming abilities, and general experience with multiple software installations. The code-free solution DeepMIB was published to help with all these aspects and with a hope to make deep learning available to a wider community of biological researchers (16). DeepMIB is a user-friendly software package that was designed to provide a smooth experience for training of convolutional neural networks (CNN) for segmentation of light and electron microscopy datasets. It is suitable for anyone with only very basic knowledge of deep learning and does not require computer programming skills.

DeepMIB comes bundled with Microscopy Image Browser (17), which is a free, open-source software package for image processing, segmentation, and quantification of microscopy datasets. Both packages are written with MATLAB, they are easy to install, and can be used either under the MATLAB environment or as a stand-alone application on Windows, macOS, or Linux.

Image segmentation in DeepMIB is organized as a step-by-step workflow, which starts with selection of a CNN architecture [2D or 3D, U-Net (18) or SegNet (19)], and definition of the most central training hyperparameters. The provided architectures are efficient and are shown to generate generalizable models even with sparse training data (20). To extend the training base, DeepMIB comes with multiple (19 for 2D, and five for 3D) augmentation filters that can be individually configured, previewed, and tuned to fulfill the needs of a specific project. The resulting CNN models can be used to predict images directly in DeepMIB or be exported to ONNX format. DeepMIB further provides the ability to test the performance of the trained model on an unseen test set with ground truth labels and evaluate the network performance using multiple metrics, such as accuracy (ACC), dice similarity coefficient (DSC) and intersection over union (IoU). The MIB software is openly available on GitHub.[5]

Multiple studies propose deep learning solutions for computational pathology (8). However, only some make their trained models openly available; even if they were, using them generally requires programming experience. In digital pathology, this is especially challenging due to the large image sizes of up to $200,000 \times 100,000$ color pixels, which makes it computationally demanding to deploy models and visualize the predictions with the WSI. Although MIB is able to run inference on the WSI level, the browser is not suitable for displaying such large images, only supports semantic segmentation models, and does not have a streamlined algorithm to exclude prediction on background glass areas. This slows viewing speed, versatility, and prediction runtime. FastPathology (21) was developed to offer a user friendly direct WSI prediction viewer to pathologists. The software is free, open-source, and focused on high-performance

---

[1]https://visiopharm.com/visiopharm-digital-image-analysis-software-features/ai-features/

[2]https://indicalab.com/halo-ai/

[3]https://www.aiforia.com/

[4]https://github.com/Project-MONAI/MONAILabel/

[5]https://github.com/Ajaxels/MIB2

computing to minimize memory usage and runtime. The software is based on the C++ library FAST (22, 23).

FastPathology enables the user to deploy deep learning methods directly from the Graphical User Interface (GUI). The software includes a rapid, pyramidal viewer for visualizing WSIs and supports overlays of segmentations. New models can be imported without implementation, by defining a FAST text pipeline that contains information about the model and how it should be handled. The software supports various inference engines i.e., TensorRT, OpenVINO, and TensorFlow (24). TensorRT enables the fastest graphical processing unit (GPU) inference, whereas OpenVINO is among the fastest central processing unit (CPU) alternatives. The recommended format is ONNX, as both OpenVINO and TensorRT support it. FastPathology is openly available on GitHub,[6] including trained models and test data.

Here we present a pipeline for developing and deploying high performance deep segmentation models for WSIs using three software packages, each specialized in different parts of the workflow (**Figure 1**). QuPath is efficient for quick annotations of WSIs, DeepMIB provides capabilities for training CNNs without programming, and FastPathology for efficient inference and visualization of full resolution model predictions with the WSI. The proposed pipeline is demonstrated on a use case of segmentation of colon epithelium and is shown to produce models that perform at a clinical acceptable accuracy and runtime level.

Example Application

The human gut mucosa comprises both non-immune and immune cells working together in a complex manner to maintain mucosal immunity. In lamina propria there are a broad range of different innate and adaptive immune cell subtypes that are separated from gut content and microbiota by a single layer of intestinal epithelial cells at the surface. These specialized epithelial cells have a pivotal role in producing mucus and antimicrobial factors, or immunomodulating cytokines involved in crosstalk between the different systems, in addition to being a physical barrier. Intermingled between the epithelial cells resides a population of intraepithelial T lymphocytes (IEL), many of which are unconventional T cells. These cells have the characteristics of both innate and adaptive immunity, and they can move and surveil the epithelium. This makes them able to respond rapidly and diverse as an effective first line defense against microbe invasion in addition to being important for maintenance of mucosal homeostasis (25, 26). Dysregulation of IELs is generally correlated to loss of mucosal barrier integrity and is implicated in the pathogenesis of several gut disorders like infections with bacteria, parasites and viruses, inflammatory processes like inflammatory bowel disease, lymphocytic colitis, and celiac disease, and possibly also tumor development (25). A lot is still unknown about the functions and clinical significance of the different IEL subtypes, and more research is needed (25, 27). Tools that provide objective and reproducible quantitative

data from tissue sections will open new doors in research and allow for new questions to be posed.

For inflammatory disorders of the GI tract that involves numerical definitions, like celiac disease or lymphocytic colitis, quantification of IEL is part of the pathologist's job. This can be done by roughly giving a visual estimate, or by manual counting of smaller areas and then make a global estimate based on that. Looking at tissue sections, the eyes are more easily drawn to the areas with the highest densities and could possibly lead to an overestimation of the number of IELs. A tool for epithelium segmentation that enables automated quantification of IELs could serve as a calibration instrument for pathologists. It can save pathologists from spending time and energy on something that can be done much more objectively by a machine. It can be of great value in research on the epithelial immune microenvironment in inflammatory and neoplastic disorders. In the present study, we have included both HE and CD3 stained images to demonstrate the potential use of this technique both for quantifying different populations of intraepithelial immune cells with the help of immunostaining and the potential (by further annotation and training) to quantify e.g., intraepithelial granulocytes directly on HE stained images. Quantification of CD3 immunostained IELs after epithelial segmentation can be achieved with high accuracy in QuPath, but is not demonstrated as part of this publication. Further developing deep learning-based models for segmentation of other important mucosal structures (e.g., lymphoid aggregates, basal plasmacytosis, specific cell types, tumors), and for other types of immunohistochemical evaluations to integrate information of protein expression, cell types and tissue structure, would vastly expand the value of this tool for research and in diagnostics.

Here, we demonstrate a use case of automatic, deep learning-based segmentation of colon epithelium with no requirements for computer programming. We further publish the resulting near pixel accurate dataset of epithelium segmentation of 140 HE stained WSIs and 111 CD3 immunostained WSIs from colon biopsies of both healthy controls and patients with active inflammatory bowel disease.

MATERIALS AND METHODS

Dataset of Endoscopic Colon Biopsies

Formalin fixed paraffin embedded (FFPE) biopsies of colonic mucosa were extracted from the NTNU/St. Olavs hospital, Trondheim University Hospital (Norway) biobank of patients with confirmed inflammatory bowel disease or healthy controls with gastrointestinal symptoms but no macroscopic- or microscopic disease. Inclusion and colonoscopies were performed at the Department of Gastroenterology and Hepatology at St. Olavs hospital, Trondheim University Hospital from 2007 to 2018. All patients gave written informed consent and ethical approvals were obtained from the Central Norway Regional Committee for Medical and Health Research Ethics (reference number 2013/212/REKMidt). Consent to publish the anonymized WSI dataset was given by REKMidt in 2021. Each database ID-number used in this

---

[6]https://github.com/AICAN-Research/FAST-Pathology

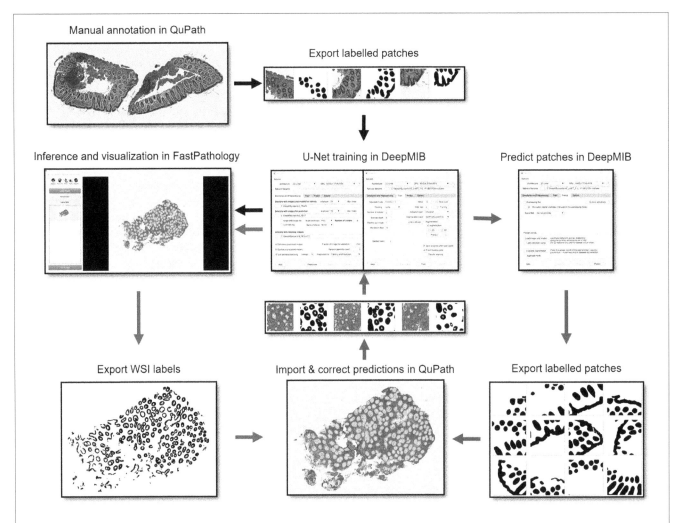

FIGURE 1 | Flowchart showing the pipeline from manual annotation in QuPath, export of labeled patches from QuPath (black arrows), CNN training in DeepMIB, expansion of the dataset by predicting unseen WSIs in DeepMIB and importing and correcting predictions in QuPath (red arrows), and final export of trained networks as ONNX-files and rapid prediction directly on WSIs in FastPathology (blue arrows).

study was changed to new anonymized IDs only containing the information "active" or "inactive" disease and whether the WSI has "HE" or "CD3" staining. The full dataset of 251 WSIs with ~31 k epithelium annotations is made openly available at DataverseNO: https://doi.org/10.18710/TLA01U (28).

FFPE sections of 4 μm were cut, mounted on slides and either stained with hematoxylin (Mayer's) and Eosin (Y) (HE) or subjected to standard pre-treatment with quenching of endogenous peroxidase and boiling in Tris EDTA pH9 for antigen retrieval before immunohistochemistry. Primary antibody for the T lymphocyte marker was mouse anti-human CD3 (M7254, clone F7.2.38, Dako Agilent, CA, USA), diluted 1:50 in antibody diluent Tris buffer with 0.025% Tween-20 and 1% BSA and incubated overnight at 4°C. Immunoreactions were visualized with the secondary antibody rabbit/mouse EnVision-HRP/DAB+ kit (K5007, Dako Agilent) and counterstaining with haematoxylin. Omission of the primary antibody was used as negative

control and sections from human peripheral lymph node as positive control.

U-Net Based Epithelial Segmentation Using QuPath and DeepMIB

The HE and CD3 immunostained slides were scanned using a Hamamatsu NanoZoomer S360 (Hamamatsu Photonics, Japan) scanner at ×40 magnification. Slides were imported into the open-source image analysis software QuPath (13). Epithelium was annotated for ~30 out of 111 CD3 stained WSIs by an experienced gastrointestinal pathologist and checked and corrected by a second pathologist. To make the images compatible with efficient training of semantic segmentation neural networks in DeepMIB, 2,048 × 2,048 pixels image tiles were exported as 4× downsampled files (from 2,048 × 2,048 pixels with 512 pixels overlap to a downsampled size of 512 × 512 pixels with 128 pixels overlap) with corresponding binary mask labels (*.png) from QuPath. Overlapping tiles were used to avoid inference errors at the edges of the patches when importing labels back into QuPath. WSIs often contain 50–90% white background, which will make the exterior class completely dominant in training. Therefore, a glass detection method was used, similarly as done in a previous study (21), and patches with <25% tissue were discarded.

Images and labels were split randomly into an 80/20% train/test split at the WSI level, such that only unseen WSIs were present in the test set. The data was then placed in separate train and test folders, each containing separate "Images" and "Labels" sub-folders.

Two semantic segmentation neural networks were used in this paper: U-Net (18) and SegNet (19). U-Net is a fully-convolutional encoder-decoder neural network initially developed for the purpose of biomedical image segmentation. U-Net is one of two available 2D semantic segmentation networks in DeepMIB which allows optimization of hyperparameters such as U-Net depth, number of filters and input patch size for each segmentation task (16). SegNet is a fully-convolutional encoder-decoder neural network where the encoder part is identical to the 13 convolutional layers in the much-used VGG16 network (19).

A SegNet network with depth of 6 layers with 32 initial filter and input patch size of 256 × 256 pixels was trained until validation loss stagnation around 5% in DeepMIB (MATLAB version 2021a, MIB version 2.8, CUDA version 11.3). The trained SegNet was then used to predict the remaining ∼70 WSIs by exporting 4× downsampled 512 × 512 image patches with 128 pixels overlap from QuPath. Patches containing <25% tissue were deleted. The resultant images with predicted label files were then loaded in DeepMIB for evaluation and the label patches saved as TIF files. The TIF files were then imported back into QuPath as annotations. Annotations were then confirmed, and errors were manually corrected in QuPath by a pathologist for the remaining WSIs to achieve a dataset of 111 WSIs. A final refinement of the dataset was done by predicting the full dataset and correcting in DeepMIB. The ∼5% patches with the lowest mean IoU scores as evaluated inside DeepMIB were exported as text-file lists and the patches could then be copied to a different folder using a Windows PowerShell script (all scripts used in this paper is made available in the NoCodeSeg GitHub repository). The worst performing image patches and their corresponding labels were then loaded and corrected in DeepMIB. A similar strategy was applied to the HE-stained dataset of 140 WSIs, using the U-Net trained on CD3 immunostained WSIs to predict and correct an initial batch of ∼30 HE-stained WSIs. Then training a U-Net on the initial batch of annotated HE-stained WSIs, applying it on the remaining HE-stained WSIs, and retraining the U-Net. The final datasets (140 HE-stained and 111 CD3 immunostained WSIs, or 6322 HE and 4323 CD3 4× downsampled 512 × 512 image patches in each dataset) were again split into an 80/20% train/test split at the WSI level, such that 36 (HE) and 21 (CD3) previously unseen WSIs were present in the test set and new networks were trained from scratch using DeepMIB to assess the performance of the software on this larger train/test set (see **Table 1**).

Finally, two CNNs, SegNet and U-Net, were then trained using DeepMIB. To achieve maximum variety of different image patches per mini batch, the number of patches DeepMIB extracts per image in a single mini batch was set to one. Initially the number of patches per image was set to the same number as the number of applied augmentations, however, this produced inferior results to using just one patch per image per mini batch. Three percent of the training set images were randomly chosen by DeepMIB for the validation set. A fixed random generator seed was used to make comparison between training different conditions more direct. Several hyperparameters were tested, such as variable input patch size (128 × 128, 256 × 256, 512 × 512), number of filters (16, 24, 32, 64), network depth (4, 5, 6, 7, 8), and the presence and absence of augmentations. Finally, U-Net and SegNet were trained for 200 epochs, which was the number of epochs required for training loss stagnation. Further global training settings were as follows: Padding: Same; Solver: Adam; Shuffle: Every-epoch; Initial learning rate: 0.00005; L2 Regularization: 0.0001; Decay rate of gradient moving average: 0.9; Decay rate of squared gradient moving average: 0.999. Augmentations used in all described trainings were performed in a blended fashion (MIB version 2.8) with a 30% probability for each augmentation to be applied to each augmented image patch during training. The fraction of images for augmentation was set to 75%, i.e., 25% of input image patches were not augmented, while 75% had a 30% chance of being augmented with either of the following augmentations [numeric limits show in brackets]: Random left-right/top-bottom reflections, random 90/270-degree rotations, random X/Y/X+Y image scaling [1.0, 1.1], random color augmentation: Hue [−0.03, 0.03], saturation [−0.05, 0.05], random intensity augmentation: brightness [−0.1, 0.1], contrast [0.9, 1.1], and zero-mean Gaussian blur with standard deviation in range [0, 0.5] (see **Supplementary Figures 1, 2**).

A selection of metrics was extracted for each patch from DeepMIB, and metrics were then averaged at the WSI-level (**Table 1**). The reported metrics were produced from calculating the WSI-level average. The following metrics were calculated: micro and macro-averaged pixel-wise accuracy, macro and weighted IoU, and class-wise DSC for the exterior Epithelium classes. U-Net proved to consistently outperform SegNet for both the HE and CD3 dataset (see **Table 1**). Initially, increasing input patch sizes were tested, with size 64 × 64, 128 × 128, 256 × 256, and 512 × 512. The available 24 GB GPU allowed a maximum batch size of 16 for a U-Net with 512 × 512 patch size, 32 filter, and depth of 6. Thus, these settings (16 batch size, 32 filter, depth 6) were kept for all the different input patch size trainings to be comparable.

Deployment in FastPathology

The best performing trained U-Net model from DeepMIB was exported to the ONNX format using the ExportONNXNetwork method from the Deep Learning Toolbox in MATLAB. As ONNX does not currently support MATLAB's implementation of the UnPooling operation in SegNet, U-Net was the only model converted to ONNX.

We defined an inference pipeline consisting of applying the trained segmentation model across the WSI in an overlapping, sliding window fashion, similarly as done in a previous study (21). The result of each patch was binarized using a threshold

TABLE 1 | Comparative accuracies on the HE stained ($n = 36$) and CD3 immunostained ($n = 21$) test sets with different hyperparameter settings for U-Net and SegNet.

Stain	Arch.	Patch size	Nr. of filt.	Depth	Batch size	MICRO Acc	MACRO Acc	MACRO IoU	Weig. IoU	Ext. DSC	Epith. DSC
HE	U-Net	512 × 512	32	6	16	**0.989**	0.972	**0.955**	**0.978**	**0.992**	**0.953**
HE	U-Net	256 × 256	32	6	16	**0.989**	**0.983**	0.938	**0.978**	**0.992**	0.920
HE	U-Net	256 × 256	32	6	32	0.988	0.978	0.936*	0.976	0.991	0.920
HE	U-Net	256 × 256	64	6	32	0.987	0.974	0.935*	0.975	0.991	0.919
HE	U-Net	128 × 128	32	6	16	0.988	**0.983**	0.932*	0.977	0.991	0.911
HE	U-Net	64 × 64	32	6	16	0.985	0.965	0.924*	0.971	0.989	0.904
HE	SegNet	512 × 512	32	6	16	0.983	0.964	0.928*	0.967	0.988	0.918
HE	SegNet	256 × 256	32	6	16	0.987	0.973	0.939*	0.974	0.991	0.927
HE	SegNet	128 × 128	32	6	16	0.979	0.964	0.904*	0.960	0.985	0.884
CD3	U-Net	512 × 512	32	6	16	**0.990**	**0.981**	**0.955**	**0.980**	**0.992**	**0.948**
CD3	U-Net	256 × 256	32	6	16	0.987	0.977	0.931*	0.974	0.990	0.911
CD3	SegNet	512 × 512	32	6	16	0.976	0.953	0.920*	0.954	0.983	0.919
CD3	SegNet	256 × 256	32	6	16	0.971	0.949	0.898*	0.945	0.979	0.889

*All metrics were reported as the mean at WSI-level. Best performing methods are highlighted in bold, for each respective metric and for each data set. The number of train/validation/test patches for each dataset was as follows: HE: (4973/154/1195); CD3 (3539/110/674). Stars indicate significant differences ($p < 0.01$) compared to the single best performing architecture within each dataset (HE and CD3 U-Net 512x512, 32 filters, 16 batch, respectively) using a two-level mixed regression model (see **Supplementary Table 1**). ARCH, Architecture; FILT, Filters; NR, Number; ACC, Accuracy; WEIG, Weighted; EXT, Exterior; IOU, Intersection over Union; DSC, Dice Similarity Coefficient; EPITH, Epithelial; HE, Hematoxylin-Eosin; CD3, T-cell lymphocyte immunomarker.*

of 0.5, before being stitched to form a tiled, pyramidal image. When inference was complete, the resulting pyramidal image was exported to the disk in the open TIFF format.

To demonstrate the performance of FastPathology, runtime experiments were conducted. Runtimes were measured for the total inference pipeline, as well as for individual pipeline components (runtimes reported are without overlapping inference). The experiments were repeated ten times for the same WSI, using three different inference engines (OpenVINO CPU, OpenVINO GPU, and TensorRT). For each metric, the average of the ten runs were reported. The source code to reproduce the experiments can be found on GitHub[7].

Computer Hardware

Runtime experiments were performed on a Razer Blade 15 Base laptop, with an Intel i7-10750H CPU @ 2.60 GHz, 32 GB RAM, an Intel UHD graphics integrated GPU, and NVIDIA RTX 2070 Max-Q (8 GB) dedicated GPU. All other analyses were performed on a Dell Precision 5820 Tower, with an Intel(R) Xeon(R) W-2155 CPU @ 3.30GHz, 96 GB RAM, and a NVIDIA Titan RTX (24 GB) dedicated GPU.

Statistical Methods

For the statistical analyses in **Table 1**; **Supplementary Table 1**, the mean IoU for each neural network architecture, for the HE and CD3 datasets separately, was compared to the best performing architecture (HE/CD3 U-Net 512 × 512, 32 filters, 16 batch). Between-architecture comparisons were performed using a two-level linear mixed regression model, where architectures were specified as level 1, image patches as level 2 and with robust variance estimates clustered by WSI and a random intercept for patch. Analyses were performed using Stata/MP 16.1 (College

Station, Texas) and the estimated mean difference is presented together with 95% CI and p-values without correction for multiple comparisons.

RESULTS

Annotation of Colon Epithelium Through Active Learning Using QuPath and DeepMIB

We performed several trainings in DeepMIB using two different CNNs (i.e., SegNet and U-Net), with a variety of hyperparameters to find the highest performance (see section U-Net Based Epithelial Segmentation Using QuPath and DeepMIB). Initially a SegNet network was trained and applied to new unannotated WSIs. Annotations were imported and manually corrected in QuPath by a pathologist. Subsequent training cycles were performed with U-Net 512 × 512 in a repetitive fashion described in **Figure 1** (DeepMIB training, inference of new WSIs and import into QuPath for correction of annotations, export for new DeepMIB training, etc.) to achieve a final dataset of 111 WSIs (see **Figure 1**). A final refinement of the annotations was done by exporting individual accuracy scores for all image patches exported from DeepMIB. This allowed sorting of the patches which was in most disagreement with the U-Net predictions (typically mean IoU scores below 0.85). The set of ∼5% worst performing patches were then loaded in DeepMIB such that a pathologist could refine the annotations directly on several hundred image patches instead of going through the whole dataset of ∼5,000–7,000 image patches. This final refinement made it possible to achieve almost pixel accurate epithelial segmentation of ∼100 WSIs. The top-performing CD3-trained network was used to repeatedly predict and correct

---

[7] https://github.com/andreped/NoCodeSeg

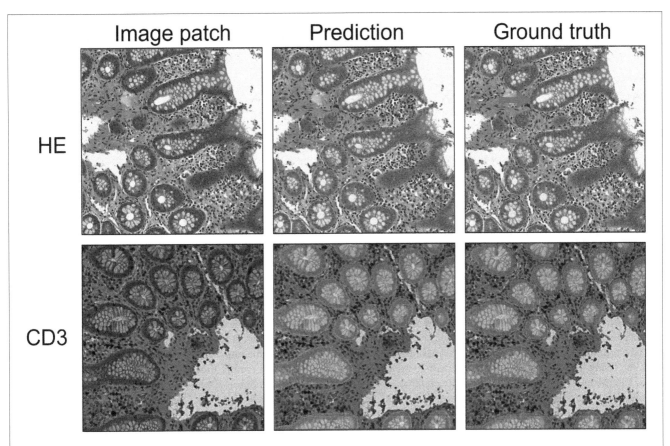

FIGURE 2 | Examples of predictions (middle column) and ground truth (right column) of epithelial segmentation (transparent green) of HE stained (top row) and CD3 immunostained (bottom row) 512 × 512-pixel image patches in DeepMIB. The arrow shows the approximate cut-offs for (filled or unfilled) minimal tubule hole size used during annotation.

the 140 HE stained WSIs, following the workflow described in **Figure 1**.

Training of Deep Semantic Segmentation of Colon Epithelium Using DeepMIB

This resulted in a final dataset of fully annotated patches, from 140 HE stained and 111 CD3 immunostained colon biopsy WSIs (see **Figure 2** for examples). The datasets were split into the two subsets: train (80%; $n = 104$ HE; $n = 90$ CD3) and test set (20%; $n = 36$ HE; $n = 21$ CD3). Two segmentation networks (i.e., U-Net and SegNet) were then trained on the final refined datasets to assess performance. We limited each training to 200 epochs and a similar global training setting (see section Materials and Methods) for comparable results (see **Table 1**). A step-by-step tutorial video demonstrating the full pipeline and for setting training hyperparameters in DeepMIB has been made available online (https://youtu.be/9dTfUwnL6zY).

For the U-Net models on the HE dataset, an increase in segmentation accuracy was observed with increasing input patch sizes from 64 × 64 (Epithelium DSC 0.904) to 512 × 512 (Epithelium DSC 0.953). This segmentation accuracy decline was statistically significant for all comparisons to the HE U-Net 512 × 512, except for HE U-Net 256 × 256

with the same number for filters (32) and batch size (16) (see **Table 1**; **Supplementary Table 1**). The best segmentation accuracy for SegNet was observed with input patch size 256 × 256 for the HE dataset (Epithelium DSC 0.927). For the CD3 dataset, the maximum segmentation accuracy was observed for 512 × 512 input patches for both U-Net and SegNet (Epithelium DSC of 0.948 and 0.919, respectively), and as was the case for the HE dataset, the larger patch input CD3 U-Net 512 × 512 performed significantly better than all the other CD3 trained architectures (see **Table 1**; **Supplementary Table 1**).

There was a negligible difference in segmentation accuracy when increasing the number of filters from 32 to 64 (Epithelium DSC 0.920 vs. 0.919) or increasing the batch size from 16 to 32 (Epithelium DSC 0.920 vs. 0.920). U-Net consistently and statistically significantly outperformed SegNet (see **Table 1**; **Supplementary Table 1**). U-Net's top segmentation accuracies of Epithelium DSC of 0.953 and 0.948 (HE and CD3, U-Net 512 × 512), were significantly better than the top performing SegNet models with Epithelium DSCs of 0.927 and 0.919 (HE SegNet 256 × 256 and CD3 SegNet 512 × 512). Further testing with different depth of the networks was also performed, but depth 6 seemed to perform consistently higher (data not shown).

TABLE 2 | Runtime measurements of different inference engines using FastPathology.

Inference engine	Processor	Patchgen. (ms)	NN input (ms)	NN inference (ms)	NN output (ms)	Patch stitcher (ms)	Export wsi tiff (ms)	Total time/wsi (s)
OpenVINO CPU	Intel i7-10750H	3.65	1.03	135.31	0.80	2.76	7.09	76.38
OpenVINO GPU	Intel UHD graphics	**3.29**	1.26	133.96	1.25	3.46	7.83	76.65
TensorRT	RTX 2070 Max-Q	5.12	**0.80**	**7.31**	**0.19**	**1.35**	**5.40**	**5.60**

The table shows means of 10 runtime experiments for the 256 × 256 pixel input patch size U-Net applied to a single representative WSI from the dataset (540 patches without overlap). Inference measurements show runtime per 256 × 256 patch in milliseconds (ms). Export of a full WSI pyramidal TIFF performed once after inference is reported in ms, and the total runtime for the full WSI (including TIFF export) is shown in seconds (s). The fastest runtimes are highlighted in bold. GEN, Generator; NN, Neural Network; WSI, Whole Slide Image.

Using our best performing 256 × 256 U-Net model, the proposed inference pipeline took ∼5.60 s to complete for the entire WSI using FastPathology (see **Table 2**). In our experience, this is well within the range for running direct inference in a clinical setting, and even the longest CPU-based inference times would be unlikely to limit the use of such algorithms by pathologists. The fastest inference engine was TensorRT, whereas using OpenVINO took ∼76.5 s (a 13.7× improvement using TensorRT). The main bottleneck of the pipeline was the neural network inference. For OpenVINO, ∼94.3% of the patch runtime was due to inference alone, whereas for TensorRT this was only ∼49.5%. Using TensorRT, our inference pipeline required ∼2.1 GB of VRAM and ∼4.2GB of RAM for running inference on a full WSI with a network trained with patch sizes of 256 × 256 pixels.

DISCUSSION

Benefits and Limitations With Using Multiple Software Solutions

The motivation of this study was to segment epithelium in a large dataset from a biobank of normal and diseased (inflammatory bowel disease) colon biopsies. We aimed to achieve this without the need for computer coding abilities, while simultaneously taking advantage of the strongest sides of available open-source software solutions. We demonstrate an open-source, free-to-use pipeline that can achieve high accuracy segmentation of histopathological WSIs available to a broad user base without the ability to write computer code. We further demonstrate the advantages of using open-source, non-proprietary software and formats that can be exchanged between these three software packages. The pipeline could be improved by incorporating all tasks into a single software solution. However, the use of several software solutions and exchange of information between them makes it possible to use more specialized open-source solutions best suited for each task—QuPath for annotations of whole slide images, DeepMIB for neural network training, and FastPathology for efficient inference and visualization of trained models. A disadvantage of such a multi-software pipeline is that it requires three separate software installations, which over time might diverge in compatibility and use different versions of auxiliary software, such as versions of CUDA.

Even though the pipeline does not require the ability to write computer code, it does require the use of some scripts, such as the

QuPath export/import scripts. This requires copy/pasting of pre-existing code, with any relevant changes to the parameters within those scripts to make the pipeline suitable for different tasks. In the near future, it is likely that this will be possible solely through the GUI in QuPath.

The epithelial segmentation accuracy was comparably high for both the best performing U-Nets on HE (DSC Epithelium 0.953) and CD3 images (DSC Epithelium 0.948), demonstrating the robustness of U-Net for this task. Segmentation accuracy was generally better with larger patch sizes (512 × 512 vs. 256 × 256 DSC Epithelium 0.953 vs. 0.920), however 256 × 256 patch size networks require much less GPU memory for training and inference. There was a statistically significant difference between the best performing architectures (HE/CD3 U-Net 512 × 512, 32 filters, 16 batch) compared to each of the other architectures in both datasets (HE and CD3). These statistically significant differences, should not, however, be automatically perceived as clinically significant different segmentation performance. Although statistically significant, the differences in mean IoU/epithelium DSC between the top performing architectures were small and may not result in clinically perceivable differences. Application of the segmentation models for downstream quantitative purposes (e.g., the number of intraepithelial lymphocytes) may more accurately address the cut-off for clinically significant performance of such models in future studies. We have not compared the segmentation accuracy of our trained models to current state-of-the-art architectures (29, 30). However, DSC scores for the epithelial class up to ∼95% on unseen test sets show little room for considerable improvement, making the U-Net segmentation accuracy for these data sets probably near state-of-the-art. It has also been argued by others (31), that there is little to gain from changing neural network architecture for semantic segmentation. The U-Net architecture presented can also easily be tuned code-free to be better suited for a specific task. The datasets are published with this paper and comparison to state-of-the-art models will therefore be possible by others.

The Dataset and Annotations

Several issues arose during annotation. Defining a pixel-accurate epithelium ground truth is difficult as several images contain artifacts (folds, blurred areas, poorly fixated tissue, stain exudates, etc.) as well as intraepithelial inclusions (e.g., granulocytes) (see **Figure 3**). These cannot be easily defined into the dichotomous categories: epithelium or exterior, as e.g., folded tissue might

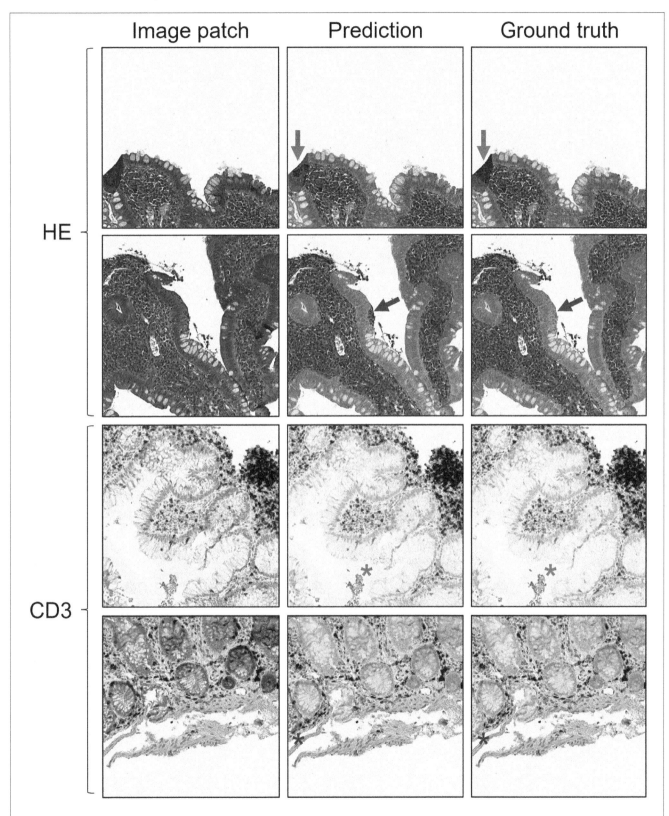

FIGURE 3 | Examples of prediction errors in difficult regions: HE stained images with folding artifacts (top row, red arrows) and granulocyte aggregates (second row, blue arrows). CD3 immunostained images with thick mucin rich epithelium (third row, red stars) and poorly fixated blurred epithelium at the edge of a patch (bottom row, blue stars). Prediction (middle column) and ground truth (right column) of epithelial segmentation are shown in transparent green. 512 × 512-pixel image patches displayed in DeepMIB.

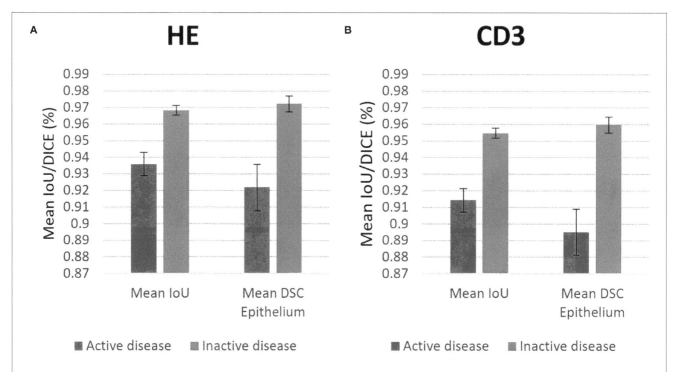

FIGURE 4 | Significant differences in prediction accuracies for the **(A)** HE stained test set WSIs ($n = 36$) with active disease ($n = 15$) vs. inactive disease ($n = 21$), and **(B)** CD3 immunostained test set WSIs ($n = 21$) with active disease ($n = 7$) and inactive disease ($n = 14$). Error bars represent 95% confidence intervals assuming normality. Two-tailed Student's T-test of active vs. inactive disease gave $p < 0.0001$ for all four comparisons.

contain both classes. Therefore, slides with more than ~10–20% artifacts were excluded from the dataset, as they contained large areas not suitable for pathological diagnostics either. Furthermore, defining intraepithelial granulocytes as part of the epithelium or not had to be individually considered, as large abscess like assemblies of granulocytes with little or no visible epithelium can obviously not be considered epithelium.

However, the clinical use of an epithelium segmentation algorithm in colon biopsies would certainly involve quantitative estimates of intraepithelial granulocytes and excluding large granulocytic abscesses during annotation also potentially diminishes the clinical value of the algorithm. Indeed, significant differences in prediction accuracies were seen for the test sets of both HE and CD3 immunostained slides between patients with active disease (with infiltration of neutrophilic granulocytes) and inactive disease (see **Figure 4**). Still, the segmentation accuracy was deemed to be at a clinically acceptable level with Epithelium DSC scores > 91% for all slides.

The cytoplasmic part of colon epithelium has a wide variation in size, particularly because of variation of mucin content. Inconsistencies in the cut-off for when mucin is no longer part of the epithelial cell and starts being part of the exterior class, was an obvious source of deviation between ground truth and predictions (see **Figure 3**). Furthermore, the cut-off between when the lumen of the colonic tubule ceases to be part of the epithelium and starts being part of the exterior class, was problematic. This was alleviated to a certain extent

by taking advantage of the power QuPath has as an annotation tool which allows running a single background thresholder pixel classifier algorithm, subsequently creating several large and small background annotations. These could subsequently be selected by a minimal size cut-off and subtracted from the epithelium annotations consistently for the entire dataset by running QuPath scripts in batch mode. A similar procedure is also possible to perform in DeepMIB using the BWThresholding tool followed by subtraction from all annotations, then a small dilation and subsequent similar erosion to fill small holes. One should be aware that this, however, might introduce merging of nearby annotations. The top row of **Figure 2** (HE segmentation results) provides a visual approximation of the maximal colonic tubule lumen sizes that are accepted as being part of the epithelium class (transparent green) or exterior class.

CONCLUSION

In this paper, we have presented a code-free pipeline for developing and deploying deep neural network segmentation models for computational pathology. The pipeline uses open, free software and enables the user to build and test state-of-the-art deep learning methods for segmentation of WSIs, without requiring any programming experience. We also demonstrate competitive results on two segmentation tasks with rapid inference of about 5 s for an entire WSI. The WSIs and annotations are also made publicly available to contribute to the active research within the field.

AUTHOR CONTRIBUTIONS

HP, AP, IBe, ER, and IBa: writing of initial draft. ER and IBa: provided data material, identified and selected patients from the biobank. ER: conducted all staining and preparation for scanning and the initial annotations of the slides. HP: iteratively improved annotations using the described QuPath/DeepMIB pipeline and performed all DeepMIB semantic segmentation trainings. AP: performed runtime experiments. AP, ES, and IBe: improved respective software to be better suited for this application. IR and EJ: supervised the structuring of the paper and code development for FastPathology/DeepMIB. MS: performed and interpreted statistical analyses comparing architectures. All authors contributed to reviewing and finalizing the manuscript.

FUNDING

This work was funded by the Research Fund for the Center for Laboratory Medicine, St. Olavs Hospital, Trondheim University Hospital, the Faculty of Medicine and Health Sciences, NTNU, the Cancer Foundation, St. Olavs Hospital, Trondheim University Hospital, and the Liaison Committee between the Central Norway Regional Health Authority and NTNU. IBe and EJ are supported by Biocenter Finland and Academy of Finland (project 1331998). Funding for open access publishing was given by NTNU University Library's Open access publishing fund.

ACKNOWLEDGMENTS

We would like to acknowledge Peter Bankhead (University of Edinburgh), Melvin Gelbard and the rest of the support team working with QuPath for continual feedback and help with sharing scripts and resolving issues with QuPath. The QuPath-related export/import scripts in the GitHub repository are inspired by their shared scripts. We thank the staff of the Gastrointestinal Endoscopy Unit, Department of Gastroenterology and Hepatology, St. Olavs Hospital, Trondheim University Hospital for support with sample collection, Bjørn Munkvold at Department of Clinical and Molecular Medicine (IKOM), NTNU for technical assistance and the Department of Pathology at St. Olavs Hospital, Trondheim University Hospital for scanning the tissue sections.

REFERENCES

1. Bulten W, Pinckaers H, van Boven H, Vink R, de Bel T, van Ginneken B, et al. Automated deep-learning system for Gleason grading of prostate cancer using biopsies: a diagnostic study. *Lancet Oncol.* (2020) 21:233–41. doi: 10.1016/S1470-2045(19)30739-9

2. Ehteshami Bejnordi B, Veta M, Johannes van Diest P, van Ginneken B, Karssemeijer N, Litjens G, et al. Diagnostic assessment of deep learning algorithms for detection of lymph node metastases in women with breast cancer. *JAMA.* (2017) 318:2199–210. doi: 10.1001/jama.2017.14585

3. Jackson SL, Frederick PD, Pepe MS, Nelson HD, Weaver DL, Allison KH, et al. Diagnostic reproducibility: what happens when the same pathologist interprets the same breast biopsy specimen at two points in time? *Ann Surg Oncol.* (2017) 24:1234–41. doi: 10.1245/s10434-016-5695-0

4. Melia J, Moseley R, Ball RY, Griffiths DF, Grigor K, Harnden P, et al. A UK-based investigation of inter- and intra-observer reproducibility of Gleason grading of prostatic biopsies. *Histopathology.* (2006) 48:644–54. doi: 10.1111/j.1365-2559.2006.02393.x

5. van der Laak J, Litjens G, Ciompi F. Deep learning in histopathology: the path to the clinic. *Nat Med.* (2021) 27:775–84. doi: 10.1038/s41591-021-01343-4

6. Jahn SW, Plass M, Moinfar F. Digital Pathology: advantages, limitations and emerging perspectives. *J Clin Med.* (2020) 9:3697. doi: 10.3390/jcm9113697

7. Djuric U, Zadeh G, Aldape K, Diamandis P. Precision histology: how deep learning is poised to revitalize histomorphology for personalized cancer care. *NPJ Precis Oncol.* (2017) 1:22. doi: 10.1038/s41698-017-0022-1

8. Srinidhi CL, Ciga O, Martel AL. Deep neural network models for computational histopathology: a survey. *Med Image Anal.* (2021) 67:101813. doi: 10.1016/j.media.2020.101813

9. Lara H, Li ZB, Abels E, Aeffner F, Bui MM, ElGabry EA, et al. Quantitative image analysis for tissue biomarker use: a white paper from the digital pathology association. *Appl Immunohistochem Mol Morphol.* (2021) 29:479–93. doi: 10.1097/PAI.0000000000000930

10. Lutnick B, Ginley B, Govind D, McGarry SD, LaViolette PS, Yacoub R, et al. An integrated iterative annotation technique for easing neural network training in medical image analysis. *Nat Mach Intell.* (2019) 1:112–9. doi: 10.1038/s42256-019-0018-3

11. Miao R, Toth R, Zhou Y, Madabhushi A, Janowczyk A. *Quick Annotator: An Open-Source Digital Pathology Based Rapid Image Annotation Tool.* arXiv:2101.02183 (2021). Available online at: https://ui.adsabs.harvard.edu/abs/2021arXiv210102183M (accessed January 01, 2021).

12. von Chamier L, Laine RF, Jukkala J, Spahn C, Krentzel D, Nehme E, et al. Democratising deep learning for microscopy with ZeroCostDL4Mic. *Nat Commun.* (2021) 12:2276. doi: 10.1038/s41467-021-22518-0

13. Bankhead P, Loughrey MB, Fernandez JA, Dombrowski Y, McArt DG, Dunne PD, et al. QuPath: open source software for digital pathology image analysis. *Sci Rep.* (2017) 7:16878. doi: 10.1038/s41598-017-17204-5

14. Schmidt U, Weigert M, Broaddus C, Myers G. Cell detection with star-convex polygons. Medical image computing and computer assisted intervention - Miccai 2018. *Pt Ii.* (2018) 11071:265–73. doi: 10.1007/978-3-030-00934-2_30

15. Moen E, Bannon D, Kudo T, Graf W, Covert M, Van Valen D. Deep learning for cellular image analysis. *Nat Methods.* (2019) 16:1233–46. doi: 10.1038/s41592-019-0403-1

16. Belevich I, Jokitalo E. DeepMIB: user-friendly and open-source software for training of deep learning network for biological image segmentation. *PLoS Comput Biol.* (2021) 17:e1008374. doi: 10.1371/journal.pcbi.1008374

17. Belevich I, Joensuu M, Kumar D, Vihinen H, Jokitalo E. Microscopy image browser: a platform for segmentation and analysis of multidimensional datasets. *PLoS Biol.* (2016) 14:e1002340. doi: 10.1371/journal.pbio.1002340

18. Ronneberger O, Fischer P, Brox T. U-Net: convolutional networks for biomedical image segmentation. Medical image computing and computer-assisted intervention. *Pt Iii.* (2015) 9351:234–41. doi: 10.1007/978-3-319-24574-4_28

19. Badrinarayanan V, Kendall A, Cipolla R. SegNet: a deep convolutional encoder-decoder architecture for image segmentation. *IEEE Trans Pattern Anal Mach Intell.* (2017) 39:2481–95. doi: 10.1109/TPAMI.2016.2644615

20. Falk T, Mai D, Bensch R, Cicek O, Abdulkadir A, Marrakchi Y, et al. U-Net: deep learning for cell counting, detection, and morphometry. *Nat Methods.* (2019) 16:351. doi: 10.1038/s41592-019-0356-4

21. Pedersen A, Valla M, Bofin AM, De Frutos JP, Reinertsen I, Smistad E. FastPathology: an open-source platform for deep learning-based research and decision support in digital pathology. *IEEE Access.* (2021) 9:58216–29. doi: 10.1109/ACCESS.2021.3072231

22. Smistad E, Bozorgi M, Lindseth F. FAST: framework for heterogeneous medical image computing and visualization. *Int J Comput Assist Radiol Surg.* (2015) 10:1811–22. doi: 10.1007/s11548-015-1158-5

23. Smistad E, Ostvik A, Pedersen A. High performance neural network inference, streaming, and visualization of medical images using FAST. *IEEE Access.* (2019) 7:136310–21. doi: 10.1109/ACCESS.2019.2942441

24. Abadi M, Agarwal A, Barham P, Brevdo E, Chen Z, Citro C, et al. *TensorFlow: Large-Scale Machine Learning on Heterogeneous Distributed Systems.* arXiv:1603.04467 (2016). Available online at: https://ui.adsabs. harvard.edu/abs/2016arXiv160304467A (accessed March 01, 2016).

25. Lutter L, Hoytema van Konijnenburg DP, Brand EC, Oldenburg B, van Wijk F. The elusive case of human intraepithelial T cells in gut homeostasis and inflammation. *Nat Rev Gastroenterol Hepatol.* (2018) 15:637–49. doi: 10.1038/s41575-018-0039-0

26. Olivares-Villagomez D, Van Kaer L. Intestinal intraepithelial lymphocytes: sentinels of the mucosal barrier. *Trends Immunol.* (2018) 39:264–75. doi: 10.1016/j.it.2017.11.003

27. Hu MD, Edelblum KL. Sentinels at the frontline: the role of intraepithelial lymphocytes in inflammatory bowel disease. *Curr Pharmacol Rep.* (2017) 3:321–34. doi: 10.1007/s40495-017-0105-2

28. Pettersen HS, Belevich I, Røyset ES, Smistad E, Jokitalo E, Reinertsen I, et al. *140 HE and 111 CD3-stained colon biopsies of active and inactivate inflammatory bowel disease with epithelium annotated: the IBDColEpi dataset Version V1) [Annotated histopathological whole slide images, Annotated histopathological image patches].* DataverseNO (2021).

29. Tao A, Sapra K, Catanzaro B. *Hierarchical Multi-Scale Attention for Semantic Segmentation.* arXiv:2005.10821 (2020). Available online at: https://ui.adsabs.harvard.edu/abs/2020arXiv200510821T (accessed May 01, 2020).

30. Yuan Y, Chen X, Chen X, Wang J. *Segmentation Transformer: Object-Contextual Representations for Semantic Segmentation.* arXiv:1909.11065 (2019). Available online at: https://ui.adsabs. harvard.edu/abs/2019arXiv190911065Y (accessed September 01, 2019).

31. Isensee F, Jaeger PF, Kohl SAA, Petersen J, Maier-Hein KH. nnU-Net: a self-configuring method for deep learning-based biomedical image segmentation. *Nat Methods.* (2021) 18:203–11. doi: 10.1038/s41592-020-01008-z

11

Extensive Tumor Profiling in Primary Neuroendocrine Breast Cancer Cases as a Role Model for Personalized Treatment in Rare and Aggressive Cancer Types

Dörthe Schaffrin-Nabe[1]*, Stefan Schuster[2], Andrea Tannapfel[3] and Rudolf Voigtmann[1]

[1] *Praxis für Hämatologie und Onkologie, Bochum, Germany,* [2] *Datar Cancer Genetics Europe GmbH, Eckersdorf, Germany,*
[3] *Institute of Pathology, Ruhr-University Bochum, Bochum, Germany*

*Correspondence:
Dörthe Schaffrin-Nabe
josten-nabe@onkologie-bochum.com

Neuroendocrine breast cancer (NEBC) is a rare entity accounting for <0.1% of all breast carcinomas and <0.1% of all neuroendocrine carcinomas. In most cases treatment strategies in NEBC are empirical in absence of prospective trial data on NEBC cohorts. Herein, we present two case reports diagnosed with anaplastic and small cell NEBC. After initial therapies failed, comprehensive tumor profiling was applied, leading to individualized treatment options for both patients. In both patients, targetable alterations of the PI3K/AKT/mTOR pathway were found, including a PIK3CA mutation itself and an STK11 mutation that negatively regulates the mTOR complex. The epicrisis of the two patients exemplifies how to manage rare and difficult to treat cancers and how new diagnostic tools contribute to medical management.

Keywords: extensive tumor profiling, rare cancer therapy, primary endocrine breast cancer, personalized treatment, targeted therapies

INTRODUCTION

Primary neuroendocrine breast cancer (NEBC) comprises a heterogeneous group of tumors with a low incidence (0.1%) among all breast cancer subtypes (1). In the literature, NEBCs are generally associated with poor long-term survival and with rapid resistance development (1–3). Therapeutic guidelines have not been established to date. The diagnosis of NEBC is often challenging as other neuroendocrine tumors, but also lung, gastrointestinal, and pancreatic cancers, need to be excluded (4, 5).

Currently, surgical intervention is the mainstay of the therapeutic approach (5, 6).

Treatment strategies are chosen dependent on Classification of Malignant Tumors (TNM) status, aggressiveness, age, general condition, and comorbidities of the patient (7). If (neo-)adjuvant chemotherapy is necessary, NEBC is being treated either analog to adenocarcinomas of the breast or SCLC (8, 9). Previously, Ki67 was used as a decision tool in NEBC; Ki67 < 15% led to a breast cancer analog therapy, i > 15% of the therapy was orientated to SCLC/neuroendocrine treatment (7). Promising results were seen when a combination of surgery, radiotherapy, and chemotherapy was applied (6).

There are no guidelines for staging and therapy in the metastatic setting, leaving the treating oncologist to opt for suitable systemic treatments (10, 11).

The development of molecular tumor profiling in recent years increasingly provides the opportunity for the use of targeted therapies, taking into account the involved activation and inhibition of the signal transduction pathways (12–14). This tool is particularly useful for rare tumors without existing therapy guidelines and for tumors that are refractory to therapy.

We want to illustrate the diagnostic and therapeutic challenges presenting the epicrisis of two patients diagnosed with NEBC in these above-mentioned situations.

PATIENT 1

The first patient was a 67-year-old female (**Figure 1**), who had a primary NEBC of the small cell subtype confirmed by histopathology. The definitive tumor stage was pT2, pN1a, L1, V0, G3, and Ki67 at 60%. She underwent modified radical mastectomy with axillary dissection and adjuvant administration of six cycles of Carboplatin and Etoposide, followed by radiotherapy. There was no indication for radiotherapy of the neurocranium as performed in SCLC.

Two years later, pronounced bilateral pleural metastasis without effusion was detected and one brain metastasis on the left occipital side was surgically removed. Both are related to the previously described NEBC. Considering micrometastases of the brain, the patient received Topotecan.

Further brain metastases, progressive lung metastasis with effusion, and metastatic spread to bone and thyroid gland were discovered by MRI 2 months afterward during ongoing chemotherapy.

Consequently, tumor profiling was performed with the exacta® test using peripheral blood to detect genetic alterations by NGS, targetable markers by immunocytochemistry staining, pharmacogenetics of tumor specific medication, and chemotherapy sensitivity testing using circulating tumor associated cells (**Table 1**) (15–17).

PATIENT 2

The second 51-year-old female patient suffered from an NEBC anaplastic large cell subtype (**Figure 2**). After breast-conserving therapy and sentinel lymphonodectomy, the definitive tumor stage was pT2, pN0, G3, Ki 67 40%, L0, V0, Pn0, ER 30%, PR neg, and Her2/neu neg. In the adjuvant setting, carboplatin and etoposide were applied with extremely poor clinical tolerability.

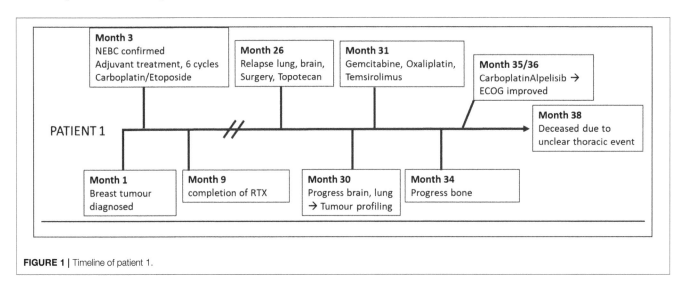

FIGURE 1 | Timeline of patient 1.

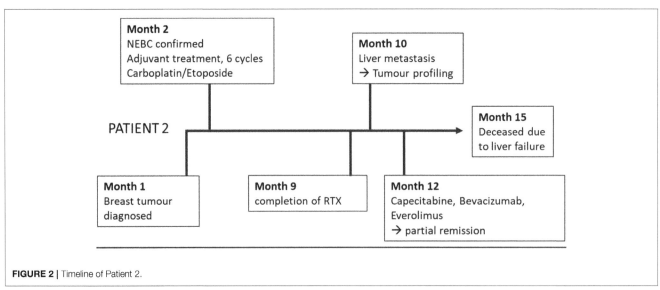

FIGURE 2 | Timeline of Patient 2.

Shortly after completion of adjuvant radiotherapy, hepatic filiae appeared in the right liver lobe. The planned atypical liver resection was rejected, because of intraoperatively detected diffuse spread into the left lobe.

Histopathologic confirmation revealed highly proliferating liver metastasis with a Ki67 of 80%, poorly differentiated, associated with the known NEBC.

Tumor profiling was performed using exacta® analysis this time based on a tumor biopsy together with a blood sample (**Table 1**). Simultaneous to this analysis, a diffuse bone metastasis with infiltration of the spinal canal with corresponding clinical signs was observed and radiotherapy was applied.

DISCUSSION

The reported aggressive scenario in both patients is consistent with high grading and high proliferation index (Ki67 > 60%). The initial chemotherapies failed and raised the question of novel therapeutic strategies. Dotatate-based PET-CT as an experimental diagnostic and therapeutic alternative was rejected (18). Both cases required the use of newly available diagnostic tools like NGS considering that recommendations for genomic alterations in specific tumor types exist, but not in NEBC or other neuroendocrine tumors (NET). At no stage, guidelines or clinical trials were available, only the individual approach was left.

In the case of the first patient, exacta® revealed an activating mutation of PIK3CA p.E545K, which is one of the most mutated genes and has been found to play a crucial role in several cancer types, but information about the incidence in NEBC is inconsistent in the literature (19–21). The PI3K/AKT/mTOR pathway is highly important for proliferation, migration, and cell survival and alterations are quite frequent in other NETs (22). The mutation, therefore, suggested a therapeutic benefit from mTOR and PIK3CA inhibition. Due to extended metastasis (pleura, neurocranium, and bone) and high Ki67, Gemcitabine and Oxaliplatin were added based on the chemosensivity result to the mTOR inhibitor Temsirolimus (16, 23). Even though the therapy was tailored to individual tumor characteristics, the patient progressed, developing new pulmonary metastasis and lymphangitis, as well as pronounced pleural effusion. No response was seen despite molecular genetic evidence, together with an upregulation at the messenger RNA (mRNA) level of AKT, an important activator of mTOR, thus, suggesting a potential benefit from mTOR inhibitors. Resistance mechanisms to mTOR inhibitors, for example, caused by disruption of the negative feedback loop between SGK1 and PI3K signaling, followed by AKT activation, could explain treatment failure (24–26). Furthermore, RHEB (RAS homolog enriched in brain) as an mTOR activator was downregulated, together with mTOR downstream activating pathway components, like eIF4B (eukaryotic initiation factor 4B) and S6 (ribosomal subunit S6 = RPS6) (27, 28).

In this case, activation of mTOR seemed to have a lesser impact concerning tumor cell proliferation. Subsequently, she underwent pleurodesis on both sides. TROP2 overexpression relating to Sacituzumab-Govitecan (29, 30), or biomarkers for immune checkpoint inhibitors, were not observed.

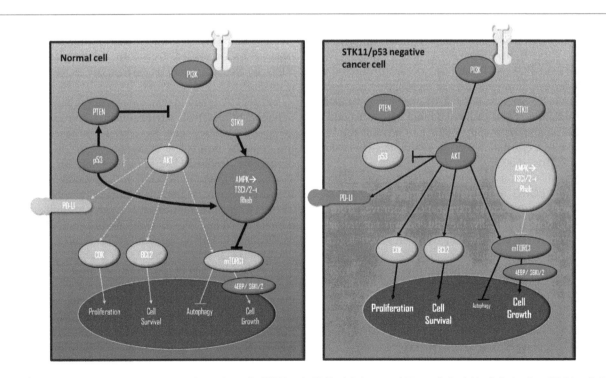

FIGURE 3 | Simplified PIK3/AKT/mTOR pathway and interactions with STK11 and p53. The left shows a wild-type cell, the right cell displays how STK11 and p53 loss of function leads to extensive proliferation/cell survival and cell growth, because of the missing negative feedbacks and activations.

TABLE 1 | Main results of the tumor profiling.

	Case 1	Case 2
Genetic Mutations/Amplifications	PIK3CA p.E545K	TP53 p.R290fs; STK11 p.Y131; NOTCH1 pQ1155; PIK3CG/D; FGFR2 amplification
Pathway Modeling (mRNA based)	Decreased DHFR signaling, increased HIF1 signaling	Increased signaling of TUBB2A, PGF, VEGFA, HIF1
Chemosensitivity Cell Death Rate [%]	Gemcitabine 72%	Gemcitabine +Carboplatin 85%
	Oxaliplatin 59%	Etoposide 79%
	Vinblastine 58%	Gemictabine 60%
	Etoposid < 25%	5-Fluoruracil 56%
	Topotecan < 25%	Carboplatin 55%
IHC Staining (PD-L1, EGFR, VEGFA, mTOR)	EGFR	-
MMR/MSI	Negative	MSI stable
Tumour Mutational Burden	0, 59 mutations/Mb blood-based	2, 21 mutations/Mb tissue based
Pharmacogenomics (altered metabolism)	ERCC1, NT5C2, UGT1A1, ABCB1	ERCC1, CYP2D6, UGT1A1, FCGR2A

Since NGS revealed PIK3CA as the only targetable alteration and AKT together with transcription factors, such as BCL2 were upregulated, it appeared that the proliferation promoting influence was not triggered via the mTOR pathway. The therapy was focused on the PIK3CA mutation, again (**Figure 3**). We evaluated intrinsic resistance factors for PIK3CA inhibitors, no PTEN loss nor amplification of FGFR1 could be detected (25, 31).

The analysis of the PI3K pathway, including the peripheral effector components involved at the molecular and mRNA levels, indicated that the use of the PI3K inhibitor Alpelisib would not suffice to inhibit the complete PI3K/AKT pathway. This assumption is supported by the fact that important components of tumor metabolism like PEPCK (phosphoenol-pyruvate-carboxykinase), cell cycle progression like CDK20, Myc, and factors of cell survival like Mcl1, Bim were not upregulated. In addition, IRS family member 4, which constitutively hyperactivates the PI3K/AKT pathway, was downregulated on the mRNA level. Components of the cross-linked oncogenic pathway, such as Rat Sarcoma Virus (RAS), were not upregulated, therefore, inhibition of this pathway did not appear promising (32). To address this issue and to take into account the high proliferation rate, a cytostatic agent was administered in analogy to the study NCT04215003, together with Alpelisib.

For the first time, a remarkable therapeutic effect was observed. From ECOG II, the patient changed toward ECOG 0 within 3 weeks, also because oxygenation improved from 57 to 70 mm/Hg. Sonographically, the effusion was not traceable anymore. Seven weeks later she suffered from an etiologically unclear thoracic pain event and died.

The second patient presented herself with hepatic progress shortly after completing adjuvant therapies. Tumor profiling was performed based on a liver biopsy together with a blood sample. An STK11p.Y131* mutation with clinical relevance was found. STK11/LKB1 mutations are reported in neuroendocrine tumors, such as large cell subtypes (33–35), but rare in breast cancers with an incidence of 0,2–1,0 % (35). STK11 alterations are associated with a lack of PDL1 expression, and the patient had a low TMB. Being MSI stable, no efficacy of checkpoint inhibitors was predicted (29).

The detected STK11mutation is considered to be a loss-of-function mutation resulting in activation of mTOR, as it is additionally induced by the detected p53 alteration (**Figure 3**). Functional loss of p53 activity can contribute to higher activities of the PI3K/AKT/mTOR pathways (36, 37).

To evaluate further the mTOR effect, we investigated additional peripheral effectors at the mRNA level.

Due to STK11 loss, the mTOR activation was most likely triggered *via* S6K1/2 (ribosomal S6 protein kinase 1/2), which was partially upregulated, stimulating proliferation by eIF4B and S6. Consequently, we applied the mTOR inhibitor, Everolimus, in this situation (35, 38–40).

Everolimus, itself, is approved by the Food and Drug Administration (FDA) for hormone receptor-positive and Her2 negative breast cancer. It is also the standard of care for NETs in National Comprehensive Cancer Network (NCCN) guidelines (41).

But mTOR inhibition as monotherapy based on allosteric inhibitors of mTORC1, like Everolimus, may lead to decreased therapeutic efficacy due to several resistance mechanisms: this could be incomplete inhibition of mTORC1, suppression of negative feedback loops, for example via increased IRS 1, which activates PI3K/AKT, ERK pathway activation, just to mention only a few of resistance factors (22, 25, 42). There is evidence of potential synergism with angiogenetic inhibitors. Taking into account the presence of upregulation of VEGFA and HIF-alpha-pathway, Bevacizumab was added to Everolimus (43–45).

Due to the highly proliferating disease and extent of metastasis, Capecitabine was administered in accordance with the test results (46). This is not surprising as Capecitabine is the standard of care to treat breast cancer, it is also mentioned in German guidelines for colorectal NETs or of NETs pancreatic origin. The therapy combination of Everolimus, Bevacizumab, and Capecitabine was well-tolerated. Imaging showed partial remission for 3 months. Then, the tumor progressed dramatically, and the patient died soon due to liver insufficiency.

Extensive Tumor Profiling in Primary Neuroendocrine Breast Cancer Cases as a Role Model...

97

CONCLUSION

To date, molecular profiling is used especially in breast, lung, colorectal, prostate, and gastric cancer (47). Here we demonstrate two patients with a rare tumor entity as a role models to illustrate the benefit to which a broader molecular tumor profiling can offer a significant contribution not only to diagnosis but also to the therapeutic regime.

Therapy-relevant mutations were uncovered, analyzing numerous tumor-relevant genes (>400) and pharmacogenomics. Specifically, the intelligent combination of immunocytochemistry/-histochemistry, chemosensitivity testing on tumor cells, DNA alterations, and expression profiles, could be detected and delivered valuable insights to tailor therapy.

Hence the rate of ineffective and cost-intensive therapies can be diminished and will improve the already available personalized, targeted therapies. Currently, application of solitary genetic testing delivers advantages only to a minority of patients (48–50). The first basket trials especially like the SHIVA trial largely failed because molecular filters were applied (48). Newer trials like the RESILIENT trial had beneficial outcomes even in late-stage patients with several previous therapies applying enhanced molecular analysis comprising also cytological features and other cancer characteristics (15).

Promising new options are especially needed for rare tumor entities, exemplified by NEBC, which remains a major diagnostic and therapeutic challenge today. From the start, there are numerous pitfalls in diagnosing NEBC, because it is itself a heterogeneous group of tumors. The rarity of this tumor type makes it imperative to apply sensitive diagnostic tools for effective treatment options.

It is also important for patients, for whom empirical therapy showed no efficiency and potential therapies based on tumor-specific profiles, respecting possible resistance mechanisms are explored. Viewed in isolation, not only the targets may be considered for the choice of therapy, but, if possible, the context of the whole pathway network together with other biomarkers too.

Questions that we need to ask, is whether the therapeutic effect justified the application of comprehensive tools in these cases. In both heavily pre-treated patients, actionable targets were discovered together with findings from ICC, chemosensitivity, and pathway modeling leading to a treatment that was well-tolerated and an improvement in the overall situation. However, both patients suffered from a highly aggressive subtype and were already in the metastatic situation where curative treatment is virtually not possible and the effects of the treatment did not last longer than a few months. Especially in rare cancers, where the prognosis is worse from the start, we should think about using tailored therapies based on comprehensive tumor characteristics earlier, because, only then, can we know whether this approach will provide a benefit. Trials to combine several rare cancer types and extensive profiling could hold the key to a successful treatment.

AUTHOR CONTRIBUTIONS

DS-N: counseling of patients, clinical management, data analysis, data interpretation, and manuscript writing. RV: counseling of patients, data interpretation, and manuscript review. AT: data interpretation and manuscript review. SS: data analysis and manuscript writing. All authors contributed to the article and approved the submitted version.

REFERENCES

1. Roininen N, Takala S, Haapasaari K-M, Jukkola-Vuorinen A, Mattson J, Heikkilä P, et al. Primary neuroendocrine breast carcinomas are associated with poor local control despite favourable biological profile: a retrospective clinical study. *BMC Cancer.* (2017) 17:72. doi: 10.1186/s12885-017-3056-4

2. Wang J, Wei B, Albarracin CT, Hu J, Abraham SC, Wu Y. Invasive neuroendocrine carcinoma of the breast: a population-based study from the surveillance, epidemiology and end results (SEER) database. *BMC Cancer.* (2014) 14:147. doi: 10.1186/1471-2407-14-147

3. Cloyd JM, Yang RL, Allison KH, Norton JA, Hernandez-Boussard T, Wapnir IL. Impact of histological subtype on long-term outcomes of neuroendocrine carcinoma of the breast. *Breast Cancer Res Treat.* (2014) 148:637–44. doi: 10.1007/s10549-014-3207-0

4. Angarita FA, Rodríguez JL, Meek E, Sánchez JO, Tawil M, Torregrosa L. Locally-advanced primary neuroendocrine carcinoma of the breast: case report and review of the literature. *World J Surg Onc.* (2013) 11:128. doi: 10.1186/1477-7819-11-128

5. Inno A, Bogina G, Turazza M, Bortesi L, Duranti S, Massocco A, et al. Neuroendocrine carcinoma of the breast: current evidence and future perspectives. *Oncologist.* (2016) 21:28–32. doi: 10.1634/theoncologist.2015-0309

6. Salemis NS. Primary neuroendocrine carcinoma of the breast: a rare presentation and review of the literature. *Intractable Rare Dis Res.* (2020) 9:233–46. doi: 10.5582/irdr.2020.03046

7. Tsai T-H, Hsieh P-P, Hong Y-C, Yeh C-H, Yu LH-L, Yu M-S. Metastatic primary neuroendocrine carcinoma of the breast (NECB). *J Cancer Res Pract.* (2018) 5:38–42. doi: 10.1016/j.jcrpr.2017.10.003

8. Oberg K. Management of neuroendocrine tumours. *Ann Oncol.* (2004) 15 Suppl 4:iv293–298. doi: 10.1093/annonc/mdh942

9. Wei X, Chen C, Xi D, Bai J, Huang W, Rong L, et al. case of primary neuroendocrine breast carcinoma that responded to neo-adjuvant chemotherapy. *Front Med.* (2015) 9:112–6. doi: 10.1007/s11684-014-0345-z

10. Trevisi E, La Salvia A, Daniele L, Brizzi MP, De Rosa G, Scagliotti GV, et al. Neuroendocrine breast carcinoma: a rare but challenging entity. *Med Oncol.* (2020) 37:70. doi: 10.1007/s12032-020-01396-4

11. Salama JK, Milano MT. Radical irradiation of extracranial oligometastases. *J Clin Oncol.* (2014) 32:2902–12. doi: 10.1200/JCO.2014.55.9567

12. Cancer Genome Atlas Network. Comprehensive molecular portraits of human breast tumours. *Nature.* (2012) 490:61–70. doi: 10.1038/nature11412

13. André F, Ciruelos E, Rubovszky G, Campone M, Loibl S, Rugo HS, et al. Alpelisib for PIK3CA-mutated, hormone receptor-positive

advanced breast cancer. *N Engl J Med.* (2019) 380:1929–40. doi: 10.1056/NEJMoa1813904

14. Lavigne M, Menet E, Tille J-C, Lae M, Fuhrmann L, Bonneau C, et al. Comprehensive clinical and molecular analyses of neuroendocrine carcinomas of the breast. *Mod Pathol.* (2018) 31:68–82. doi: 10.1038/modpathol.2017.107

15. Nagarkar R, Kohi S, Hirata K, Goggins M, Sato N. Encyclopedic tumor analysis for guiding treatment of advanced, broadly refractory cancers: results from the RESILIENT trial. *Oncotarget.* (2019) 10:27188. doi: 10.18632/oncotarget.27188

16. Crook T, Gaya A, Page R, Limaye S, Ranade A, Bhatt A, et al. Clinical utility of circulating tumor-associated cells to predict and monitor chemo-response in solid tumors. *Cancer Chemother Pharmacol.* (2020) 87:197–205. doi: 10.1007/s00280-020-04189-8

17. Crook T, Patil D, Gaya A, Plowman N, Limaye S, Ranade A, et al. Improved treatment outcomes by using patient specific drug combinations in mammalian target of rapamycin activated advanced metastatic cancers. *Front Pharmacol.* (2021) 12:631135. doi: 10.3389/fphar.2021.631135

18. Terlević R, Perić Balja M, Tomas D, Skenderi F, Krušlin B, Vranic S, et al. Somatostatin receptor SSTR2A and SSTR5 expression in neuroendocrine breast cancer. *Ann Diagn Pathol.* (2019) 38:62–6. doi: 10.1016/j.anndiagpath.2018.11.002

19. Ang D, Ballard M, Beadling C, Warrick A, Schilling A, O'Gara R, et al. Novel mutations in neuroendocrine carcinoma of the breast: possible therapeutic targets. *Appl Immunohistochem Mol Morphol.* (2015) 23:97–103. doi: 10.1097/PDM.0b013e3182a40fd1

20. McCullar B, Pandey M, Yaghmour G, Hare F, Patel K, Stein M, et al. Genomic landscape of small cell carcinoma of the breast contrasted to small cell carcinoma of the lung. *Breast Cancer Res Treat.* (2016) 158:195–202. doi: 10.1007/s10549-016-3867-z

21. Marchiò C, Geyer FC, Ng CK, Piscuoglio S, De Filippo MR, Cupo M, et al. The genetic landscape of breast carcinomas with neuroendocrine differentiation: Genetics of neuroendocrine breast cancer. *J Pathol.* (2017) 241:405–19. doi: 10.1002/path.4837

22. Yang J, Nie J, Ma X, Wei Y, Peng Y, Wei X. Targeting PI3K in cancer: mechanisms and advances in clinical trials. *Mol Cancer.* (2019) 18:26. doi: 10.1186/s12943-019-0954-x

23. Burstein HJ, Mangu PB, Somerfield MR, Schrag D, Samson D, Holt L, et al. American society of clinical oncology clinical practice guideline update on the use of chemotherapy sensitivity and resistance assays. *JCO.* (2011) 29:3328–30. doi: 10.1200/JCO.2011.36.0354

24. Li Z, Yang Z, Passaniti A, Lapidus RG, Liu X, Cullen KJ, et al. positive feedback loop involving EGFR/Akt/mTORC1 and IKK/NF-kB regulates head and neck squamous cell carcinoma proliferation. *Oncotarget.* (2016) 7:31892–906. doi: 10.18632/oncotarget.7441

25. Rozengurt E, Soares HP, Sinnet-Smith J. Suppression of feedback loops mediated by PI3K/mTOR induces multiple overactivation of compensatory pathways: an unintended consequence leading to drug resistance *Mol Cancer Ther.* (2014) 13:2477–88. doi: 10.1158/1535-7163.MCT-14-0330

26. Vellai T. How the amino acid leucine activates the key cell-growth regulator mTOR. *Nature.* (2021) 596:192–4. doi: 10.1038/d41586-021-01943-7

27. Li S, Kong Y, Si L, Chi Z, Cui C, Sheng X, et al. Phosphorylation of mTOR and S6RP predicts the efficacy of everolimus in patients with metastat renal cell carcinoma. *BMC Cancer.* (2014) 14:376. doi: 10.1186/1471-2407-14-376

28. Rutkovsky AC, Yeh ES, Guest ST, Findlay VJ, Muise-Helmericks RC, Armeson K, et al. Eukaryotic initiation factor 4E-binding protein as an oncogene in breast cancer. *BMC Cancer.* (2019) 19:491. doi: 10.1186/s12885-019-5667-4

29. Vranic S, Palazzo J, Sanati S, Florento E, Contreras E, Xiu J, et al. Potential novel therapy targets in neuroendocrine carcinomas of the breast. *Clin Breast Cancer.* (2019) 19:131–6. doi: 10.1016/j.clbc.2018.09.001

30. Bardia A, Mayer IA, Diamond JR, Moroose RL, Isakoff SJ, Starodub AN, et al. Efficacy and safety of Anti-Trop-2 antibody drug conjugate sacituzumab govitecan (IMMU-132) in heavily pretreated patients with metastatic triple-negative breast cancer. *JCO.* (2017) 35:2141–8. doi: 10.1200/JCO.2016.70.8297

31. Xie Y, Su N, Yang J, Tan Q, Huang S, Jin M, et al. FGF/FGFR signaling in health and disease. *Sig Transduct Target Ther.* (2020) 5:181. doi: 10.1038/s41392-020-00222-7

32. Khan AQ, Kuttikrishnan S, Siveen KS, Prabhu KS, Shanmugakonar M, Al-Naemi HA, et al. RAS-mediated oncogenic signaling pathways in human malignancies. *Semin Cancer Biol.* (2019) 54:1–13. doi: 10.1016/j.semcancer.2018.03.001

33. Rekhtman N, Pietanza MC, Hellmann MD, Naidoo J, Arora A, Won H, et al. Next-generation sequencing of pulmonary large cell neuroendocrine carcinoma reveals small cell carcinoma–like and non–small cell carcinoma–like subsets. *Clin Cancer Res.* (2016) 22:3618–29. doi: 10.1158/1078-0432.CCR-15-2946

34. Derks JL, Leblay N, Thunnissen E, van Suylen RJ, den Bakker M, Groen HJM, et al. Molecular subtypes of pulmonary large-cell neuroendocrine carcinoma predict chemotherapy treatment outcome. *Clin Cancer Res.* (2018) 24:33–42. doi: 10.1158/1078-0432.CCR-17-1921

35. Parachoniak CA, Rankin A, Gaffney B, Hartmaier R, Spritz D, Erlich RL, et al. Exceptional durable response to everolimus in a patient with biphenotypic breast cancer harboring an STK11variant. *Cold Spring Harb Mol Case Stud.* (2017) 3:a000778. doi: 10.1101/mcs.a000778

36. Levine AJ, Puzio-Kuter AM. The control of the metabolic switch in cancers by oncogenes and tumor suppressor genes. *Science.* (2010) 330:1340–4. doi: 10.1126/science.1193494

37. Nakanishi A, Kitagishi Y, Ogura Y, Matsuda S. The tumor suppressor PTEN interacts with p53 in hereditary cancer (review). *Int J Oncol.* (2014) 44:1813–9. doi: 10.3892/ijo.2014.2377

38. Laderian B, Mundi P, Fojo TE, Bates S. Emerging therapeutic implications of stk11mutation: case series. *Oncol.* (2020) 25:733–7. doi: 10.1634/theoncologist.2019-0846

39. Han D, Li S-J, Zhu Y-T, Liu L, Li M-X. LKB1/AMPK/mTOR signaling pathway in non-small-cell lung cancer. *Asian Pac J Cancer Prev.* (2013) 14:4033–9. doi: 10.7314/APJCP.2013.14.7.4033

40. Akeno N, Miller AL, Ma X, Wikenheiser-Brokamp KA. p53 suppresses carcinoma progression by inhibiting mTOR pathway activation. *Oncogene.* (2015) 34:589–99. doi: 10.1038/onc.2013.589

41. Shah MH, Goldner WS, Halfdanarson TR, Bergsland E, Berlin JD, Halperin D, et al. NCCN guidelines insights: neuroendocrine and adrenal tumors, version 2.2018. *J Natl Compr Canc Netw.* (2018) 16:693–702. doi: 10.6004/jnccn.2018.0056

42. Formisano L, Napolitano F, Rosa R, D'Amato V, Servetto A, Marciano R, et al. Mechanisms of resistance to mTOR inhibitors. *Crit Rev Oncol Hematol.* (2020) 147:102886. doi: 10.1016/j.critrevonc.2020.102886

43. Marton I, Knezevic F, Ramic S, Milosevic M, Tomas D. Immunohistochemical expression and prognostic significance of HIF-1α and VEGF-C in neuroendocrine breast cancer. *Anticancer Res.* (2012) 32:5227–32.

44. Pal K, Madamsetty VS, Dutta SK, Wang E, Angom RS, Mukhopadhyay D. Synchronous inhibition of mTOR and VEGF/NRP1 axis impedes tumor growth and metastasis in renal cancer. *NPJ Precis Oncol.* (2019) 3:31. doi: 10.1038/s41698-019-0105-2

45. Hobday TJ, Qin R, Reidy-Lagunes D, Moore MJ, Strosberg J, Kaubisch A, et al. Multicenter phase II trial of temsirolimus and bevacizumab in pancreatic neuroendocrine tumors. *JCO.* (2015) 33:1551–6. doi: 10.1200/JCO.2014.56.2082

46. Sabanathan D, Eslick GD, Shannon J. Use of neoadjuvant chemotherapy plus molecular targeted therapy in colorectal liver metastases: a systematic review and meta-analysis. *Clin Colorectal Cancer.* (2016) 15:e141–7. doi: 10.1016/j.clcc.2016.03.007

47. Mosele F, Remon J, Mateo J, Westphalen CB, Barlesi F, Lolkema MP, et al. Recommendations for the use of next-generation sequencing (NGS) for patients with metastatic cancers: a report from the ESMO precision medicine working group. *Annals Oncol.* (2020) 31:1491–505. doi: 10.1016/j.annonc.2020.07.014

48. Le Tourneau C, Delord J-P, Gonçalves A, Gavoille C, Dubot C, Isambert N, et al. Molecularly targeted therapy based on tumour molecular profiling versus conventional therapy for advanced cancer (SHIVA): a multicentre, open-label, proof-of-concept, randomised, controlled phase 2 trial. *Lancet Oncol.* (2015) 16:1324–34. doi: 10.1016/S1470-2045(15)00188-6

49. Tsimberidou A-M, Hong DS, Ye Y, Cartwright C, Wheler JJ, Falchook GS, et al. Initiative for molecular profiling and advanced cancer therapy (IMPACT): an md anderson precision medicine study. *JCO Precis Oncol.* (2017) 2017:10. doi: 10.1200/PO.17.00002

50. Jovelet C, Ileana E, Le Deley M-C, Motte N, Rosellini S, Romero A, et al. Circulating cell-free tumor DNA analysis of 50 genes by next-generation sequencing in the prospective MOSCATO trial. *Clin Cancer Res.* (2016) 22:2960–8. doi: 10.1158/1078-0432.CCR-15-2470

12

Dissecting and Reconstructing Matrix in Malignant Mesothelioma through Histocell-Histochemistry Gradients for Clinical Applications

Marcelo Luiz Balancin[1†], Camila Machado Baldavira[1†], Tabatha Gutierrez Prieto[1],
Juliana Machado-Rugolo[1,2], Cecília Farhat[1], Aline Kawassaki Assato[1],
Ana Paula Pereira Velosa[3], Walcy Rosolia Teodoro[3], Alexandre Muxfeldt Ab'Saber[1],
Teresa Yae Takagaki[4] and Vera Luiza Capelozzi[1*]

[1] Laboratory of Genomics and Histomorphometry, Department of Pathology, University of São Paulo Medical School (USP), São Paulo, Brazil, [2] Health Technology Assessment Center (NATS), Clinical Hospital (HCFMB), Medical School of São Paulo State University (UNESP), Botucatu, Brazil, [3] Rheumatology Division of the Hospital das Clinicas da Faculdade de Medicina da Universidade de São Paulo, FMUSP, São Paulo, Brazil, [4] Division of Pneumology, Instituto do Coração (Incor), University of São Paulo Medical School (USP), São Paulo, Brazil

*Correspondence:
Vera Luiza Capelozzi
vera.capelozzi@fm.usp.br

† These authors have contributed equally to this work and share first authorship

Background: Malignant pleural mesotheliomas (MM) are known for their heterogenous histology and clinical behavior. MM histology reveals three major tumor cell populations: epithelioid, sarcomatoid, and biphasic. Using a dissecting approach, we showed that histochemical gradients help us better understand tumor heterogeneity and reconsider its histologic classifications. We also showed that this method to characterize MM tumor cell populations provides a better understanding of the underlying mechanisms for invasion and disease progression.

Methods: In a cohort of 87 patients with surgically excised MM, we used hematoxylin and eosin to characterize tumor cell populations and Movat's pentachrome staining to dissect the ECM matrisome. Next, we developed a computerized semi-assisted protocol to quantify and reconstruct the ECM in 3D and examined the clinical association between the matricellular factors and patient outcome.

Results: Epithelioid cells had a higher matrix composition of elastin and fibrin, whereas, in the sarcomatoid type, hyaluronic acid and total collagen were most prevalent. The 3D reconstruction exposed the collagen I and III that form channels surrounding the neoplastic cell blocks. The estimated volume of the two collagen fractions was 14% of the total volume, consistent with the median estimated area of total collagen (12.05 mm^2) for epithelioid MM.

Conclusion: Differential patterns in matricellular phenotypes in MM could be used in translational studies to improve patient outcome. More importantly, our data raise the possibility that cancer cells can use the matrisome for disease expansion and could be effectively targeted by anti-collagen, anti-elastin, and/or anti-hyaluronic acid therapies.

Keywords: malignant mesothelioma, Movat's pentachrome stain, Picrosirius, immunohistochemistry, prognosis

INTRODUCTION

Malignant mesothelioma (MM) is a rare malignancy characterized by its aggressive growth, local invasion, and strong etiologic relationship to asbestos exposure. MM arises from serosal mesothelial cells, mesodermal derivative cells that exhibit both epithelial and mesenchymal features (1). Different clinical trials have investigated the striking differences in behavior and response to therapy in MM patients, some often suggest that this heterogeneity may emerge from the presence of different cell populations in a single tumor (2). The heterogeneous and aggressive nature of this tumor often lead to a poor prognosis for these patients. Therefore, it is crucial that we improve our comprehension of MM heterogeneity in its several aspects to develop new therapeutic protocols that can improve survival.

Tumor heterogeneity can be investigated at the intra-tumor and inter-tumor levels and contemplates not only tumor cell populations but also their microenvironments. There are currently three major histological MM types: epithelioid, biphasic (epithelioid-sarcomatoid), and sarcomatoid. The nonmalignant cells in the tumor microenvironment are, in turn, called the stroma and include blood vessels, immune cells, fibroblasts, signaling molecules, and the extracellular matrix (ECM) (3). Regarding the latter, it is worth noting that the ECM core matrisome can be broken down into fibrillar collagen types (such as types I), proteoglycans (such as hyaluronic acid), and glycoproteins (such as elastin) (4).

Previous histological observations made by pathologists identified two juxtaposed tumor cell populations (epithelioid and sarcomatoid) in MM. To further explore this question, our group adopted a dissecting approach to decompose each bulk MM histochemistry profile into a combination of these two cell populations. This novel approach quantifies different cell populations in a single tumor and avoids a strict subtype signature based on subjective hierarchical classifications that fail to take into account intermediate phenotypes and show intrinsic limitations when investigating intra-tumor heterogeneity. We also used bioinformatics to decompose and reconstruct MM profiles. This new method to classify the pathology is a step forward toward an improved comprehension of the underlying behavior of MM when different cell populations coexist in the same tumor. Moreover, this technique can have critical clinical applications and implications for prognosis and therapeutic strategies.

PATIENTS AND METHODS

Patient's Selection and Clinicopathologic Review

This retrospective study was conducted using data from institutions linked to the Hospital das Clínicas Complex of the Faculty of Medicine of the University of São Paulo (HC-FMUSP)–including the Central Institute (Division of Pathological Anatomy, DAP), the Heart Institute (InCOR, Laboratory of Pathological Anatomy) and the Cancer Institute of the State of São Paulo (ICESP)–and was approved by their Ethics Committees (protocol number: 2,394,571).

A search for the word "mesothelioma" led our group to 246 cases treated between 2008 and 2018 in the three institutions—75 at InCOR, 59 at HC-FMUSP, and 112 at ICESP. However, not all cases identified in the search were MM cases, since the word "mesothelioma" was sometimes used in the comments section of differentiated diagnoses, as well as in reports related to benign mesotheliomas, their variants (papillary, well-differentiated cystic), and cytological exams. Other cases were dismissed due to their blocks not being found or having been removed for external review or because they did not meet the proposed inclusion criteria. The final sample totaled 87 cases (35.4% of the initial search), as shown in **Supplementary Figure 1**.

All blocks and slides of the cases initially found (246) were requested from the pathology files for review by two experienced pathologists in Thoracic and Pulmonary Pathology (VLC and MLB). The review compared the diagnosis and findings reported in the anatomopathological reports, including the immunohistochemical test, with the original slides. When the slides were lightened or showed preservation artifacts due to temporal wear, they were considered unsuitable for reassessment, and new cuts or immunohistochemical reactions were performed.

Moreover, these reviews used the diagnostic criteria reported in the World Health Organization (WHO) update of 2021 (5). MM cases were histologically classified by their predominant tumor cell population – epithelioid or sarcomatoid. The nuclear features, as described by Kadota et al. (6), are illustrated in **Supplementary Figure 2**. All cases had their immunohistochemical profile reviewed–and expanded when necessary–to ensure a minimum of two positive and two negative markers for MM, as proposed by the WHO (7, 8). Positivity was expected to fall between 80 and 100% for D2-40 and between 70 and 93% for WT1, whereas negativity was expected to fall between 95 and 100% for both D2-40 and MOC31. In case of any remaining uncertainty, the pathologists expanded the panel, evaluated it with the BAP1, and individualized each characterization according to the clinical context on a case-by-case basis.

We extracted clinical data from the original anatomopathological reports, imaging examination reports, surgical reports, and patient charts. Asbestos exposure was inferred from indirect data such as residential location and registered employment history. We also used search engines to search for each patient's name online, looking for indexing, litigations, or any association with groups of former workers in the asbestos industries. Next, we staged pleural mesotheliomas according to the clinical-pathological model of the 8th edition of the AJCC/UICC (8), whereas extrapleural cases were staged according to the patient's medical record. Overall survival (OS) was defined as the time interval between the date of histopathological diagnosis and the outcome event (death or end of segment, if alive) and was obtained from death records at a registry office or at a death verification service. If no death records were identified, the time of the last follow-up was

TABLE 1 | Clinical characteristics of patients with malignant mesothelioma.

Characteristic	Number (%)
Age (years)*	
Median (range)	60 (35–92)
Sex, *n* (%)	
Male	59 (67.8%)
Female	28 (32.2%)
Asbestos exposure, *n* (%)	
No	43 (49.4%)
Yes	44 (50.6%)
Stage[†] III/IV	87 (100%)
Treatment, *n* (%)	
Surgery	62 (71.3%)
Chemotherapy	25 (28.7%)
Overall Survival, median*	21.6 months
Status*	
Alive	35 (41.7%)
Died	52 (58.3%)

*Some cases lacked follow-up information: Age [3]; Overall Survival [16]; Status [3]. †Per International Association for the Study of Lung Cancer (IASLC) criteria (7).

calculated based on the last consultation or laboratory tests in the computerized hospital system.

Table 1 summarizes the clinical-pathological and epidemiologic data of these patients.

Morphological Sample Assessmeny
Construction of Tissue Microarray (TMA)

We chose the TMA investigation model based on the currently available literature, including studies of immune response (9–11). Before to construct the model, we carefully examined the hematoxylin and eosin (HE) stained slides to assure that areas epithelioid and sarcomatoid were present. Then, three cylinders of 1.0 mm in diameter containing the epithelioid areas and three cylinders containing sarcomatoid areas, were noted on the original corresponding HE slides and paraffin blocks (named as "donor" blocks) and then extracted and transported to receiver paraffin blocks using the precision mechanized equipment MTA1 (Manual Tissue Microarrayer, Beecher Instruments, USA). Each cylinder was positioned in the receiver block according to a previously prepared map, with a 0.3 mm spacing between samples (**Supplementary Figure 3**). Each case produced six cylinders distributed in duplicate in the receiver block, aiming to minimize a possible sampling bias resulting from physical losses and/or representativeness inherent to the TMA technology. Next, the TMA blocks were submitted to serial 3 μm-thick cuts in a manual microtome (Leica Instruments, Germany), each cut made in a single session to avoid losses with trimming. As a result, each block produced 70 sections that were then distributed on a marked slide embedded in paraffin and stored in a dark box at−20°C to preserve the antigenicity of the samples. The built TMAs are illustrated in **Supplementary Figure 4**.

Histochemistry

Each MM TMA had one of its sections stained using the Modified Russell-Movat's pentachrome stain adopted by the FMUSP biotechnics sector (12). **Supplementary Table 1** lists the evaluable connective elements and their respective color tones. **Supplementary Figure 5** illustrates the elements of Movat's pentachrome stain under evaluation. We also subjected the paraffin blocks with a representative surgical specimen to a Picrosirius histochemical staining and visualized it under polarized light under 90 degrees for indirect identification of type I fibers (coarser in appearance, in shades ranging from yellowish to reddish) and type III fibers (more delicate and greenish) (13, 14).

Scanning and Image Capture of Histology Slides

Histology slides for brightfield viewing (HE, Movat, Picrosirius) were scanned in a Pannoramic 250 scanner (3DHistech, Budapest, Hungary), under a 40x objective (Plan-Apochromat, 40x/NA0.95, Zeiss, Germany), with a resulting pixel density of 0.185 μm2. The resulting files, saved in mirax format, were stored on an external hard disk with a 2 TB capacity, with redundant copies on a secondary disk for data security. For visualization, we used the proprietary software Panoramic Viewer (3DHistech) and QuPath open platform, version 0.2.0-m4 (Centre for Cancer Research & Cell Biology, University of Edinburgh, Edinburgh, Scotland). For scientific documentation and acquisition of microscopy images under polarized light, we used Zeiss Axiocam 512 scientific camera (Zeiss, Germany) coupled to a Zeiss Axioscope A1 optical microscope with x40 and x63 N-Planochromatic objectives (Zeiss) under the Zen 3.0 (Zeiss) software to acquire brightfield and polarized light images.

Computerized Semi-assisted Quantification

We used the QuPath analysis visualization software in a semi-assisted manner. This platform had been previously validated in other studies (15), and we followed the protocol suggested by their authors (16). After the data was uploaded to the software, QuPath normalized the slide vectors, "dissecting" epithelioid and sarcomatoid areas, corrected them by automated sample detection, delineating them (**Supplementary Figure 6**), and computer them as cellularity (**Supplementary Figures 7, 8**). We then quantified the Movat's stain in epithelioid and sarcomatoid areas associating the Trainable Weka Segmentation (TWS) machine learning tool ("Waikato Environment for Knowledge Segmentation") (17) and the ImageJ software (National Institute of Health, USA). Next, a training set was created by an experienced pathologist (MLB) consisting of 18 images of 100 x 100 pixels extracted from the general sample. These images are representative of "ideal" areas (ground truth), representing the components highlighted in this coloration: fibrin, collagen matrix, hyaluronic acid, elastic fibers (**Supplementary Figure 9**). The correspondence of each of these elements was "taught" to the system through slide annotations, algorithms, trial and error, correction to its adequacy, and validation. Once the training set had been validated, the algorithm grouped all spots into separate images. This group segmentation resulted in 8-bit colored images censored by the previously designated color codes. Next, these images were again validated by a pathologist (MLB) and finally quantified by component under the optical threshold in the ImageJ software. The final measurements of cellularity, hyaluronic acid, fibrin, elastin, and total collagen in epithelioid and sarcomatoid populations obtained from the three cylinders in the TMA were averaged and directly calculated on the QuPath software. A final single patient value was expressed as the percentage per mm^2, and then transferred to individual patients to determine OS and risk of death as final endpoint. Moreover, heterogeneity among the different cylinders from a same patient occurred mimicking the scenario of MM, a heterogeneous tumor. Albeit this heterogeneity, the predominant histoarchitecture was considered.

Three-Dimensional Reconstruction and 3D Collagen Printing

Type I and III collagen fibers were reconstructed using the Picrosirius histological staining, a technique based on the azo pigment Sirius Red F 3B in saturated picric acid, as described by Junqueira et al. (18). The purpose of this reconstruction method was to create a 3D visualization of the patterns found in collagen networks made up of Col fibers type I and III. We chose not to individualize them to better understand the spatial distribution between the neoplastic cell blocks. Other collagen types that could not be stained with Picrosirius were not reconstructed because the method was chosen for its affordability. In this coloration, when viewed under polarized light with a brightfield optical microscope, Col I fibers are identified as thick, reddish, or orange-colored fibers, whereas Col III fibers are thin and greenish. **Supplementary Figure 10** is a photomicrograph that highlights the observed patterns of staining with or without polarized microscopy. In the absence of polarization, all collagen fibers had a reddish color, contrasting with the yellowish tones of the cytoplasm and muscle tissue. It was only under the use of polarized light that, as previously mentioned, the different fiber refringence patterns, conformations, and color patterns between Col I and III emerged. Also, lower magnification showed their architectural distribution as ECM components, with different patterns of fiber distribution: Col (I) was organized in thicker orange and reddish fibers, whereas Col (III) fibers were thin and greenish.

The collagen reconstruction involved the use of a destructive microscopy technique (19) where ten 3μm sequential cuts are made in the paraffin blocks of surgical specimens containing viable tumor cell representation and ECM. All the block slices are then stained using the Picrosirius red technique in a single session to avoid technique variations. Next, their images are captured using a brightfield optical microscope (Zeiss Axioscope A1, Zeiss), with 4x (N-Achroplan NA: 0.15, Zeiss), 20x (N-Achroplan, NA: 0.45, Zeiss) and 63x (Achroplan, NA: 0.56, Zeiss) magnification, polarizer, and led light source. The camera employed in this study was a scientific camera with a 12-megapixel, 1-inch CCD sensor, Axiocam 512 (Zeiss). The images were captured in multiple magnitudes, sequentially, at the same point on all slides, and the image files were saved in the proprietary format of the Zen 3.0 capture software (Zeiss) ".czi" and exported in uncompressed ".tif" format, with 100%

quality. For the collagen reconstruction, we used the images captured under polarization and under 4 and 20x objectives. The next step was to align the images digitally. First, an image grouping (stack) was imported into the Fiji software and transposed to 8-bit in grayscale. We then applied the optical threshold (threshold) of the Otsui method to highlight Col I and III fibers and aligned them using the TrakEM2 (20) plugin, choosing the stack alignment option, without deformations, in the proposed configurations, with the affine transformation method. After a visual validation of the alignment, the resulting images were exported in ".tif" format. For the three-dimensional visualization, we used the Fiji software's 3D viewer and the 3D Slicer software (version 4.10.2 r28257) (21). We first imported the previously treated ".tif" images into the 3D Slicer software and defined a virtual spacing of 5 mm in the voxel metadata configuration for z-axis visualization. Then we established a similar optical threshold to the one used for collagen fibers through the threshold option, defined the plane filling, and carried out the smoothing treatment. Finally, the Fiji software viewer created the final 3D visualization and exported it to ".stf" format in 1.9 gigabytes files. **Supplementary Figure 11** illustrates the image resulting from the reconstructions by Fiji (A) and 3D Slicer (B) software. With this file, the next step was to prepare it for 3D printing, reducing the image's vertices and triangles. Since the original image had 30966169 vertices and 61915216 triangles, stored in 2.88 gigabytes, the resolution of the triangles was reduced to achieve printability, without loss of quality in the perception of the reconstruction. To do so, we used Autodesk Meshmixer (Autodesk, USA) (22, 23) to create a ".stl" file of 18.8 megabytes containing 116,147 vertices and 234,066 triangles, with dimensions of 100.00 x 65,713 x 22.203 mm. In addition, the model was simplified by excluding loose stitches, that is, those without connection to other stitches, and rounding of the ends for printing, as illustrated in **Supplementary Figure 12**. Once adjusted for printing, the model was submitted to the Craftcloud website[1] for printing on a resin printer with a resolution of 0.05 mm.

Data Analysis

The statistical analysis was performed using SPSS v18 (Chicago, IL, USA) for Windows. We assessed the relationship between quantitative variables using Student's t-test and used an analysis of variance to correlate the color patterns. The paired-sample t-test and general linear model were used to test the relationship between one continuous variable and several others. All patients were clustered for similar expression levels between the five morphometric variables (tumor cellularity, hyaluronic acid, fibrin, elastic fibers, and total collagen) on an R statistical software using the pvclust package which provides a bootstrap agglomerative hierarchical clustering option. Clusters with similar expressions of the five variables were analyzed for risk of death and survival time. The risk of death was obtained by logistic regression. The total accumulated survival time was calculated by

---

[1] www.craftcloud.com, Germany

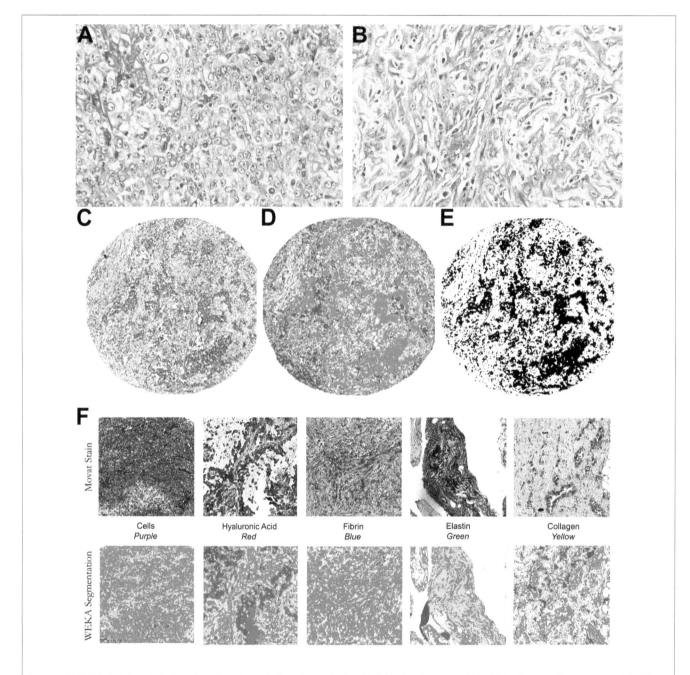

FIGURE 1 | Histological characterization of a malignant mesothelioma (MM) cohort. Epithelioid **(A)** and sarcomatoid **(B)** MM stained by HE. Input images **(C)**, TMA spot stained by modified Russell-Movat staining; **(D,E)** output of the Weka segmentation and of the threshold segmentation for data extraction by coloration. **(F)** Input and output images of the Weka segmentation, showing areas of segmented fundamental truths.

the Kaplan-Meier method and analyzed by the log-rank test. A P-value of two seams <0.05 was considered statistically significant for all tests.

RESULTS

Table 1 summarizes the clinical characteristics of patients who were mostly male (67.8%) at a median age of 60 years. All patients were stage III/IV, 71.3% had undergone surgical resection, and 28.7% had received chemotherapy. 50.6% of patients reported prior exposure to asbestos. 58.3% of patients died after disease progression.

Histological examinations found two contrasting tumor cell populations (epithelioid and sarcomatoid) in the MM cohort stained with Movat's pentachrome for cellularity and overall matrix characterization (**Figure 1**). The epithelioid population

TABLE 2 | Differences in the decomposed extracellular matrix factors between the epithelioid and sarcomatoid cell populations in MM.

	Epithelioid Cell Population	Sarcomatoid Cell Population	P-value*
Cellularity (mean cell number/mm²)	71.14	53.22	0.0001
Hyaluronic acid (area fraction/mm²)	6.57	10.73	0.05
Fibrin (area fraction/mm²)	4.13	1.29	0.0001
Elastin (area fraction/mm²)	6.08	2.30	0.0001
Total collagen (area fraction/mm²)	12.05	32.71	0.0001

*The t-test was used to detect differences in continuous variables between groups of the tumor cell population. P-value ≤ 0.05 was considered statistically significant.

showed a prominent tumor cellularity involvement in the dense hyaluronic acid matrix. In contrast, the sarcomatoid tumor cell population had modest tumor cellularity and hyaluronic acid area fraction.

Table 2 brings the distribution of the matrix components in the epithelioid and sarcomatoid tumor cell populations of MM. A closer evaluation of the ECM through the elements of Movat's pentachrome stain showed two distinct profiles: the epithelioid cell population had a higher mean cell density (1.33 times higher than sarcomatoid), with higher matrix composition of elastic fibers (2.64 times higher), and fibrin (3.2 times higher). Conversely, hyaluronic acid, a non-fibrillary element of ECM, and total collagen were predominant in the sarcomatoid tumor cell population (1.63 and 2.71 times higher, respectively). **Figure 2** uses four plots to compare the expression of matrix elements, including cellularity (**Figure 2A**), hyaluronic acid (**Figure 2B**), fibrin (**Figure 2C**), and total collagen (**Figure 2D**), between epithelioid and sarcomatoid tumor populations. The box plots in **Figure 2A** demonstrate a relatively strong relationship between cellularity and epithelioid tumor cell population ($P = 0.0001$), whereas the boxes in **Figures 2B,D** show a strong relationship between the sarcomatoid tumor population and hyaluronic acid and total collagen ($P = 0.05$ and $P = 0.0001$, respectively).

The three-dimensional reconstruction of the ECM based on Picrosirius made Col I and III more visible; the estimated volume of the two collagen fractions was 14% of the total volume in the chosen block, consistent with the median estimated volume of total Col (12.05) for epithelioid tumor population (**Figure 3**). The digital model was simplified to allow for three-dimensional printing and remove disjointed structures. As a result, **Figure 4** shows features that were not observed by the two-dimensional brightfield optical microscopy, such as channels formed by Col fibers surrounding the neoplastic cell blocks. While the digital model showed cellular channel areas between collagen fibers, the printed model made ECM more tangible, as illustrated in **Figure 4B**.

After the univariate analysis showed which morphometric variables differed significantly between epithelioid and sarcomatoid tumor cell population in MM (tumor cellularity, hyaluronic acid, fibrin, elastic fibers, and total collagen), we grouped these variables in hierarchical cluster analyses independent of clinicopathological variables and identified three clusters of patients: 24 subjects in cluster 1 (CL I), 13 in cluster 2 (CL II), and 50 in cluster 3 (CL III). **Figure 5** shows the

cluster dendrogram separating the three groups by dispersion similarities. CL I included tumors with a high area fraction of hyaluronic acid (13.03/mm2) and total collagen (25.48/mm2) compared to CL II (1.97 and 3.30/mm2, respectively) and CL III (5.43 and 11.90/mm2, respectively) (**Figure 6**); this cluster coincided with sarcomatoid tumor cell population histology. In contrast, CL II had tumors with a high area fraction of fibrin (9.82/mm2), and elastin (15.37/mm2) than CL I (0.97 and 2.63/mm2, respectively), and CL III (3.36 and 4.41/mm2, respectively); suggesting a biphasic tumor cell population in CL II–that is, one that includes both epithelioid and sarcomatoid cell types (**Figure 6**). Finally, CL III was made of tumors with a high number of cells/mm2 (74.89 cells/mm2) compared to CL I (57.89/mm²) and CL II (69.54/mm²) and coincided with the epithelioid tumor cell population histology (**Figure 6**).

In **Supplementary Table 2**, **Supplementary Figure 13** are shown the association between the three clusters classification with the final histotype (epithelioid, biphasic or sarcomatoid) resulting from pathological classification. Interestingly, cluster analysis recognizes with strong significance three different subsets in epithelioid MM classified only by histology (X^2; $P = 0.02$).

Considering that BAP1 is a surrogate marker for the presence of BAP1 gene alterations, clusters classification was compared with BAP1 protein status. The distribution of BAP1 protein was positive in 17 (22%) epithelioid-sarcomatoid and 3 (3.9%) epithelioid histotypes (**Supplementary Table 3**, **Supplementary Figure 14**; X^2; $P = 0.48$).

Table 3 shows the independent association between these clusters and survival probability in MM. CL II had three times the probability for better overall response (OR = 3.462, 95% CI = 1.115–10.746, $P = 0.032$).

Figure 7 shows overall survival data compared cluster classification with those resulting from the histopathological classification of the cases into the three major histotypes. The median overall survival between the cases classification was respectively 30.1 vs. 37.6 for CIII and epithelioid histotype, 44.4 vs. 34.4 for CII and epithelioid-sarcomatoid histotype and 23.3 into three major histotypes was 11.4 months for CL I, 5.5 months for CL II, and 25.1 months for CL III. And 30.1 vs. 11.26 for CI and sarcomatoid histotype. Clearly, the clusters tended to separate patients into three groups with distinctly different average survival times compared to histological classification, as illustrated by Kaplan-Meier curves in **Figures 7A,B**. CL III appears as the top curve. By contrast, those in CL II and I

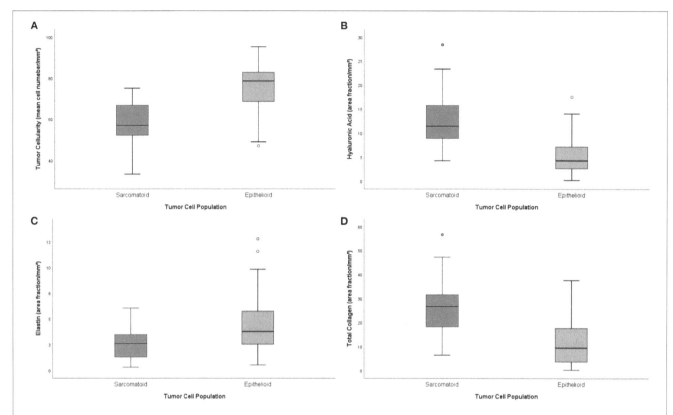

FIGURE 2 | Boxplots of the distribution of matrix elements [cellularity **(A)**, hyaluronic acid **(B)**, fibrin **(C)** and total collagen **(D)**] between the epithelioid and sarcomatoid groups.

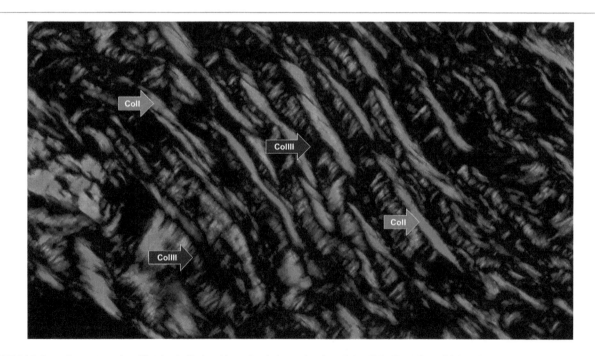

FIGURE 3 | Collagen fiber patterns I and III stained with picrosirius red and observed under polarized light. Type I fibers (thick and reddish fibers) and type III (thin and greenish fibers) are indicated by the arrows (red and green, respectively) (Picrosirius under polarized light, 630x).

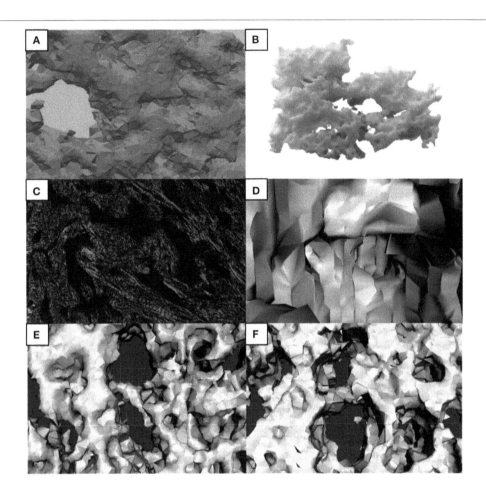

FIGURE 4 | Morphological characteristics observed under conventional microscopy and identified in the 3D model. **(A)** Simplified 3D model; **(B)** 3D printed model; **(C)** 2D microphotography–Picrosirius; **(D)** Features in the 3D model, such as the communicating channels pointed; **(E,F)** are the equivalent of the thick central septa of **(C)**, seen from different angles in the 3D model.

overlapped (bottom curves), respectively ($P < 0.01$; by Log Rank test).

DISCUSSION

Our study described histologic studies of MM, the different tumor cell populations in these samples, and their extracellular matrix components. We then suggested a complementary way to describe MM behavior using Movat's pentachrome stain and the TWS bioinformatics approach [IP1].

Movat's pentachrome was described in 1955 as a histochemical technique to highlight multiple components of the connective tissue compartment (24); in 1972, it was modified by Russell (12), who optimized the technique. The pentachrome adds elements with different colors, such as Verhoeff, sodium thiosulfate, acetic acid, alcian blue, Scarlet orcein with acid fuchsin, and safro-alcohol solutions. This histochemistry staining technique produces massive image datasets when observed under an optical microscope. However, to quantitatively evaluate the images, researchers frequently need to manually annotate the components of interest, a time-consuming procedure. To overcome this problem, the TWS works as a machine learning tool that studies a restricted number of manual observations and creates a list of classifier elements to slice the remaining data automatically (17). The TWS approach breaks down different MM profiles–each made of a distinct combination of tumor features–and reconstructs them according to the different cell populations found in the samples, as well as their non-tumoral extracellular matrix. This approach also minimizes the number of requirements assessed in various MM histological subtypes and is driven by the occurrence of epithelioid and sarcomatoid morphologies in different proportions within MM. TWS can also cluster the samples through unsupervised segmentation learning schemes and can be tailored to employ user-designed image features or classifiers. Both Movat's pentachrome stain and the TWS depend on the premise that distinct morphological phenotypes correspond to distinct molecular phenotypes. Therefore, we infer that the dissecting approach may influence the potential improvement of clinical management in terms of prognosis or therapeutic plan.

Along these lines, our results highlight several crucial points, namely: the combination of different tumor cell components,

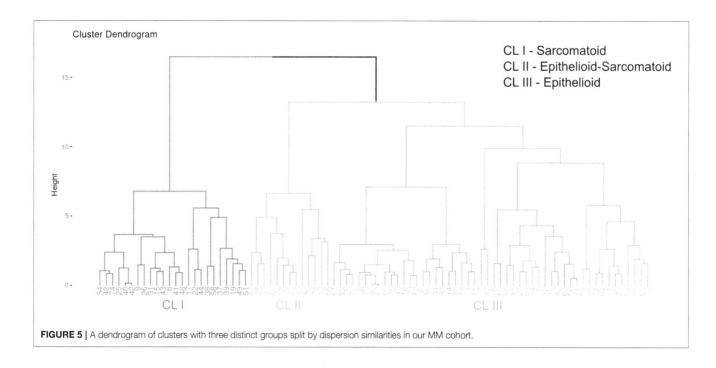

FIGURE 5 | A dendrogram of clusters with three distinct groups split by dispersion similarities in our MM cohort.

their relationship with their microenvironment, their association with patient survival, and their possible contribution to defining new therapeutic strategies. Using a similar approach, Mäkelä et al. (25) reported the prognostic value of fibroblast foci and inflammation in idiopathic pulmonary fibrosis. In an elegant study, Jones and colleagues applied an integrated micro-CT and Movat's stain to dissect the morphology of fibroblast foci in 3D and reveal a collection of heterogeneous structures, suggesting previously unrecognized plasticity, in contrast to the 2D tissue standard pathology of sections (26). Blum et al. (27) employed WISP, a deconvolution method, to show that different morphological phenotypes in MM correspond to distinct transcriptome phenotypes. More recently, Jargidar et al. (28) tested epithelioid, biphasic and sarcomatoid MM cell types *in vitro* and found that fibronectin (FN) and homologous cell-derived extracellular matrix (hcd-ECM) treated substratum differentially affected the above phenotypes; 3D MM spheroid invasion was higher in fibronectin-collagen matrices in the epithelioid and biphasic cells, while 3D cell cultures of epithelioid and sarcomatoid MM cells in fibronectin-collagen showed a higher contractility compared to hcd-ECM-collagen. Collectively, these results support our findings that histological subtypes are remarkably consistent with the MM-derived epithelioid-like, biphasic-like, and sarcomatoid-like tumor cell populations. Using thresholds to discriminate these populations, we can equally recapitulate all former tumor classification systems. We suggest that our method offers a more objective solution for describing MM subtypes, in contrast with discrete classification systems based either on morphology or molecular parameters to modulate stratified clinical trials. We also believe that precision medicine may benefit from the finely tuned information provided here to establish, for instance,

drug combinations and dosages that target different tumor cell compartments.

To understand the relationship between different tumor cell populations and their matricellular factors in MM progression, we used a three-stage design. First, we used histochemistry and a computerized semi-assisted quantification system to characterize the ECM matrisome (fibrin, hyaluronic acid, elastin, and collagen) in both epithelioid and sarcomatoid tumor cell populations. Second, the components that showed significant differences between epithelioid and sarcomatoid populations, regardless of any clinicopathological variables, were grouped according to the similarities produced in high-throughput protein analyses and used to characterize different subgroups of MM. Third, we examined the clinical association between different tumor-matricellular factors in TMAs built from 87 patients with surgically excised MM. Finally, we showed that this more subtle way of characterizing different tumor cell populations and stroma context provides a better understanding of the clinical behavior of MM.

However, some major points still require further investigations. The first important question that remains unanswered pertains to the significance of the high area fraction of fibrin and elastosis found in the ECM of the epithelioid cell population when compared to the sarcomatoid population. The behavior of individual cells is dictated by the forces exerted on them by the surrounding ECM (29), and the physical attachments that connect the cell interior to the ECM (30). During oncogenesis, the tumor stroma is changed, suffering modifications in its biochemical and viscoelastic properties, including elastic fibers (31). The ECM in solid tumors is stiffened, and as the tumor mass grows, it induces tumor hypoxia and cellular injury due to the increased interstitial pressure (32) modulating tumor cell phenotype (33). It has also been

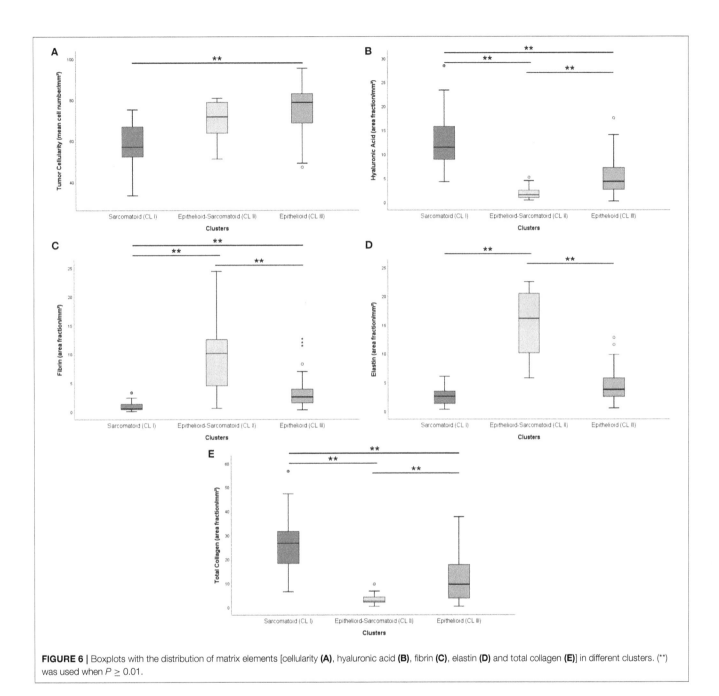

FIGURE 6 | Boxplots with the distribution of matrix elements [cellularity **(A)**, hyaluronic acid **(B)**, fibrin **(C)**, elastin **(D)** and total collagen **(E)**] in different clusters. (******) was used when $P \geq 0.01$.

established that the stiffened ECM is not an inactive bioproduct of cellular dedifferentiation but rather a dynamic contributor of tumor growth and progression (33). Augmented ECM stiffness and increasing core matrisome factors also disrupt stroma morphogenesis, thus helping develop a specific malignant phenotype in tumor cell populations (34). To understand the dynamic nature of the ECM and the functional consequences of ECM changes as tumor tissues develop and remodel, we can use the classic concept of tissue regeneration, repair, and remodeling (3Rs) as an example (35). In the repair stage, edema, cytokines, and growth factors originating from the opening of endothelial cells' tight junctions lead to a "fibrillar" network composed of

plasma proteins, such as fibrinogen and fibrin (36). These plasma proteins intermingle to form a crossed-linked gel which works as a temporary scaffold for cellular regeneration after injury (37). Thereby, the provisional matrix confers a framework and substrate for other cells, such as fibroblasts, which characterizes the remodeling stage. In MM, this substrate modulates the typical phenotype of the epithelioid tumor cell population in contact with this matrix.

Among the components studied, elastin helps define the rigidity and elasticity of the regular ECM, while fibrin forms the scaffold to support neoplastic cells (38). Elastin, one of the longest-lived proteins (39), is highly present in tissues subjected

TABLE 3 | Unconditional logistic regression exploring the independent association of clusters categorization and survival risk.

	B	S.E.	Sig.	Exp(β)	95% C.I. for Exp(β)	
					Inferior	Superior
Cluster 3 (Reference)			0.064			
Cluster 1	0.143	0.684	0.834	1.154	0.302	4.406
Cluster 2	1.242	0.578	0.032	3.462	1.115	10.746
Constant	−1.099	0.436	0.012	0.333		

B, coefficient for survival; S.E, standard error; Sig., significance; Exp (β), risk of B coefficient; C.I., confidence interval.

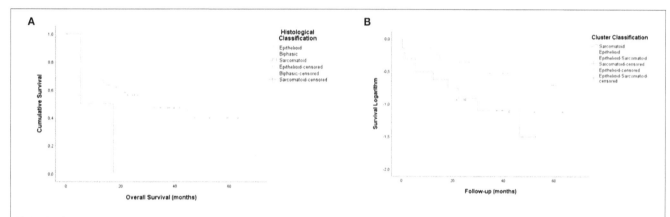

FIGURE 7 | Kaplan-Meier curves showing different average survival times between the three clusters groups with those resulting from the histopathological classification of the cases into the three major histotypes (**B,A,** Log rank, 5.1 vs. 2.52; *P* < 0.01 vs. *P* = 0.28).

to high mechanical stresses and demands recurrent cycles of extension and contraction such as the skin, lungs, tendons, or arteries (40). During oncogenesis, tropoelastin degradation leads to the release of elastokines, bioactive elastin-derived peptides. Elastokines modulate tumor cell phenotype by exciting several properties of tumor cells, including a higher expression and secretion of proteases that powerfully stimulate tumor cell migration and matrix invasion (41). It has been reported that elastokines have intense chemotactic activity on malignant melanoma cells, and their presence in distant organs might contribute to metastasis (42). Elastokines have also been shown to promote *in vitro* proliferation of glioblastoma cells (43) and astrocytoma human cell lines (44), as well as murine melanoma cell lines (45). Using the Elastin van Gieson (EVG) stain, Al Abri et al. (46) reported that the amount of elastosis varied in different breast cancer cell populations and could be considered a surrogate marker for estrogen positivity and HER2/neu negativity in breast cancer patients. Using a similar approach, Kardam et al. (47) quantitatively evaluated elastic fibers stained by Verhoeff–Van Gieson in oral squamous cell carcinoma and found different grades of elastosis involved in disease progression.

The second question that should be further investigated involves the hyaluronic acid (HA) and total collagen densely present in the ECM of sarcomatoid tumor cell populations, contrasting with only a minor area fraction in the stroma of epithelioid populations. In short, HA is a ubiquitous connective tissue glycosaminoglycan synthesized by HA synthase enzymes

(48) that supports matrix stability and tissue hydration. HA is also known to self-associate to form fibers (cables), networks, and stacks (36). At the cell surface, HA forms a huge pericellular matrix or "coat" named "glycocalyx," which plays several critical roles, from morphology and mechanochemical functions to cellular cycle regulation and motility (49). This cell coat allows the cells to change shape and facilitates cell division and migration (50), which explains why it was more highly expressed in the sarcomatoid tumor cell population. It has also been reported that ECM cytoskeleton components have both tumor-suppressing and tumor-promoting capacities, and depending on its molecular weight, HA may work as either a tumor suppressor or a tumor promoter (49). As previously demonstrated by Tian et al. (51), naked mole-rat's tumor resistance involves the presence of a unique HA with high molecular mass as a major component in their ECM. This HA with high molecular mass signals through the CD44 receptor and triggers the expression of crucial tumor suppressor genes, promoting a hypersensitive cell-cycle arrest, a usual mechanism of tumor suppression (52). Conversely, high levels of small HA oligosaccharides are associated with poor prognosis in several tumors such as colorectal, breast, and prostate cancer (53– 55). Collectively, these data contribute to understanding our findings of a greater amount of HA in MM sarcomatoid cell populations. HA interactions are prominent in diseases such as cancer and affect events that promote tumor cell phenotypes with higher invasion and metastasis rates (56). In fact, changes in cell shape are one of well-proved methods that cancer cells use

to overcome mechanical barriers and thus competently invade restricted networks (57).

Interestingly, interactions between HA molecules and fibrillar collagen types seem to modulate the mechanical function of the collagen and modify the contractile forces produced by fusiform sarcomatoid cells (58). Moreover, the release of mechanical forces in collagen fibers, which seems to be dependent upon the synthesis and secretion of HA, have been linked to myofibroblast loss (59), suggesting that pericellular HA may thus promote myofibroblast survival and, consequently, collagen synthesis. In the current study, we observed inhomogeneities in 3D collagen matrices that reflected the mechanical phenotype of the matrices. We also observed an adjustment between pore size and stiffness, a critical factor for invasion (60, 61). Therefore, we successfully gained insights about structural cytoskeletons and mechanical properties of the tumor stroma, as these support the invasion of the sarcomatoid tumor cell population.

Finally, a third important question that should be addressed in future research relates to the need of a more accurate diagnosis of MM. MM has gained importance because of its association with exposure to asbestos, which has become more prevalent in recent years. However, the current fear of litigation in MM diagnoses has implications in prognosis and therapeutic protocols. The difficulties regarding MM are also intensified beyond the usual problem of anaplasia by its many subtypes and underlying substrate dimorphism (62). While knowledge of the more frequent histologic patterns has improved diagnosis precision, a great deal of inter observer subjectivity remains necessary (63). In this context, the use of a clustering method to collect more objective data is desirable. When we compared how the three clusters correlated with the final histotype (epithelioid, biphasic or sarcomatoid) resulting from pathological classification, we found that cluster analysis recognizes with strong significance three different subsets inside of epithelioid MM classified only by histology. We also found that the distribution of BAP1 protein was positive in 17 (22%) epithelioid-sarcomatoid, speculating a better behavior for those patients? Moreover, comparison between survival curves obtained with cluster and histopathological classification showed that histochemistry evaluation of matrix refined the prognostic information, suggesting that both procedures should be combined in the routine practice. Interestingly, our cluster analysis identified three groups of MM with prognostic implications: CL II (low risk of death), CL I (intermediate risk of death) and CL III (high risk of death). Overall, our results showed that the decreased risk of death in CL II patients was characterized by an epithelioid-sarcomatoid (biphasic) tumor cell population. In fact, these patients had a three times higher chance of survival than patients in CL I (epithelioid) and CL III (sarcomatoid). The reasons for this difference may be linked to a better balance between components that favor invasion (elastin, HA and collagen) and those that act as a barrier (cellularity).

In summary, these developing mechanisms help investigators to better characterize the phenotypes and functional mechanisms of tumors that express different cell populations. The characterization of distinct cell populations using specific biomarkers, microdissection, or single cell analysis is an incredibly exciting field with many questions that are yet to be answered. To contribute to these efforts, our study tests new methods of analyzing MM tumor cell populations and complements the description of MM behavior by integrating different tumor cells population and their extracellular matrix components. Notably, our findings may help guide more personalized treatments for MM patients and help develop novel targeted therapies, while also highlighting new ways for other researchers to investigate MM treatments.

AUTHOR CONTRIBUTIONS

VC and MB: conception and design. VC, MB, and CB: writing, review and editing. VC, MB, CB, AV, and WT: data analysis and interpretation. VC, MB, CB, and CF: statistical analysis. MB, AKA, and AMA: provision of study materials or patients. VC: administrative support. All authors: final approval of manuscript.

ACKNOWLEDGMENTS

We are grateful to Ms. Esmeralda Miristeni Eher, Ms. Sandra de Morais Fernezlian, Ms. Kelly Cristina Soares Bispo, and Ms. Cassia Arruda for their expertise on histochemical protocols.

REFERENCES

1. Batra H, Antony VB. Pleural mesothelial cells in pleural and lung diseases. *J Thorac Dis.* (2015) 7:964–80. doi: 10.3978/j.issn.2072-1439.2015.02.19
2. Yap TA, Aerts JG, Popat S, Fennell DA. Novel insights into mesothelioma biology and implications for therapy. *Nat Rev Cancer.* (2017) 17:475–88. doi: 10.1038/nrc.2017.42
3. Joyce JA, Fearon DT. T cell exclusion, immune privilege, and the tumor microenvironment. *Science.* (2015) 348:74–80. doi: 10.1126/science.aaa6204
4. Naba A, Clauser KR, Ding H, Whittaker CA, Carr SA, Hynes RO. The extracellular matrix: tools and insights for the "omics" era. *Matrix Biol.* (2016) 49:10–24. doi: 10.1016/j.matbio.2015.06.003
5. *Thoracic Tumours, WHO Classification of Tumours.* Avaialbe online at: https://tumourclassification.iarc.who.int/welcome/ (accessed August 26, 2021).
6. Kadota K, Suzuki K, Colovos C, Sima CS, Rusch VW, Travis WD, et al. A nuclear grading system is a strong predictor of survival in epitheloid diffuse malignant pleural mesothelioma. *Mod Pathol.* (2012) 25:260–71. doi: 10.1038/modpathol.2011.146
7. Husain AN, Colby TV, Ordóñez NG, Allen TC, Attanoos RL, Beasley MB, et al. Guidelines for pathologic diagnosis of malignant mesothelioma 2017 update of the consensus statement from the international mesothelioma interest group. *Arch Pathol Lab Med.* (2018) 142:89–108. doi: 10.5858/arpa.2017-0124-RA
8. Nicholson AG, Tsao MS, Travis WD, Patil DT, Galateau-Salle F, Marino M, et al. Eighth edition staging of thoracic malignancies: implications for the reporting pathologist. *Arch Pathol Lab Med.* (2018) 142:645–61. doi: 10.5858/arpa.2017-0245-RA

9. Kao SC, Lee K, Armstrong NJ, Clarke S, Vardy J, van Zandwijk N, et al. Validation of tissue microarray technology in malignant pleural mesothelioma. *Pathology.* (2011) 43:128–32. doi: 10.1097/PAT.0b013e328342016c

10. Thapa B, Salcedo A, Lin X, Walkiewicz M, Murone C, Ameratunga M, et al. The immune microenvironment, genome-wide copy number aberrations, and survival in mesothelioma. *J Thorac Oncol.* (2017) 12:850–9. doi: 10.1016/j.jtho.2017.02.013

11. Chee SJ, Lopez M, Mellows T, Gankande S, Moutasim KA, Harris S, et al. Evaluating the effect of immune cells on the outcome of patients with mesothelioma. *Br J Cancer.* (2017) 117:1341–8. doi: 10.1038/bjc.2017.269

12. Russell HK. A modification of Movat's pentachrome stain. *Arch Pathol.* (1972) 94:187–91.

13. Lattouf R, Younes R, Lutomski D, Naaman N, Godeau G, Senni K, et al. Picrosirius red staining: a useful tool to appraise collagen networks in normal and pathological tissues. *J Histochem Cytochem.* (2014) 62:751–8. doi: 10.1369/0022155414545787

14. Montes GS, Krisztán RM, Shigihara KM, Tokoro R, Mourão PA, Junqueira LC. Histochemical and morphological characterization of reticular fibers. *Histochemistry.* (1980) 65:131–41. doi: 10.1007/BF00493161

15. Loughrey MB, Bankhead P, Coleman HG, Hagan RS, Craig S, McCorry AMB, et al. Validation of the systematic scoring of immunohistochemically stained tumour tissue microarrays using QuPath digital image analysis. *Histopathology.* (2018) 73:327–38. doi: 10.1111/his.13516

16. Bankhead P, Loughrey MB, Fernández JA, Dombrowski Y, McArt DG, Dunne PD, et al. QuPath: open source software for digital pathology image analysis. *Sci Rep.* (2017) 7:16878. doi: 10.1038/s41598-017-17204-5

17. Arganda-Carreras I, Kaynig V, Rueden C, Eliceiri KW, Schindelin J, Cardona A, et al. Trainable Weka Segmentation: a machine learning tool for microscopy pixel classification. *Bioinformatics.* (2017) 33:2424–6. doi: 10.1093/bioinformatics/btx180

18. Junqueira LC, Bignolas G, Brentani RR. Picrosirius staining plus polarization microscopy, a specific method for collagen detection in tissue sections. *Histochem J.* (1979) 11:447–55. doi: 10.1007/BF01002772

19. Livingston DP, Tuong TD, Gadi SR, Haigler CH, Gelman RS, Cullen JM. 3D volumes constructed from pixel-based images by digitally clearing plant and animal tissue. *J Microsc.* (2010) 240:122–9. doi: 10.1111/j.1365-2818.2010.03393.x

20. Cardona A, Saalfeld S, Schindelin J, Arganda-Carreras I, Preibisch S, Longair M, et al. TrakEM2 software for neural circuit reconstruction. *PLoS ONE.* (2012) 7:e38011. doi: 10.1371/journal.pone.0038011

21. Fedorov A, Beichel R, Kalpathy-Cramer J, Finet J, Fillion-Robin JC, Pujol S, et al. 3D Slicer as an image computing platform for the quantitative imaging network. *Magn Reson Imaging.* (2012) 30:1323–41. doi: 10.1016/j.mri.2012.05.001

22. Schubert C, van Langeveld MC, Donoso LA. Innovations in 3D printing: a 3D overview from optics to organs. *Br J Ophthalmol.* (2014) 98:159–61. doi: 10.1136/bjophthalmol-2013-304446

23. Schmidt R, Ratto M. Design-to-fabricate: maker hardware requires maker software. *IEEE Comput Graph Appl.* (2013) 33:26–34. doi: 10.1109/MCG.2013.90

24. Movat HZ. Demonstration of all connective tissue elements in a single section; pentachrome stains. *AMA Arch Pathol.* (1955) 60:289–95.

25. Mäkelä K, Mäyränpää MI, Sihvo HK, Bergman P, Sutinen E, Ollila H, et al. Artificial intelligence identifies inflammation and confirms fibroblast foci as prognostic tissue biomarkers in idiopathic pulmonary fibrosis. *Hum Pathol.* (2021) 107:58–68. doi: 10.1016/j.humpath.2020.10.008

26. Jones MG, Fabre A, Schneider P, Cinetto F, Sgalla G, Mavrogordato M, et al. Three-dimensional characterization of fibroblast foci in idiopathic pulmonary fibrosis. *JCI Insight.* (2016) 1:e86375. doi: 10.1172/jci.insight.86375

27. Blum Y, Meiller C, Quetel L, Elarouci N, Ayadi M, Tashtanbaeva D, et al. Dissecting heterogeneity in malignant pleural mesothelioma through histo-molecular gradients for clinical applications. *Nat Commun.* (2019) 10:1333. doi: 10.1038/s41467-019-09307-6

28. Jagirdar RM, Papazoglou ED, Pitaraki E, Kouliou OA, Rouka E, Giannakou L, et al. Cell and extracellular matrix interaction models in benign mesothelial and malignant pleural mesothelioma cells in 2D and 3D in-vitro. *Clin Exp Pharmacol Physiol.* (2021) 48:543–52. doi: 10.1111/1440-1681.13446

29. Paszek MJ, Weaver VM. The tension mounts: mechanics meets morphogenesis and malignancy. *J Mammary Gland Biol Neoplasia.* (2004) 9:325–42. doi: 10.1007/s10911-004-1404-x

30. Discher DE, Janmey P, Wang YL. Tissue cells feel and respond to the stiffness of their substrate. *Science.* (2005) 310:1139–43. doi: 10.1126/science.1116995

31. Bissell MJ, Hines WC. Why don't we get more cancer? a proposed role of the microenvironment in restraining cancer progression. *Nat Med.* (2011) 17:320–9. doi: 10.1038/nm.2328

32. Stylianopoulos T, Martin JD, Snuderl M, Mpekris F, Jain SR, Jain RK. Coevolution of solid stress and interstitial fluid pressure in tumors during progression: implications for vascular collapse. *Cancer Res.* (2013) 73:3833–41. doi: 10.1158/0008-5472.CAN-12-4521

33. Leight JL, Drain AP, Weaver VM. Extracellular matrix remodeling and stiffening modulate tumor phenotype and treatment response. *Annu Rev Cancer Biol.* (2017) 1:313–34. doi: 10.1146/annurev-cancerbio-050216-034431

34. Paszek MJ, Zahir N, Johnson KR, Lakins JN, Rozenberg GI, Gefen A, et al. Tensional homeostasis and the malignant phenotype. *Cancer Cell.* (2005) 8:241–54. doi: 10.1016/j.ccr.2005.08.010

35. Singer AJ, Clark RA. Cutaneous wound healing. *N Engl J Med.* (1999) 341:738–46. doi: 10.1056/NEJM199909023411006

36. Wight TN. Provisional matrix: a role for versican and hyaluronan. *Matrix Biol.* (2017) 60-61:38–56. doi: 10.1016/j.matbio.2016.12.001

37. Schultz GS, Wysocki A. Interactions between extracellular matrix and growth factors in wound healing. *Wound Repair Regen.* (2009) 17:153–62. doi: 10.1111/j.1524-475X.2009.00466.x

38. Tracy LE, Minasian RA, Caterson EJ. Extracellular matrix and dermal fibroblast function in the healing wound. *Adv Wound Care.* (2016) 5:119–36. doi: 10.1089/wound.2014.0561

39. Petersen E, Wågberg F, Angquist KA. Serum concentrations of elastin-derived peptides in patients with specific manifestations of atherosclerotic disease. *Eur J Vasc Endovasc Surg.* (2002) 24:440–4. doi: 10.1053/ejvs.2002.1750

40. Scandolera A, Odoul L, Salesse S, Guillot A, Blaise S, Kawecki C, et al. The elastin receptor complex: a unique matricellular receptor with high anti-tumoral potential. *Front Pharmacol.* (2016) 7:32. doi: 10.3389/fphar.2016.00032

41. Donet M, Brassart-Pasco S, Salesse S, Maquart FX, Brassart B. Elastin peptides regulate HT-1080 fibrosarcoma cell migration and invasion through an Hsp90-dependent mechanism. *Br J Cancer.* (2014) 111:139–48. doi: 10.1038/bjc.2014.239

42. Pocza P, Süli-Vargha H, Darvas Z, Falus A. Locally generated VGVAPG and VAPG elastin-derived peptides amplify melanoma invasion via the galectin-3 receptor. *Int J Cancer.* (2008) 122:1972–80. doi: 10.1002/ijc.23296

43. Hinek A, Keeley FW, Callahan J. Recycling of the 67-kDa elastin binding protein in arterial myocytes is imperative for secretion of tropoelastin. *Exp Cell Res.* (1995) 220:312–24. doi: 10.1006/excr.1995.1321

44. Jung S, Hinek A, Tsugu A, Hubbard SL, Ackerley C, Becker LE, et al. Astrocytoma cell interaction with elastin substrates: implications for astrocytoma invasive potential. *Glia.* (1999) 25:179–89. doi: 10.1002/(sici)1098-1136(19990115)25:2<179::aid-glia8>3.0.co;2-b

45. Devy J, Duca L, Cantarelli B, Joseph-Pietras D, Scandolera A, Rusciani A, et al. Elastin-derived peptides enhance melanoma growth in vivo by upregulating the activation of Mcol-A (MMP-1) collagenase. *Br J Cancer.* (2010) 103:1562–70. doi: 10.1038/sj.bjc.6605926

46. Al Abri S, Al Rawahi A, Rao L. Elastosis in breast cancer as a surrogate marker for estrogen receptor positivity. *Oman Med J.* (2021) 36:e247. doi: 10.5001/omj.2021.60

47. Kardam P, Mehendiratta M, Rehani S, Kumra M, Sahay K, Jain K. Stromal fibers in oral squamous cell carcinoma: a possible new prognostic indicator? *J Oral Maxillofac Pathol.* (2016) 20:405–12. doi: 10.4103/0973-029X.190913

48. Pierce GF, Vande Berg J, Rudolph R, Tarpley J, Mustoe TA. Platelet-derived growth factor-BB and transforming growth factor beta 1 selectively modulate glycosaminoglycans, collagen, and myofibroblasts in excisional wounds. *Am J Pathol.* (1991) 138:629–46.

49. Evanko SP, Tammi MI, Tammi RH, Wight TN. Hyaluronan-dependent pericellular matrix. *Adv Drug Deliv Rev.* (2007) 59:1351–65. doi: 10.1016/j.addr.2007.08.008

50. Bohaumilitzky L, Huber AK, Stork EM, Wengert S, Woelfl F, Boehm H, et al. Trickster in disguise: hyaluronan's ambivalent roles in the matrix. *Front Oncol.* (2017) 7:242. doi: 10.3389/fonc.2017.00242

51. Tian X, Azpurua J, Ke Z, Augereau A, Zhang ZD, Vijg J, et al. INK4 locus of the tumor-resistant rodent, the naked mole rat, expresses a functional p15/p16 hybrid isoform. *Proc Natl Acad Sci U S A.* (2015) 112:1053–8. doi: 10.1073/pnas.1418203112

52. Hanahan D, Weinberg RA. Hallmarks of cancer: the next generation. *Cell.* (2011) 144:646–74. doi: 10.1016/j.cell.2011.02.013

53. Schmaus A, Bauer J, Sleeman JP. Sugars in the microenvironment: the sticky problem of HA turnover in tumors. *Cancer Metastasis Rev.* (2014) 33:1059–79. doi: 10.1007/s10555-014-9532-2

54. Ropponen K, Tammi M, Parkkinen J, Eskelinen M, Tammi R, Lipponen P, et al. Tumor cell-associated hyaluronan as an unfavorable prognostic factor in colorectal cancer. *Cancer Res.* (1998) 58:342–7.

55. Anttila MA, Tammi RH, Tammi MI, Syrjänen KJ, Saarikoski SV, Kosma VM. High levels of stromal hyaluronan predict poor disease outcome in epithelial ovarian cancer. *Cancer Res.* (2000) 60:150–5.

56. Toole BP. Hyaluronan promotes the malignant phenotype. *Glycobiology.* (2002) 12:37R—42. doi: 10.1093/glycob/12.3.37R

57. Baskaran JP, Weldy A, Guarin J, Munoz G, Shpilker PH, Kotlik M, et al. Cell shape, and not 2D migration, predicts extracellular matrix-driven 3D cell invasion in breast cancer. *APL Bioeng.* (2020) 4:026105. doi: 10.1063/1.5143779

58. Allison DD, Wight TN, Ripp NJ, Braun KR, Grande-Allen KJ. Endogenous overexpression of hyaluronan synthases within dynamically cultured collagen gels: Implications for vascular and valvular disease. *Biomaterials.* (2008) 29:2969–76. doi: 10.1016/j.biomaterials.2008.04.005

59. Hinz B, Gabbiani G. Mechanisms of force generation and transmission by myofibroblasts. *Curr Opin Biotechnol.* (2003) 14:538–46. doi: 10.1016/j.copbio.2003.08.006

60. Lang NR, Skodzek K, Hurst S, Mainka A, Steinwachs J, Schneider J, et al. Biphasic response of cell invasion to matrix stiffness in three-dimensional biopolymer networks. *Acta Biomater.* (2015) 13:61–7. doi: 10.1016/j.actbio.2014.11.003

61. Wisdom KM, Adebowale K, Chang J, Lee JY, Nam S, Desai R, et al. Matrix mechanical plasticity regulates cancer cell migration through confining microenvironments. *Nat Commun.* (2018) 9:4144. doi: 10.1038/s41467-018-06641-z

62. Kannerstein M, Churg J, Magner D. Histochemistry in the diagnosis of malignant mesothelioma. *Ann Clin Lab Sci.* (1973) 3:207–11.

63. Ascoli V. Pathologic diagnosis of malignant mesothelioma: chronological prospect and advent of recommendations and guidelines. *Ann Ist Super Sanita.* (2015) 51:52–9. doi: 10.4415/ANN_15_01_09

13

Opportunities and Challenges for Machine Learning in Rare Diseases

Sergio Decherchi [1†], Elena Pedrini [2†], Marina Mordenti [2†], Andrea Cavalli [1,3] and Luca Sangiorgi [2]*

[1] *Computational and Chemical Biology, Fondazione Istituto Italiano di Tecnologia, Genoa, Italy,* [2] *Department of Rare Skeletal Disorders, IRCCS Istituto Ortopedico Rizzoli, Bologna, Italy,* [3] *Department of Pharmacy and Biotechnology (FaBiT), Alma Mater Studiorum – University of Bologna, Bologna, Italy*

Correspondence:
Marina Mordenti
marina.mordenti@ior.it

[†] *These authors have contributed equally to this work and share first authorship*

Rare diseases (RDs) are complicated health conditions that are difficult to be managed at several levels. The scarcity of available data chiefly determines an intricate scenario even for experts and specialized clinicians, which in turn leads to the so called "diagnostic odyssey" for the patient. This situation calls for innovative solutions to support the decision process *via* quantitative and automated tools. Machine learning brings to the stage a wealth of powerful inference methods; however, matching the health conditions with advanced statistical techniques raises methodological, technological, and even ethical issues. In this contribution, we critically point to the specificities of the dialog of rare diseases with machine learning techniques concentrating on the key steps and challenges that may hamper or create actionable knowledge and value for the patient together with some on-field methodological suggestions and considerations.

Keywords: machine learning, rare disease, disease registry, open data, clinical decision support system

INTRODUCTION

A rare disease (RD) is defined as a low-prevalence condition that affects fewer than one in 2,000 people. Due to the frequent lack of knowledge and treatment (which makes them also known as "orphan diseases"), they represent a real emerging global public health priority. So far 6,000–7,000 distinct RDs have been recognized, affecting 4–6% of the European population, and 300 million persons globally (1). From a clinical perspective, RDs are extremely heterogeneous and complex, often characterized by different clinical subtypes and overlapping phenotypic manifestations. Although most of the RDs are classified as "genetic diseases," (2, 3) the causes remain unclear for many of them, making the identification of therapies troublesome.

Different from other clinical fields, RDs are often lacking specific and adequate public health policies and can be considered as a real health system challenge. Difficult and delayed diagnosis (with diagnostic processes taking many years and unnecessary costs), unknown molecular mechanisms, lack of specific treatments, and scattered patient data are all responsible for the difficulty in both taking care of these patients and setting up research activities. This makes RDs a major public health problem, and many challenges hamper the development of therapies. In addition, they are often neglected by major public and industrial funding with a limited interest of pharmaceutical companies (4, 5).

Overall, RDs are responsible for enormous healthcare costs, just for the difficulties in diagnosis and their often serious health degenerative consequences. To reduce RDs healthcare costs and to optimize the assistance of patients, new effective treatments are required, making it necessary to promote research with new strategies. Recent advances in next-generation sequencing (NGS) have already represented a great opportunity (6); in particular, whole exome or whole genome approaches have strongly improved the diagnosis and shortened the "diagnostic odyssey" (7), also helping in the molecular characterization of diseases. Data coming from many other innovative technologies such as advanced imaging techniques, multiomics, gait analyses, and others (depending on the clinical field) represent an invaluable source of information too. As a result of all these new approaches and technologies, there is a huge amount of available data (never collected before) to be managed and analyzed according to privacy regulations, still with a limited sample set (number of patients). This scenario is a big data one in the omics component, but not in terms of the sample size.

As an innovative discipline for data modeling, machine learning (ML) is becoming a great opportunity. ML is a branch of artificial intelligence (AI) rooted in statistics that learns from data (the examples) and then performs predictions on new unseen data. By using specific algorithms, and typically large datasets, the goal is to use available data to make classifications or predictions in general, uncovering not previously discovered key insights, which will potentially drive the decision on the diagnosis and treatment options of a patient.

During the last two decades, AI and ML have been characterized by an unprecedented development, also supported by empowered computational means (i.e., graphical processing units). However, to further improve their applicability in healthcare challenges, it is essential to consider the compatibility of RDs specificities with respect to ML approaches. In the following, we critically discuss the role of the two key ingredients of any ML attempt namely, the data and the methods (and their interplay) (8). We discuss in detail diseases registries, genuinely public datasets, and lastly, methodological approaches, and ML challenges for RDs. **Figure 1** summarizes a prototypical pipeline for the data flow in a clinical decision support system.

DISEASE REGISTRIES

By definition, a registry is "an organized system that uses observational study methods to collect uniform data (clinical and other) to evaluate specified outcomes for a population defined by a particular disease, condition, or exposure, and that serves one or more predetermined scientific, clinical or policy purposes" (9). Among different registries, the disease registry represents the pivotal tool in supporting RD research and care, since the primary aims are collection, analysis, and dissemination of information on a group of people defined by a particular disease (10).

Many stakeholders recognize the crucial role of a high-quality registry and uniformity in data collection, particularly for networking activities. In 2015, the European Medicines Agency

has established a patient registry initiative to promote registry data collection and reuse for postauthorization safety study and postauthorization effectiveness study (11). Moreover, 24 European Reference Networks (ERNs) [wanted by the European Commission (EC)] were installed in 2017 to facilitate the discussion on complex or RDs that require highly specialized treatment and concentrated knowledge (2014/286/EU). The EC defined specific criteria for ERNs, encouraging the research and epidemiological surveillance through shared patient registries (12–14).

Nonetheless, the RDs domain may greatly benefit from data pooling, since information on orphan patients is frequently scattered across different hospitals and institutions (14, 15). To promote the merging of standardized data, the European Rare Diseases Platform has released the "Set of common data elements for Rare Diseases Registration" produced by a Working Group coordinated by the Joint Research Center. In addition, the semantic compatibility of phenotypic data captured within a registry can be ensured by the implementation of ontologies, standards, and dictionaries, like Human Phenotype Ontology (16) and ORPHAcode. The process to make registry data findable, accessible, interoperable, and reusable (FAIR) surely increases the quality of information, but at the same time enhances the potential extensive use of the captured data to improve research and to promote patient health. The FAIR principles allow data sharing, including tools and workflows, from different registries using the same syntax (12, 17, 18).

Moreover, some legal and ethical obstacles can afflict data pooling, restricting the range of action of the registry. The sharing of personal and clinical data, even pseudonymized, presents privacy issues. The European General Data Privacy Regulation (GDPR; EU Regulation 2016/679) allows data-free movement, even if the sensitive nature of phenotypic information requires a rigorous balancing between data protection to avoid mistreatment and the data accessibility to promote accurate research networking activities. Accordingly, a solid framework that addresses privacy issues and ethical and social implications becomes mandatory.

All the mentioned approaches, put in place to pursue the establishment of a high-quality disease registry, were the grounds on which our group has created and implemented five RD registries. These registries realized aiming both care and research purposes, address four skeletal orphan disorders (Multiple Osteochondromas, Osteogenesis Imperfecta, Ollier-Maffucci Diseases, Ehlers-Danlos syndrome), and one oncological rare condition (Li-Fraumeni syndrome). All of them rely on a web-based platform, genotype-phenotype data integration (GeDI) platform, established on a relational database. GeDI was created considering the JRC "Set of common data elements for Rare Diseases Registration," as well as highly recommended ontologies (HPO, ORPHAcode, HGVS, and ICF), and following GDPR and privacy requirements.

Until a few years ago, the phenotypic information was not considered big (19), but with the evolution in terms of standardization and FAIRness, the consequent simplification in data merged across healthcare providers, and the integration among different data sources transformed clinical data into

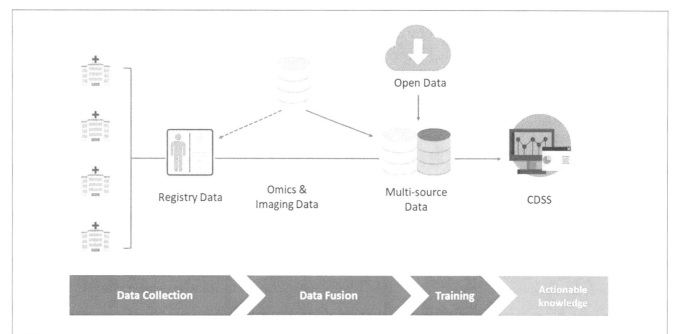

FIGURE 1 | A prototypical data flow pipeline in the clinical decision support system (CDSS) dedicated to rare diseases (RDs). Omics and imaging data can either be integrated from different sources or be collected as part of disease registry data. Data are then fed to the learning engine and the results are provided through a CDSS GUI interface.

new types of big files. The primary and essential investigation of skeletal disorders is imaging data, ranging from traditional X-Rays and ultrasounds, through hybrid imaging such as positron emission tomography/MRI (PET/MRI) up to innovative instruments like high-resolution peripheral quantitative CT (HR-pQCT) (20). These data are increasingly needed to support the diagnostic process, to longitudinally follow-up disease evolution, and to promote translational research. The integration of imaging data with all other detailed phenotypic information is becoming mandatory to obtain a complete overview of patient manifestations. Similarly, the rapid advancement in NGS approaches and the parallel explosion of bioinformatics has revolutionized the research on RDs, reinforcing the understanding of biological pathways and pathomechanisms (21, 22). The accompaniment of NGS and imaging data to deep phenotyping is a fundamental enrichment for rare skeletal disease research. The analysis of that notable amount of data requires *ad hoc* computational solutions, like ML approaches (23).

The rarity of orphan patients, despite the presence of registries, still has an impact on ML analyses highly, hence then open data can highly contribute to support the modeling attempt.

OPEN DATA

As clearly stated by Cohen, "medical artificial intelligence is particularly data-hungry" (24); nonetheless, the demand is limited by the reduced availability of trusted and reliable biomedical data (25). Public or open datasets must respond

to three main criteria: online availability, the absence of costs, and reusability (26). Public data may represent a solution, considering that they create value in multiple heterogeneous areas (healthcare, city security, savings, etc.); therefore, numerous worldwide countries have implemented governmental open data sites (27) to increase findability and accessibility.

The open data role in biomedical research is widely recognized and scientists boost public sharing of resources at an increasing speed. Free access to data would expedite research and open new opportunities in scientific research, improving care and treatment; nevertheless, some substantial pitfalls and issues still exist (28).

The first limitation is represented by the lack of harmonization principles governing data (28) and the presence of multiple standards is a known concern on data sharing and biomedical information reuse (23). Common "languages," in terms of formats and ontologies, are continually being improved for innovative data types (i.e., omics), but compatibility among sources is affected by the variability of standards (when present) on many other data elements and related metadata (i.e., phenotyping) (23).

Another challenging point is the reliability of public data (29). This aspect can include a variety of subtopics that carries costs, like the unavailability of ongoing quality control, the lack of updating of datasets, the absence of support for potential users and the need of highly specialized human resources.

The final and critical point is the use of open data for rare conditions. This peculiar scenario amplifies the aforementioned concerns. At the same time, the need for public data is clear in paving the way for prompt diagnosis, innovative treatments, personalized care, and research activities (23).

MACHINE LEARNING FOR RARE DISEASES

Machine learning, as already anticipated, is a wide and largely heterogeneous subfield of computer science that in the last 20 years has evolved toward a consolidated and largely usefu discipline. In ML, one is interested in building a robust and predictive model, which for instance, within a certain degree of accuracy, can predict a class (classification) or find patterns on data (i.e., groups *via* clustering). In the first case, when applied to clinical data, one often talks of diagnosis prediction, and in the second, it is often about the stratification of patients. Many other learning paradigms are available and despite the ubiquitous success achieved in many applications ranging from engineering problems to the life science, the systematic application of ML methods to clinical practice is still relatively modest albeit starting to be present in clinical decisions support systems (30–33 There are many reasons that hamper the widespread diffusion of ML in the clinic, and in the case of RDs, this scenario is amplified by several specificities (34, 35), which, however, the scientific community is addressing *via* methods, protocols, and technologies in general.

In the RD, the most important limitation in building meaningful predictive models, either supervised or agnostic, with respect to *a priori* labeling, is the data collection process (36 38). Although deep learning models typically require thousand of samples to converge to robust solutions, shallow (i.e., limited parameters) models still require in the order of hundreds of samples to build acceptably robust models. It should be stressed that ML aims at building predictive models, in other words, models that can be used out-of-sample. While it could be considered sufficient for a qualitative analysis having a limited sample size and/or finding associations as in epidemiological studies (39), in the ML case, there is a more ambitious modeling attempt that is deemed to fail if working in a very restrictive small sample regime.

To deal with the small sample regime, the machine literature provides several possibilities: one may use available data possibly extending the collection outside the disease of interest to collect unlabeled examples (40–42), one can inherit from similar models [transfer learning (43)] to just fine-tune the model and lastly, one could even imagine a data augmentation strategy (44), that is finding ways to populate the dataset with new artificially built samples.

The strategy of collecting more unlabeled data is widely applicable as it requires gathering more data from possibly more controls or even more from diseases different from the current disease under analysis. This is particularly relevant for rare diseases where many patients with "uncertain" diagnosi can be present; collecting this additional unlabeled data can give interesting information about the manifold where data live.

On the other side, data augmentation, possibly through ingenious generative techniques (45), can be another original

way to face the data scarcity problem. In this second case, however, it is more difficult to assess the reliability of this modeling. First, generative networks often need a large amount of data to be trained, and second, inferring new data based on a manifold implicitly learned on few data may lead to a partial tautology rendering the overall strategy perilous.

The small sample regime, despite being probably the most impactful and first problem to be faced when dealing with the RD field, is not however the only point to be carefully addressed when modeling such data. Despite the wide success of deep learning paradigms in big data scenarios (to be precise big sample sizes), they often deliver not easily interpretable models. To allow the clinician to understand the meaning of a classification result, it is, therefore, necessary to resort to possibly less complex but explainable models (46). At a technical level, this brings to the scene chiefly linear models [possibly sparse ones (47)] and non-linear rule-based models, such as decision trees (48) or switching neural networks (49) for instance.

The availability and effectiveness of explainable models still are necessary, but not sufficient conditions to determine robust and explainable models. Indeed, explainable models are valuable when the explanation that they deliver is stable and robust inside the domain they deal with (assuming the same learning method) and across learning algorithms, ideally. This means that feature weighting/extraction must be a stable process to allow the clinician to get a value from the obtained results; this far from the trivial problem is feature stability, something we recently discussed for epidemiological data (50). Albeit often neglected in practice, this problem is relevant particularly when coupled with the small regime of RDs (50) and sample sizes in general; unsupervised feature selection techniques can mitigate this issue (50).

However, when dealing with features it can be relevant to consider the fairness (51). In other words, when determining a disease condition possibly "confounding" factors, such as gender and social status should be protected features, that is *a priori* one postulates that the gender or another feature to be protected cannot determine the disease (or any other) outcome. While this view today is quite uncommon, yet in clinical ML, for sensitive disease or particular case-dependent conditions could be of utility and necessary to protect specific patient characteristics to avoid discriminations and exacerbate iniquities.

Feature sets (clinical or omics) are associated inevitably with costs and time. Getting an X-ray is different from other diagnostic tools, possibly not standard, such as for instance, collective lipidomic signatures through mass Spectrometry (52). As these features set links with different time and cost profiles, feature selection is particularly challenging as one would like to maintain the representation power of possibly costly non-standard features, while at the same time maintaining a fast and inexpensive diagnostic tool. These contrasting forces together with, again, the small data regime call for proper solutions that allow obtaining a quantitative compromise (a multiobjective optimization problem) between accuracy, explainability, and cost/time effectiveness of the selected clinical or omics data necessary for diagnosis.

It is hence evident that the delivery of knowledge has several, sometimes tight, prerequisites which if not met cannot allow any meaningful analysis; while methods development is fundamental to the ML field, it is tantamount clear that in clinical ML for RD the data is the undiscussed protagonist.

A last key aspect is the privacy preserving issue that, for Europe, translates into GDPR compliance, as already mentioned. Historically, ML methodologies have been devised having in mind all the data resident in the same local storage; this is something largely unmet by the clinical reality where each hospital/research center has its own dataset/registry not in sync typically with a central shared, common repository. This situation is the absolute standard for clinical ML and RDs share this liability. The need to maintain privacy and avoiding to move a significant amount of data inspired what is now commonly under the name of federated ML (53). In this learning paradigm, data is resident on the original data infrastructure and on the network, only parameters are shared. Federated ML requires a specific rethinking of algorithms; this is a beneficial stimulus to the community, but still requires both a theoretical and programming effort to redesign and reimplement theoretically sound and well-established mathematical methodologies. It is promising that for instance in Europe, this need for federation has been largely and overall correctly perceived by the policymaker through initiatives like Gaia-X (54) which have the specific objective of creating a trustable, distributed, and federated data sharing infrastructure. Interestingly, very recently, the Swarm distributed learning paradigm (55) has been pushed as a further development of federated learning, offering the explicit capability of nodes of avoiding relying on a central repository of learning parameters, thus creating an effective collective swarm of collaborating agents. This technology also involves decentralized data structures as the blockchain and represents a very interesting protocol to deal safely with privacy concerns.

CONCLUSIONS

In this contribution, we have discussed what ML has to deal with in trying to effectively face the RD issue to grant robust,

usable, and actionable knowledge to the clinician. While several points are shared with the more general realm of the clinical machine learning, RDs pose specific challenges and for instance, present an unusual big data regime, in which one has potentially a huge omics data but still for a limited number of patients, thus bringing the typical bioinformatics scenario of several features, small samples. The proof-of-time of ML solutions will have to deal with the discussed specificities, and the solution is inevitably a well-concerted mix of rigorous math, trusted and privacy preserving technologies, and chiefly standardization for data curation and federation.

AUTHOR CONTRIBUTIONS

SD, EP, and MM contributed to conception and design of this mini-review. They were deeply involved in all the steps of the manuscript preparation, references collection and evaluation of the contest. They have drafted the article and participated in all the steps of its revising. AC has participated to paper design and supported the other authors in structuring the manuscript. He has critically revised the manuscript during the drafting process. LS has contributed to conception and design of this mini-review and he supported all the activities. He has participated step by step at the revising process with concrete suggestions and integrations. All the authors approved the final version for publication and agreed to be accountable for all aspects of the work in ensuring that questions related to the accuracy or integrity of any part of the work are appropriately investigated and resolved.

ACKNOWLEDGMENTS

Three of the authors of this publication are members of the European Reference Network for rare BONe Diseases - http://ernbond.eu/. This work was partially supported by grant from Fondazione del Monte di Bologna e Ravenna for the project Intelligenza artificiale e registri di patologia: un approccio innovativo nella ricerca di biomarcatori diagnostici/prognostici nelle fragilità ossee (PRWEB: 730262) and by grant POR FESR 2014-2020 for the project SUPER: Supercomputing Unified Platform - Emilia-Romagna (PRWEB: 730251).

REFERENCES

1. Nguengang Wakap S, Lambert DM, Olry A, Rodwell C, Gueydan C, Lanneau V, et al. Estimating cumulative point prevalence of rare diseases: analysis of the orphanet database. *Eur J Hum Genet.* (2020) 28:165–73. doi: 10.1038/s41431-019-0508-0

2. Sernadela P, González-Castro L, Carta C, van der Horst E, Lopes P, Kaliyaperumal R, et al. Linked registries: connecting rare diseases patient registries through a semantic web layer. *Biomed Res Int.* (2017) 2017:8327980. doi: 10.1155/2017/8327980

3. Ekins S. Industrializing rare disease therapy discovery and development. *Nat Biotechnol.* (2017) 35:117–8. doi: 10.1038/nbt.3787

4. Stoller JK. The challenge of rare diseases. *Chest.* (2018) 153:1309–14. doi: 10.1016/j.chest.2017.12.018

5. Ahmed MA, Okour M, Brundage R, Kartha RV. Orphan drug development: the increasing role of clinical pharmacology. *J Pharmacokinet Pharmacodyn.* (2019) 46:395–409. doi: 10.1007/s10928-019-09646-3

6. Fernandez-Marmiesse A, Gouveia S, Couce ML. NGS technologies as a turning point in rare disease research, diagnosis and treatment. *Curr Med Chem.* (2018) 25:404–32. doi: 10.2174/0929867324666170718101946

7. Boycott KM, Hartley T, Biesecker LG, Gibbs RA, Innes AM, Riess O, et al. A diagnosis for all rare genetic diseases: the horizon and

the next frontiers. *Cell.* (2019) 177:32–7. doi: 10.1016/j.cell.2019.02.040

8. Roh Y, Heo G, Whang SE. A survey on data collection for machine learning: a big data – ai integration perspective. *IEEE Transac Knowl Data Eng.* (2021) 33:1328–47. doi: 10.1109/TKDE.2019.2946162

9. Gliklich RE, Leavy MB, Dreyer NA, eds. *Registries for Evaluating Patient Outcomes: A User's Guide.* 4th ed. Rockville, MD: Agency for Healthcare Research and Quality (US) (2020).

10. Zaletel M, Kralj M. Methodological guidelines and recommendations for efficient and rational governance of patient registries. National Institute of Public Health. *Ljubljana.* (2015). doi: 10.1093/eurpub/ckv169.006

11. McGettigan P, Alonso Olmo C, Plueschke K, Castillon M, Nogueras Zondag D, Bahri P, et al. Patient registries: an underused resource for medicines evaluation: operational proposals for increasing the use of patient registries in regulatory assessments. *Drug Saf.* (2019) 42:1343–51. doi: 10.1007/s40264-019-00848-9

12. Kodra Y, Weinbach J, Posada-de-la-Paz M, Coi A, Lemonnier SL, van Enckevort D, et al. Recommendations for improving the quality of rare disease registries. *Int J Environ Res Public Health.* (2018) 15:1644. doi: 10.3390/ijerph15081644

13. Ali SR, Bryce J, Smythe C, Hytiris M, Priego AL, Appelman-Dijkstra NM, et al. Supporting international networks through platforms for tandardized data collection-the European registries for rare endocrine conditions (EuRRECa) model. *Endocrine.* (2021) 71:555–60. doi: 10.1007/s12020-021-02617-0

14. Opladen T, Gleich F, Kozich V, Scarpa M, Martinelli D, Schaefer F, et al. U-IMD: the first unified European registry for inherited metabolic diseases. *Orphanet J Rare Dis.* (2021) 16:95. doi: 10.1186/s13023-021-01726-3

15. Laverty A, Jaffé A, Cunningham S. Establishment of a web-based registry for rare (orphan) pediatric lung diseases in the United Kingdom: the BPOLD registry [published correction appears in Pediatr Pulmonol. *Pediatr Pulmonol.* (2008) 43:451–6. doi: 10.1002/ppul.20783

16. Köhler S, Vasilevsky NA, Engelstad M, Foster E, McMurry J, Aymé S, et al. The human phenotype ontology in 2017. *Nucleic Acids Res.* (2017) 45:D865–76. doi: 10.1093/nar/gkw1039

17. Wilkinson MD, Dumontier M, Aalbersberg IJ, Appleton G, Axton M, Baak A, et al. The FAIR guiding principles for scientific data management and stewardship [published correction appears in Sci Data. *Sci Data.* (2016) 3:160018. doi: 10.1038/sdata.2016.18

18. Dos Santos Vieira B, Groenen K, 't Hoen PAC, Jacobsen A, Roos M, Kaliyaperumal R, et al. Applying the FAIR data principles to the registry of vascular anomalies (VASCA). *Stud Health Technol Inform.* (2020) 271:115–6. doi: 10.3233/SHTI200085

19. Delude CM. Deep phenotyping: the details of disease. *Nature.* (2015) 527:S14–5. doi: 10.1038/527S14a

20. Giraudo C, Kainberger F, Boesen M, Trattnig S. Quantitative imaging in inflammatory arthritis: between tradition and innovation. *Semin Musculoskelet Radiol.* (2020) 24:337–54. doi: 10.1055/s-0040-1708823

21. Johnston L, Thompson R, Turner C, Bushby K, Lochmuller H Straub V. The impact of integrated omics technologies for patients with rare diseases. *Exp Opin Orphan Drugs.* (2016) 11:1211–9. doi: 10.1517/21678707.2014.974554

22. Danielsson K, Mun LJ, Lordemann A, Mao J, Lin CH. Next-generation sequencing applied to rare diseases genomics. *Expert Rev Mol Diagn.* (2014) 14:469–87. doi: 10.1586/14737159.2014.904749

23. Rubinstein YR, Robinson PN, Gahl WA, Avillach P, Baynam G, Cederroth H, et al. The case for open science: rare diseases. *JAMIA Open.* (2020) 3:472–86. doi: 10.1093/jamiaopen/ooaa030

24. Cohen IG, Mello MM. Big data, big tech, and protecting patient privacy. *JAMA.* (2019) 322:1141–2. doi: 10.1001/jama.2019.11365

25. Nielsen SS, Krasnik A, Rosano A. Registry data for cross-country comparisons of migrants' healthcare utilization in the EU: a survey study of availability and content. *BMC Health Serv Res.* (2009) 9:210. doi: 10.1186/1472-6963-9-210

26. Chignard S. *A Brief History of Open Data.* (2013). Available online at: http://parisinnovationreview.com/articles-en/a-brief-history-of-open-data (accessed June 23, 2021).

27. Kobayashi S, Kane TB, Paton C. The privacy and security implications of open data in healthcare. *Yearb Med Inform.* (2018) 27:41–47. doi: 10.1055/s-0038-1641201

28. Conrado DJ, Karlsson MO, Romero K, Sarr C, Wilkins JJ. Open innovation: towards sharing of data, models and workflows. *Eur J Pharm Sci.* (2017) 109S:S65–71. doi: 10.1016/j.ejps.2017.06.035

29. Wilhelm EE, Oster E, Shoulson I. Approaches and costs for sharing clinical research data. *JAMA.* (2014) 311:1201–02. doi: 10.1001/jama.2014.850

30. Berner E. *Clinical Decision Support Systems. Theory and Practice. Health Informatics Series.* New York, NY: Springer (2007).

31. Faviez C, Chen X, Garcelon N, Neuraz A, Knebelmann B, Salomon R, et al. Diagnosis support systems for rare diseases: a scoping review. *Orphanet J Rare Dis.* (2020) 15:94. doi: 10.1186/s13023-020-01374-z

32. Svenstrup DT. *FindZebra – Using Machine Learning to Aid Diagnosis of Rare Diseases. DTU Computer.* Kongens Lyngby: DTU Compute (2018).

33. Long E, Lin H, Liu Z, Wu X, Wang L, Jiang J et al. An artificial intelligence platform for the multihospital collaborative management of congenital cataracts. *Nat Biomed Eng.* (2017) 1:0024. doi: 10.1038/s41551-016-0024

34. Schaefer J, Lehne M, Schepers J, Prasser F, Thun S. The use of machine learning in rare diseases: a scoping review. *Orphanet J Rare Dis.* (2020) 15:145. doi: 10.1186/s13023-020-01424-6

35. Brasil S, Pascoal C, Francisco R, Dos Reis Ferreira V, Videira PA, Valadão AG. Artificial intelligence (AI) in rare diseases: is the future brighter? *Genes.* (2019) 10:978. doi: 10.3390/genes10120978

36. Garcelon N, Neuraz A, Benoit V, Salomon R, Kracker S, Suarez F, et al. Finding patients using similarity measures in a rare diseases-oriented clinical data warehouse: Dr. Warehouse and the needle in the needle stack. *J Biomed Inform.* (2017) 73:51–61. doi: 10.1016/j.jbi.2017.07.016

37. Mitani AA, Haneuse S. Small data challenges of studying rare diseases. *JAMA Netw Open.* (2020) 3:e201965. doi: 10.1001/jamanetworkopen.2020.1965

38. Li X, Yu L, Jin Y, Fu CH, Xing L, Heng PH. Difficulty-aware meta-learning for rare disease diagnosis. In: Martel AL, Abolmaesumi P, Stoyanov D, et al, editors. *Medical Image Computing and Computer Assisted Intervention – MICCAI 2020: 23rd International Conference, Lima, Peru, October 4–8, 2020, Proceedings, Part I.* Cham: Springer (2020). p. 357–66.

39. Nitta H, Yamazaki S, Omori T, Sato T. An introduction to epidemiologic and statistical methods useful in environmental epidemiology. *J Epidemiol.* (2010) 20:177–84. doi: 10.2188/jea.je20100010

40. Weston J, Collobert R, Sinz F, Bottou L, Vapnik V. *Inference with the Universum. In Proceedings of the 23rd International Conference on Machine Learning (ICML '06).* New York, NY: Association for Computing Machinery (2006). p. 1009–16.

41. Bisio F, Decherchi S, Gastaldo P, Zunino R. Inductive bias for semi-supervised extreme learning machine. In: Cao J, Mao K, Cambria E, Man Z, Toh KA, editors. *Proceedings of ELM-2014 Volume 1. Proceedings in Adaptation, Learning and Optimization.* Cham: Springer (2015).

42. Decherchi S, Ridella S, Zunino R, Gastaldo P, Anguita D. Using unsupervised analysis to constrain generalization bounds for support vector classifiers. *IEEE Trans Neural Netw.* (2010) 21:424–38. doi: 10.1109/TNN.2009.2038695

43. Zhuang F, Qi Z, Duan K, Xi D, Zhu Y, Zhu H, et al. A comprehensive survey on transfer learning. *Proc IEEE.* (2021) 109:43–76. doi: 10.1109/JPROC.2020.3004555

44. Wong, SC, Gatt A, Stamatescu V, McDonnell MD. *Understanding Data Augmentation for Classification: When to Warp? International Conference on Digital Image Computing: Techniques and Applications (DICTA).* Gold Coast (2016).

45. Cui L, Biswal S, Glass LM, Lever G, Sun J, Xiao C. *CONAN: Complementary Pattern Augmentation for Rare Disease Detection. Proceedings of the AAAI Conference on Artificial Intelligence.* Palo Alto, CA (2020). p. 614–21.

46. Holzinger A. From machine learning to explainable AI. In: *World Symposium on Digital Intelligence for Systems and Machines (DISA)* Košice: Piscataway (2018).

47. Zou H, Hastie T. Regularization and variable selection via the elastic net. *J Royal Stat Soc.* (2005) 67:301–20. doi: 10.1111/j.1467-9868.2005.00503.x

48. Bae JM. The clinical decision analysis using decision tree. *Epidemiol Health.* (2014) 36:e2014025. doi: 10.4178/epih/e2014025

49. Mordenti M, Ferrari E, Pedrini E, Fabbri N, Campanacci L, Muselli M, et al. Validation of a new multiple osteochondromas classification through switching neural networks. *Am J Med Genet A.* (2013) 161A:556–60. doi: 10.1002/ajmg.a.35819

50. Pestarino L, Fiorito G, Polidoro S, Vineis P, Cavalli A, Decherchi S. *On the Stability of Feature Selection in Multiomics Data. International Joint Conference on Neural Networks 2021 – IJCNN 2021* (2021).

51. McCradden MD, Joshi S, Mazwi M, Anderson JA. Ethical limitations of algorithmic fairness solutions in health care machine learning. *Lancet Digit Health.* (2020) 2:e221–3. doi: 10.1016/S2589-7500(20)30065-0

52. Nygren H, Seppänen-Laakso T, Castillo S, Hyötyläinen T, Orešič M. Liquid chromatography-mass spectrometry (LC-MS)-based lipidomics for studies of body fluids and tissues. *Meth Mol Biol.* (2011) 708:247–57.doi: 10.1007/978-1-61737-985-7_15

53. Rieke N, Hancox J, Li W, Milletarì F, Roth HR, Albarqouni S, et al. The future of digital health with federated learning. *NPJ Digit Med.* (2020) 3:119. doi: 10.1038/s41746-020-00323-1

54. *GAIA-X: A Federated Data Infrastructure for Europe.* Available online at: http://www.data-infrastructure.eu/GAIAX/Navigation/EN/Home/home. html (accessed June 24, 2021).

55. Warnat-Herresthal S, Schultze H, Shastry KL, Manamohan S, Mukherjee S, Garg V, et al. Swarm learning for decentralized and confidential clinical machine learning. *Nature.* (2021) 594:265–70. doi: 10.1038/s41586-021-03583-3

14

CK5/6 and GATA3 Defined Phenotypes of Muscle-Invasive Bladder Cancer: Impact in Adjuvant Chemotherapy and Molecular Subtyping of Negative Cases

Florestan J. Koll[1,2,3]*, Alina Schwarz[4], Jens Köllermann[4], Severine Banek[1], Luis Kluth[1], Clarissa Wittler[1], Katrin Bankov[4], Claudia Döring[4], Nina Becker[3,4], Felix K.H. Chun[1], Peter J. Wild[2,4,5] and Henning Reis[4]*

[1] Department of Urology, University Hospital Frankfurt, Goethe University, Frankfurt, Germany, [2] Frankfurt Cancer Institute (FCI), University Hospital, Goethe University, Frankfurt, Germany, [3] University Cancer Center (UCT) Frankfurt, University Hospital, Goethe University, Frankfurt, Germany, [4] Dr. Senckenberg Institute of Pathology, University Hospital Frankfurt, Frankfurt, Germany, [5] Frankfurt Institute for Advanced Studies, Frankfurt, Germany

*Correspondence:
Florestan J. Koll
florestanjohannes.koll@kgu.de
Henning Reis
Henning.reis@kgu.de

Introduction and Objective: Identifying patients that benefit from cisplatin-based adjuvant chemotherapy is a major issue in the management of muscle-invasive bladder cancer (MIBC). The purpose of this study is to correlate "luminal" and "basal" type protein expression with histological subtypes, to investigate the prognostic impact on survival after adjuvant chemotherapy and to define molecular consensus subtypes of "double negative" patients (i.e., without expression of CK5/6 or GATA3).

Materials and Methods: We performed immunohistochemical (IHC) analysis of CK5/6 and GATA3 for surrogate molecular subtyping in 181 MIBC samples. The mRNA expression profiles for molecular consensus classification were determined in CK5/6 and GATA3 (double) negative cases using a transcriptome panel with 19.398 mRNA targets (HTG Molecular Diagnostics). Data of 110 patients undergoing radical cystectomy were available for survival analysis.

Results: The expression of CK5/6 correlated with squamous histological subtype (96%) and expression of GATA3 was associated with micropapillary histology (100%). In the multivariate Cox-regression model, patients receiving adjuvant chemotherapy had a significant survival benefit (hazard ratio [HR]: 0.19 95% confidence interval [CI]: 0.1– 0.4, $p < 0.001$) and double-negative cases had decreased OS (HR: 4.07; 95% CI: 1.5–10.9, $p = 0.005$). Double negative cases were classified as NE-like (30%), stroma-rich (30%), and Ba/Sq (40%) consensus molecular subtypes and displaying different histological subtypes.

Conclusion: Immunohistochemical-based classification was associated with histological subtypes of urothelial MIBC. IHC markers like CK5/6 and GATA3 that are used in pathological routine could help to identify patients with basal and luminal tumor characteristics. However, a two-sided classification system might not sufficiently reflect the heterogeneity of bladder cancer to make treatment decisions. Especially the group of IHC-double negative cases, as further analyzed by mRNA expression profiling, are a heterogeneous group with different implications for therapy.

Keywords: bladder cancer, molecular subtyping, immunohistochemistry, adjuvant chemotherapy, double negative, consensus classification

INTRODUCTION

Bladder cancer (BCa) is the second most common genitourinary malignancy with about 570,000 new cases worldwide every year (1). About 25% of patients present with the muscle-invasive disease at the time of diagnosis and >90% of cases are urothelial carcinomas. The current standard of care for muscle invasive BCa (MIBC) is radical cystectomy with pelvic lymphadenectomy. However, relapse rates after surgery are high and 5-year overall survival (OS) rates are about 43% for pT3-tumors and 25% if the tumor has spread to local lymph nodes (2, 3). Cisplatin-based adjuvant chemotherapy may prolong survival rates and should be offered to patients with pT3/4 and/or pN + tumors (4). Patient selection for adjuvant chemotherapy is based on pathological tumor stage and chemo-eligibility, but no biomarker-based selection criteria for cisplatin-based chemotherapies exist or are included in current guidelines (4). The predictive biomarker-based decisions are needed to identify potential responders to chemotherapy and those that would be unnecessarily exposed to adjuvant therapy toxicities.

In recent years, genomic sequencing techniques have advanced, leading to comprehensive genomic characterization of BCa cohorts. This led to transcriptomic-based molecular subtyping of cancers and drove our understanding of BCa biology (5–9). It has been proposed that patients with basal tumors benefit most of neoadjuvant chemotherapy (NAC), whereas luminal tumors have a better prognosis regardless of the application of NAC (10, 11). However, contradictory results have been published and different nomenclatures, definitions, numbers of molecular subtypes, and inter-/intra-tumoral heterogeneity of BCa have hindered prospective validation and clinical translation.

To facilitate the clinical implementation of subtyping into clinical routine, immunohistochemical (IHC) markers that refer to "basal" and "luminal" molecular subtypes have been proposed (12–14). Guo et al. reported that IHC-staining with GATA3 and CK5/6 can classify the BCa correctly in over 80% of the cases into luminal and basal molecular subtypes. However, it remains unclear to which molecular subtype tumors without GATA3, nor CK5/6 expression (double negative) can be assigned.

In the present study, we explore IHC markers as surrogate markers for molecular subtyping, correlations with histologic subtypes, and impact on survival with adjuvant chemotherapy in a mono-institutional cystectomy cohort of urothelial MIBC. In addition, we performed RNA-sequencing of the group of "double negative" cases (CK5/6 and GATA3 negative), which are a heterogenous group on the molecular level.

MATERIALS AND METHODS

Cohort

Tissue/tumor samples and patient data used in this study were provided by the University Cancer Center Frankfurt (UCT). The written informed consent was obtained from all patients and the study was approved by the institutional review boards of the UCT and the ethical committee at the University Hospital Frankfurt (project-number: SUG-6-2018 and UCT-53-2021) which was conducted according to local and national regulations and according to the Declaration of Helsinki.

A total of 186 FFPE tissue samples from 181 patients with MIBC treated at the Department of Urology, University Hospital Frankfurt from 2010 to 2020 were retrieved from the archive of the Senckenberg Biobank of the Senckenberg Institute of Pathology.

Clinico-pathological and follow-up data were gathered from medical charts and records of the University Cancer Center and independently reviewed by two authors.

Histopathology of all cases was systematically re-reviewed by two experienced genitourinary pathologists according to current WHO-criteria (15). Histological subtypes were reported if at least 10% of tumor showed subtype histology including pure and mixed tumors.

Immunohistochemical Analysis

For construction of the tissue microarray (TMA), one tissue core (diameter 1 mm) of a representative tumor area was taken from a "donor" block and was arranged in a new "recipient" block using the TMA Grandmaster (3DHISTECH, Budapest, Hungary).

Hematoxylin and eosin stain slides were automatically developed on a Tissue-Tek Prisma Plus staining device (Sakura Finetek, Torrance, CA, United States). All IHC-analyses were conducted using the DAKO Omnis staining system (Agilent, Santa Clara, CA, United States) with the DAKO FLEX-Envision Kit (Agilent) according to manufacturer's instruction. We performed staining of CK5/6 (Clone: D5/16 B4; ready-to-use kit; Dako/Agilent, Santa Clara, CA, United States) and GATA3 (Clone: L50-823; ready-to-use kit; Cell Marque, Rocklin, CA, United States). IHC "double negative" was defined as negative for expression of CK5/6 and GATA3 and "double positive" was defined as positive for expression of CK5/6 as well as GATA3.

Stained slides were scanned with the Pannoramic slide scanner (3DHISTECH, Budapest, Hungary). The quantitative analysis of IHC was annotated by two genitourinary pathologists. TMA cores with either absence of representative tumor tissue or presence of staining artifacts were excluded from the analysis.

RNA Isolation and Molecular Subtype Calling

A 1 mm punch was taken from the FFPE blocks of a representative tumor area with at least 50% tumor content. RNA was isolated using the "truXTRAC FFPE total NA Kit–Column" (Covaris, Woburn, MA, United States) and RNA-concentration was measured by using the QuantiFluor RNA System (Promega, Madison, WI, United States) according to the manufacturer's protocol. The mRNA expression of 19,398 mRNA targets was determined using the HTG Transcriptome Panel (HTG Molecular Diagnostics, Tucson, AZ, United States) on Illumina NextSeq 550 system (Illumina, San Diego, CA, United States). Gene counts were normalized using median normalization and log2-transformed for further analysis. Sequencing data have been uploaded to the Gene Expression Omnibus (GSE198607). IHC double negative samples were defined as negative for CK5/6 and GATA3 in IHC analyses and classified according to the six molecular consensus classes of MIBC using the R-based consensus MIBC classification tool and the Bioconductor-package for R (6).

Statistical Analysis

We performed descriptive statistics of all data.

For the survival analysis, only patients with radical cystectomy in "curative intent" ($n = 110$) were included to create a homogenous cohort. In total, 71 patients that did not fulfill this requirement were excluded, i.e., no radical cystectomy, with primary metastatic disease, NAC or missing follow up data. We defined the OS as main endpoint of interest, which was defined as time interval between surgery and death. Secondary endpoint was disease-free survival (DFS), defined as time interval between surgery and death due to BCa or recurrence.

Kaplan–Meier method was used to estimate and illustrate survival probabilities. We used uni- and multivariable Cox's proportional hazards models to estimate the hazard ratio (HR) and corresponding 95% confidence interval (CI) for covariates for OS and DFS. All tests were two-tailed, and a significance level of $\alpha = 5\%$ was used. The statistical analyses were performed using the R Statistical Software (Version 4.1) and R Studio (Version 2021.09.1 + 372).

RESULTS

Patient Characteristics

Overall, we included specimen of 181 patients with MIBC on the TMA. Samples were obtained from transurethral resection of the bladder (TURB) in 86 (47.5%) cases and from cystectomy in 95 (52.5%) cases. The median age was 71 years (IQR: 62–78). A total of 140 (77%) patients were male and 41 (23%) were female. The clinico-pathological details of the cohort are summarized in **Table 1**.

Immunohistochemical-Classification

176 TMA-Spots were evaluable for the IHC-status of CK5/6 and GATA 3. Cases were classified into CK5/6 positive, GATA3 positive, "double negative" or "double positive" (representative images in **Figure 1**). CK5/6 positive cases were significantly associated with female gender (63% of tumors of female patients had CK5/6 expression vs. 37% tumors of male patients had CK5/6 expression, $p = 0.004$). CK5/6 positivity correlated with squamous histological subtype (24 of 25 cases [96%] had positive CK5/6 expression), whereas all 9 micropapillary cases were negative for the basal marker CK5/6 and positive for GATA 3 ($p < 0.0001$). All cases with neuroendocrine subtype were double negative. Twelve cases with other histological subtypes were negative for CK5/6, positive for GATA3 in 6 cases (one sarcomatoid, three plasmacytoid, one undifferentiated [giant cell], one glandular), double negative in 4 cases (one clear cell, one sarcomatoid, one undifferentiated [giant cell], one lymphoepithelial), and double positive in 2 cases (one sarcomatoid, one undifferentiated [giant cell]). Correlation of gender, tumor stage, age, and histology subtype with the two IHC markers are shown in **Table 2**.

Survival Analysis

We assessed survival rates of 110 patients with adequate follow up that received radical cystectomy in curative intend. Median follow-up was 66 months (IQR: 34–98 months). In this group, 35 patients received at least two cycles of adjuvant chemotherapy. **Table 3** shows patients characteristics, tumor stage, and IHC markers for patients with and without adjuvant chemotherapy.

Tumor and lymph node stage as well as the application of adjuvant chemotherapy were significantly associated with OS (**Figure 2** and **Supplementary Figures 1, 2**). The 12-month OS and DFS rates were 49% and 41 without and 77 and 62% with adjuvant chemotherapy, respectively.

In the total cohort, neither IHC markers (CK5/6, GATA3) nor the histological subtype were significantly associated with OS or DFS (**Table 4** and **Supplementary Figure 3**). After stratification for patients receiving only the cystectomy vs. patients receiving an adjuvant chemotherapy, expression of CK5/6 had a HR of

TABLE 1 | Clinico-pathological details of 181 patients on the TMA analyzed for histological subtype of urothelial carcinoma and immunohistochemistry.

Median Age (IQR)		71 (62–78)
Gender	Male	140 (77%)
	Female	41 (23%)
Max. tumor-Stage	pT2	87 (48%)
	pT3	67 (37%)
	pT4	27 (15%)
Histological subtype on TMA spot	NOS	131 (72%)
	Squamous	25 (14%)
	Micropapillary	9 (5%)
	Neuroendocrine	4 (2%)
	Sarcomatoid	3 (2%)
	Plasmacytoid	3 (2%)
	Other (1 lymphoepithelial, 1 clear cell, 1 glandular, 3 giant cell)	6 (3%)

IQR, interquartile range; NOS, not otherwise specified; TMA, tissue micro array.

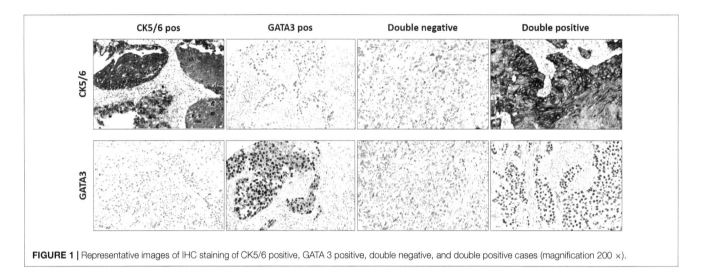

	CK5/6 pos	GATA3 pos	Double negative	Double positive
CK5/6				
GATA3				

FIGURE 1 | Representative images of IHC staining of CK5/6 positive, GATA 3 positive, double negative, and double positive cases (magnification 200 ×).

TABLE 2 | Association of clinic-pathological findings with the IHC-markers CK5/6 and GATA3.

		n (%)	CK5/6 positive (n = 32)	GATA3 positive (n = 81)	Double negative (n = 17)	Double positive (n = 46)	p
Age	<70	73 (41%)	15 (47%)	29 (36%)	9 (53%)	20 (44%)	0.5
	≥70	103 (59%)	17 (53%)	52 (64%)	8 (47%)	26 (15%)	
Gender	Male	135 (77%)	23 (72%)	67 (83%)	16 (94%)	29 (63%)	**0.021**
	Female	41 (23%)	9 (28%)	14 (17%)	1 (6%)	17 (37%)	
Max. Tumor-Stage	pT2	83 (47%)	11 (34%)	45 (56%)	8 (47%)	19 (41%)	0.138
	pT3	66 (38%)	18 (56%)	23 (28%)	5 (29%)	20 (44%)	
	pT4	27 (15%)	3 (10%)	13 (16%)	4 (24%)	7 (15%)	
Histological subtype	NOS	127 (72%)	18 (59%)	65 (80%)	10 (59%)	34 (74%)	**<0.0001**
	Squamous	25 (14%)	14 (44%)	1 (1%)	0	10 (22%)	
	Micropapillary	9 (5%)	0	9 (11%)	0	0	
	Neuroendocrine	3 (2%)	0	0	3 (18%)	0	
	Sarcomatoid	3 (2%)	0	1 (1%)	1 (6%)	1 (2%)	
	Plasmacytoid	3 (2%)	0	3 (4%)	0	0	
	Undifferentiated (giant cell)	3 (2%)	0	1 (1%)	1 (6%)	1 (2%)	
	Glandular	1 (0.6%)	0	1 (1%)	0	0	
	Clear cell	1 (0.6%)	0	0	1 (6%)	0	
	Lymphoepithelial	1 (0.6%)	0	0	1 (6%)	0	

A total of 176 spots were evaluated. The p-values were calculated using Pearson–Chi square test. NOS, not otherwise specified. Bold values indicate significant differences with p-values < 0.05.

0.4 (95% *CI*: 0.2–1.2, $p = 0.09$) in the adjuvant chemotherapy group. A multivariate cox-regression model adjusting for tumor and lymph node (LN) stage, adjuvant chemotherapy, and IHC-staining is shown in **Figure 3**. In addition to tumor- and LN stage, the double negative cases were associated with an increased risk of death (*HR*: 4.07; 95% *CI*: 1.5–10.9, $p = 0.005$). Adjuvant chemotherapy was associated with the survival benefit (*HR*: 0.19; 95% *CI*: 0.10–0.36, $p < 0.001$). The multivariate cox-regression model for DFS is shown in the **Supplementary Material**.

Molecular Analysis of CK5/6 and GATA3 Negative Cases

Ten double negative cases were analyzed using the HTG Transcriptome Panel and molecular subtypes were determined according to the consensus classification of Kamoun et al. (6).

Three cases were classified as stroma-rich, three as NE-like and four as Ba/Sq. **Table 5** shows molecular subtypes with histological subtype and pathological stage. The Ba/Sq cases showed heterogeneous histology with lymphoepithelial, undifferentiated (giant cell) and sarcomatoid subtypes. According to the UNC classification system, all cases were classified as basal (8). And according to the TCGA classification system, cases were classified as basal-squamous and neuronal (5). Representative HE-stained pictures of histological subtype and their molecular subtype are shown in **Figure 4**.

DISCUSSION

This study shows a high concordance of an IHC-subclassification based on the two markers CK5/6 and GATA3 with histological

TABLE 3 | Characteristics of patients with and without adjuvant chemotherapy.

		CE only $n = 75$	Adjuvant Chemotherapy $n = 35$	p
Age (IQR)		72 (64.25–76.75)	60 (52.75–71)	
Age	<71	32 (43%)	26 (74%)	**0.002**
	≥71	43 (57%)	9 (26%)	
Gender	Male	59 (79%)	28 (80%)	1.0
	Female	16 (21%)	7 (20%)	
Stage Max.	pT2	23 (31%)	5 (14%)	0.12
	pT3	37 (49%)	24 (69%)	
	pT4	15 (20%)	6 (17%)	
Lymph node status	pN0	42 (56%)	13 (37%)	0.084
	pN1 + pNx	33 (44%)	22 (63%)	
R-Status	R0	60 (80%)	28 (80%)	1.0
	R1/R2/Rx	15 (20%)	7 (20%)	
Histological subtype	NOS	57 (77%)	23 (66%)	0.39
	Squamous	8 (11%)	4 (11%)	
	Micropapillary	5 (7%)	2 (6%)	
	Neuroendocrine	1 (1%)	2 (6%)	
	Other	3 (4%)	4 (11%)	
Type of chemotherapy	Gem/Cis		28 (80%)	
	Gem/Carbo		4 (11%)	
	Platin/Etoposid		2 (6%)	
	other		1 (3%)	
Recurrence	No	54 (72%)	18 (51%)	0.058
	Yes	21 (28%)	17 (49%)	
CK5/6 + GATA3	CK5/6 pos	14 (19%)	5 (15%)	0.45
	GATA 3 pos	36 (48%)	13 (38%)	
	Double neg	7 (9%)	6 (18%)	
	Double pos	18 (24%)	10 (29%)	

CE, cystectomy; NOS, not otherwise specified; Gem/Cis, gemcitabine/cisplatin; Gem/Carbo, gemcitabine/carboplatin; R-Status, resection status. Bold values indicate significant differences with p-values < 0.05.

subtypes in MIBC. Double negative patients without expression of CK5/6 nor GATA3 had decreased OS rates. Subtyping of double negative cases revealed a histological and molecular heterogeneous subgroup. Strengths of our study are the

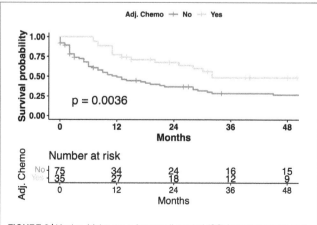

FIGURE 2 | Kaplan–Meier curve for overall survival (OS) for patients with and without adjuvant chemotherapy.

pathological re-review of all cases, evaluation of standardized IHC-staining, the use of a broad transcriptome panel for molecular phenotyping, and the analysis of adjuvant chemotherapy in a clinically well-annotated cohort of patients with MIBC.

The use of molecular subtyping to guide the selection of systemic therapies has been proposed for NAC and immune checkpoint inhibitors (7, 10, 16). However, contradictory results published in the past years and the diversity of molecular subtype taxonomy until the publication of the consensus classification have hindered the use and clinical translation (6, 17–19). Data to provide guidance to select patients for adjuvant chemotherapy based on molecular subtypes are sparse.

It has been suggested that CK5/6 and GATA3 expression can identify basal and luminal molecular subtypes in 80–90% of cases which could be a useful tool in routine pathological assessments to identify the basic molecular subtypes of BCa (12). Other studies using more markers confirmed a good correlation of IHC-based subtyping with gene expression-based subtypes (determined by targeted NanoString panels), but still with a risk of differing classification in about 15–20% of cases (13, 20).

Our results show that CK5/6 expression was associated with squamous histological subtype and female gender, which

TABLE 4 | Univariate cox-regression model for histological subtype and IHC-markers CK5/6 and GATA3 stratified for patients with and without adjuvant chemotherapy.

		Total cohort (n = 110)	p	Adjuvant chemotherapy (n = 35)	p	CE only (n = 75)	p
Histological subtype on TMA	NOS	Reference		Reference		Reference	
	Squamous	0.8 (0.3–1.7)	0.5	0.4 (0.06–3.4)	0.6	0.9 (0.4–2.2)	0.9
	Micropapillary	1.2 (0.5–3.1)	0.7	2.9 (0.6–13.1)	0.2	0.89 (0.3–2.9)	0.9
	Neuroendocine	0.9 (0.2–4.1)	0.9	1.8 (0.2–14.1)	0.6	NA	
	Other	0.7 (0.3–1.9)	0.5	0.9 (0.2–4.2)	0.9	0.8 (0.2–3.5)	0.8
CK56	Pos	0.9 (0.5–1.4)	0.5	0.4 (0.2–1.2)	0.09	1.1 (0.7–1.9)	0.7
GATA3	Pos	0.8 (0.5–1.3)	0.3	0.7 (0.3–1.8)	0.4	0.8 (0.4–1.4)	0.4
CK56 + GATA3	CK56 pos	Reference		Reference			
	GATA3 pos	1.0 (0.5–2.0)	0.9	1.9 (0.4–8.8)	0.4	0.9 (0.4–1.8)	0.71
	Double neg	1.6 (0.7–3.7)	0.3	0.3 (0.5–16.7)	0.2	1.7 (0.6–4.7)	0.31
	Double pos	1.0 (0.5–2.1)	1.0	1.1 (0.1–5.0)	0.8	1.3 (0.6–2.8)	0.59

CE, cystectomy; NOS, not otherwise specified.

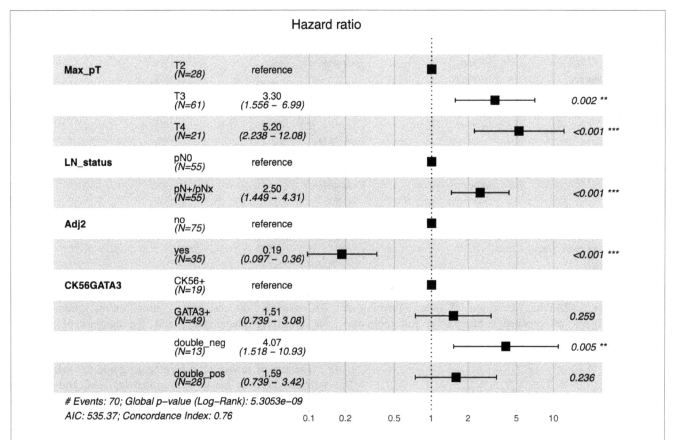

FIGURE 3 | Multivariate cox-regression model for OS adjusting for tumor and LN stage, adjuvant chemotherapy, and the IHC-markers CK5/6 and GATA3. Number of events: 70; Global p-value (Log Rank): 5.3053e-09. LN, lymph node; Adj2, at least two cycles of adjuvant chemotherapy. **p < 0.05; ***p < 0.001.

is in concordance with published data (6, 13). The same applies to the positive correlation between GATA3-expression and micropapillary histological subtype. Four cases with neuroendocrine histological subtype were double negative in IHC-analyses.

To test the two-marker-based IHC-classification for its predictive value of chemotherapy efficacy, we performed analyses in the cohort of adjuvant-treated patients. We are aware, that our survival analyses, which demonstrated a significant

benefit for patients receiving adjuvant chemotherapy, hold the risk of selection bias since patients receiving chemotherapy were younger and kidney function or comorbidities were not considered. However, when analyzing only patients receiving chemotherapy, none of the markers predicted survival, but cases expressing the basal marker CK5/6 tend to have improved survival with adjuvant chemotherapy, with the level of significance missed (*HR* 0.42 95% *KI* 0.15–1.2, *p* = 0.09). These results are in line with the available data for NAC

TABLE 5 | Description of double negative cases analyzed for mRNA expression profiles, including histological subtypes on TMA and whole slide, and molecular subtypes according to the consensus, UNC, and TCGA (5) classifier.

Patient	Age at surgery	Gender	Max. pT stage	LN metastases	Predominant histological subtype on TMA	Histological subtype on whole slide	Adjuvant chemotherapy	Consensus class	UNC subtype	TCGA subtype
001_069	68	m	3b	Yes	Lymphoepithelial	Lymphoepithelial	Yes	Ba/Sq	Basal	Basal_squamous
001_004	71	m	4a	No	Undifferentiated/Giant cell	Undifferentiated/Giant cell	No	Ba/Sq	Basal	Basal_squamous
001_033	71	m	3b	Yes	NOS	NOS + Squamous	No	Ba/Sq	Basal	Basal_squamous
001_039	60	m	2b	Yes	Sarcomatoid	Sarcomatoid	Yes	Ba/Sq	Basal	Basal_squamous
001_012	57	m	4b	Yes	NOS	NOS	Yes	Stroma-rich	Basal	Basal_squamous
001_040	78	m	4a	Yes	NOS	NOS	Yes	Stroma-rich	Basal	Basal_squamous
001_065	70	m	4a	No	NOS	NOS + Pseudoglandular	No	Stroma-rich	Basal	Neuronal
001_021	62	m	3b	No		Neuroendocrine	Yes	NE-like	Basal	Neuronal
001_050	62	m	3b	Yes	Neuroendocrine	Neuroendocrine	Yes	NE-like	Basal	Neuronal
001_071	67	m	2b	No	Neuroendocrine	Neuroendocrine	No	NE-like	Basal	Neuronal

Ba/Sq, basal/squamous; m, male; NE, neuroendocrine; NOS, not otherwise specified; UNC, University of North Carolina; TCGA, the cancer genome atlas.

proposing that patients with basal-like tumors respond better to chemotherapy, whereas luminal-like tumors have an inferior response to chemotherapy.

For the neoadjuvant setting, Seiler and colleagues developed a single-sample genomic subtyping classifier to subdivide patients into four groups revealing that patients with basal tumors had the most improvement in OS with NAC compared with surgery alone (10). More recent studied showed similar results for non-luminal tumors (11, 20). Contrary results from Sjödahl and colleagues as well as Taber and colleagues, however, indicated that basal tumors less frequently respond to NAC and according to Kamoun and colleagues, the consensus molecular subtypes do not correlate with response to NAC (6, 17, 18). Therefore, further research will have to clarify the role of molecular subtypes as predictive markers of chemotherapy efficacy.

In addition to the findings in cases with IHC expression of at least one marker, we detected a subgroup of double negative cases without expression of CK5/6 or GATA3. The cohort seems to be of biological significance, as patients in this group had an increased risk of death in multivariate analysis. This finding has recently been described also by other groups (13, 14). However, no detailed molecular analyses were reported, as no full transcriptomic analyses were performed (12, 13). We, therefore, conducted further molecular analyses of the double negative group using an mRNA transcriptome panel covering approximately 19,300 targets, thus enabling us to call consensus class molecular subtypes.

Double negative cases tended to be molecularly basal-like according to the UNC classifier but are more heterogenous than a two tailed-classification can represent. Three molecular subtypes (Ba/Sq, stroma-rich, neuronal) and five histological subtypes (NOS, neuroendocrine, sarcomatoid, undifferentiated/giant cell, lymphoepithelioma-like) were present in this group. This highlights the heterogeneity of double negative cases and implicates that a more complex system than a two-tailed classification might be needed for more individualized treatment decisions. For example, the (molecular and histological) neuroendocrine subtype is known to have a poor prognosis and thus should be treated aggressively with upfront chemotherapy and might be responsive to immune checkpoint inhibition (4, 16). On the other hand, the lymphoepithelioma-like subtype of urothelial carcinoma is associated with a more favorable prognosis and might be more responsive to immune checkpoint inhibition as proposed by the results of the PURE-1 trial (21, 22). The well-known fact of intra-tumoral heterogeneity in urothelial BCa adds to these facts.

The limitations of our study are the retrospective design and the low number of molecular analyses. Due to low numbers, we did not include patients receiving NAC in our survival analysis. Selecting patients for NAC, which is the recommended treatment for MIBC, might be of higher clinical relevance than for adjuvant chemotherapy. In addition, we performed two IHC-marker analyses only to surrogate basal and luminal molecular subtypes. However, this was intentionally done to create comparability with the literature. Other studies using more markers for protein-based subtyping reported similar

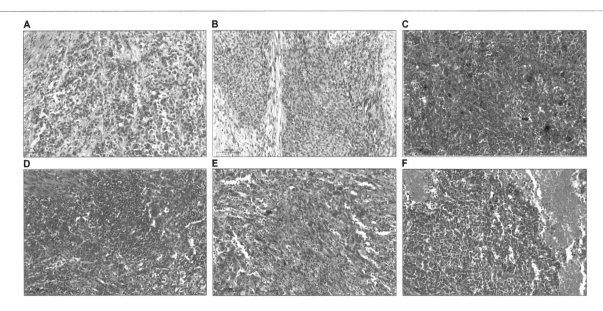

FIGURE 4 | Representative pictures of different histological subtypes on the whole slides classified as double negative in tissue micro array (TMA)-analysis and their molecular consensus subtypes. **(A)** Histological subtype: NOS; molecular Subtype: Stroma-rich. **(B)** Histological subtype: NOS (+ squamous on whole slide); molecular subtype: Ba/Sq. **(C)** Histological subtype: poorly differentiated/giant cell; molecular subtype: Ba/Sq. **(D)** Histological subtype: lymphoepithelial; molecular subtype: Ba/Sq. **(E)** Histological subtype: sarcomatoid; molecular subtype: Ba/Sq. **(F)** Histological subtype: neuroendocrine; molecular subtype: NE-like. Ba/Sq, basal/squamous; NE, neuroendocrine; NOS, not otherwise specified.

results with high concordance of histological subtypes and IHC, but also demonstrated that protein-based subtyping did not predict survival in population-based cystectomy cohorts (13, 19). Thus, the question remains if a limited protein-based assessment of surrogate markers for molecular subtypes can serve as a predictor for chemotherapy response or if mRNA-expression profiles are necessary for adequate determination of molecular subtypes or other markers like immune cell infiltration are necessary for patient selection (18). So far, the histopathological staging remains the most important prognostic factor (23). However, efforts to bring the results of the large transcriptomic studies into a clinical routine are underway (24).

In conclusion, we demonstrated that an IHC-based classification was associated with histological subtypes of urothelial MIBC. Although IHC markers used in pathological routine might help to identify patients with basal and luminal tumor characteristics, a two-sided classification system might not sufficiently reflect the heterogeneity of BCa to guide treatment decisions. Especially the group of IHC-double negative cases is a heterogeneous group with different implications for therapy.

AUTHOR CONTRIBUTIONS

FK, HR, and PW contributed to conception and design of the study. FK, LK, SB, CW, AS, and KB organized the database and samples. AS, NB, KB, JK, HR, and PW performed data curation and formal analysis. FK and CD performed the statistical analysis and analysis of sequencing data. AS, NB, and KB performed IHC. FK wrote the first draft of the manuscript. HR, PW,

and FC performed review and editing of the manuscript and supervision. All authors contributed to manuscript revision, read, and approved the submitted version.

REFERENCES

1. Sung H, Ferlay J, Siegel RL, Laversanne M, Soerjomataram I, Jemal A, et al. Global cancer statistics 2020: GLOBOCAN estimates of incidence and mortality worldwide for 36 cancers in 185 countries. *CA.* (2021) 71:209–49. doi: 10.3322/caac.21660

2. Hautmann RE, Gschwend JE, de Petriconi RC, Kron M, Volkmer BG. Cystectomy for transitional cell carcinoma of the bladder: results of a surgery only series in the neobladder era. *J Urol.* (2006) 176:486–92.

3. Stein JP, Lieskovsky G, Cote R, Groshen S, Feng AC, Boyd S, et al. Radical cystectomy in the treatment of invasive bladder cancer: long-term results in 1,054 patients. *J Clin Oncol.* (2001) 19:666–75. doi: 10.1200/JCO.2001.19.3.666

4. Witjes JA, Bruins HM, Cathomas R, Comperat EM, Cowan NC, Gakis G, et al. European association of urology guidelines on muscle-invasive and metastatic bladder cancer: summary of the 2020 guidelines. *Eur Urol.* (2021) 79:82–104.

5. Robertson AG, Kim J, Al-Ahmadie H, Bellmunt J, Guo G, Cherniack AD, et al. Comprehensive molecular characterization of muscle-invasive bladder cancer. *Cell.* (2017) 171:540–56.e25.

6. Kamoun A, de Reynies A, Allory Y, Sjodahl G, Robertson AG, Seiler R, et al. A consensus molecular classification of muscle-invasive bladder cancer. *Eur Urol.* (2019) 77:420–33.

7. Choi W, Porten S, Kim S, Willis D, Plimack ER, Hoffman-Censits J, et al. Identification of distinct basal and luminal subtypes of muscle-invasive bladder cancer with different sensitivities to frontline chemotherapy. *Cancer Cell.* (2014) 25:152–65. doi: 10.1016/j.ccr.2014.01.009

8. Damrauer JS, Hoadley KA, Chism DD, Fan C, Tiganelli CJ, Wobker SE, et al. Intrinsic subtypes of high-grade bladder cancer reflect the hallmarks of breast cancer biology. *Proc Natl Acad Sci USA.* (2014) 111:3110–5. doi: 10.1073/pnas.1318376111

9. Sjodahl G, Lauss M, Lovgren K, Chebil G, Gudjonsson S, Veerla S, et al. A molecular taxonomy for urothelial carcinoma. *Clin Cancer Res.* (2012) 18:3377–86. doi: 10.1158/1078-0432.CCR-12-0077-T

10. Seiler R, Ashab HAD, Erho N, van Rhijn BWG, Winters B, Douglas J, et al. Impact of molecular subtypes in muscle-invasive bladder cancer on predicting response and survival after neoadjuvant chemotherapy. *Eur Urol.* (2017) 72:544–54. doi: 10.1016/j.eururo.2017.03.030

11. Lotan Y, de Jong JJ, Liu VYT, Bismar TA, Boorjian SA, Huang HC, et al. Patients with muscle-invasive bladder cancer with nonluminal subtype derive greatest benefit from platinum based neoadjuvant chemotherapy. *J Urol.* (2021) 207:541–50. doi: 10.1097/JU.0000000000002261

12. Guo CC, Bondaruk J, Yao H, Wang Z, Zhang L, Lee S, et al. Assessment of luminal and basal phenotypes in bladder cancer. *Sci Rep.* (2020) 10:9743. doi: 10.1038/s41598-020-66747-7

13. Weyerer V, Stoehr R, Bertz S, Lange F, Geppert CI, Wach S, et al. Prognostic impact of molecular muscle-invasive bladder cancer subtyping approaches and correlations with variant histology in a population-based mono-institutional cystectomy cohort. *World J Urol.* (2021) 39:4011–9. doi: 10.1007/s00345-021-03788-1

14. Bejrananda T, Kanjanapradit K, Saetang J, Sangkhathat S. Impact of immunohistochemistry-based subtyping of GATA3, CK20, CK5/6, and CK14 expression on survival after radical cystectomy for muscle-invasive bladder cancer. *Sci Rep.* (2021) 11:21186. doi: 10.1038/s41598-021-00628-5

15. Moch H, Ulbright TM, Reuter VE. *WHO Classification of Tumours of the Urinary System and Male Genital Organs.* Lyon: International Agency for Research on Cancer (2016).

16. Kim J, Kwiatkowski D, McConkey DJ, Meeks JJ, Freeman SS, Bellmunt J, et al. The cancer genome atlas expression subtypes stratify response to checkpoint inhibition in advanced urothelial cancer and identify a subset of patients with high survival probability. *Eur Urol.* (2019) 75:961–4. doi: 10.1016/j.eururo.2019.02.017

17. Sjodahl G, Abrahamsson J, Holmsten K, Bernardo C, Chebil G, Eriksson P, et al. Different responses to neoadjuvant chemotherapy in urothelial carcinoma molecular subtypes. *Eur Urol.* (2021) 81:523–32.

18. Taber A, Christensen E, Lamy P, Nordentoft I, Prip F, Lindskrog SV, et al. Molecular correlates of cisplatin-based chemotherapy response in muscle invasive bladder cancer by integrated multi-omics analysis. *Nat Commun.* (2020) 11:4858.

19. Kollberg P, Chebil G, Eriksson P, Sjodahl G, Liedberg F. Molecular subtypes applied to a population-based modern cystectomy series do not predict cancer-specific survival. *Urol Oncol.* (2019) 37:791–9. doi: 10.1016/j.urolonc.2019.04.010

20. Font A, Domenech M, Benitez R, Rava M, Marques M, Ramirez JL, et al. Immunohistochemistry-based taxonomical classification of bladder cancer predicts response to neoadjuvant chemotherapy. *Cancers (Basel).* (2020) 12:1784. doi: 10.3390/cancers12071784

21. Amin MB. Histological variants of urothelial carcinoma: diagnostic, therapeutic and prognostic implications. *Mod Pathol.* (2009) 22(Suppl. 2):S96–118. doi: 10.1038/modpathol.2009.26

22. Necchi A, Raggi D, Gallina A, Madison R, Colecchia M, Luciano R, et al. Updated results of PURE-01 with preliminary activity of neoadjuvant pembrolizumab in patients with muscle-invasive bladder carcinoma with variant histologies. *Eur Urol.* (2020) 77:439–46. doi: 10.1016/j.eururo.2019.10.026

23. Morera DS, Hasanali SL, Belew D, Ghosh S, Klaassen Z, Jordan AR, et al. Clinical parameters outperform molecular subtypes for predicting outcome in bladder cancer: results from multiple cohorts including TCGA. *J Urol.* (2020) 203:62–72. doi: 10.1097/JU.0000000000000351

24. Olah C, Hahnen C, Nagy N, Musial J, Varadi M, Nyiro G, et al. A quantitative polymerase chain reaction based method for molecular subtype classification of urinary bladder cancer-Stromal gene expressions show higher prognostic values than intrinsic tumor genes. *Int J Cancer.* (2021) 150:856–67. doi: 10.1002/ijc.33809

15

Up-to-Date Pathologic Classification and Molecular Characteristics of Intrahepatic Cholangiocarcinoma

Taek Chung[1] and Young Nyun Park[2]*

[1] Department of Biomedical Systems Informatics, Yonsei University College of Medicine, Seoul, South Korea, [2] Department of Pathology, Graduate School of Medical Science, Brain Korea 21 Project, Yonsei University College of Medicine, Seoul, South Korea

Correspondence:
Young Nyun Park
young0608@yuhs.ac

Intrahepatic cholangiocarcinoma (iCCA) is an aggressive primary liver malignancy with an increasing incidence worldwide. Recently, histopathologic classification of small duct type and large duct type iCCA has been introduced. Both these types of tumors exhibit differences in clinicopathological features, mutational profiles, and prognosis. Small duct type iCCA is composed of non-mucin-producing cuboidal cells, whereas large duct type iCCA is composed of mucin-producing columnar cells, reflecting different cells of origin. Large duct type iCCA shows more invasive growth and poorer prognosis than small duct type iCCA. The background liver of small duct type iCCA often shows chronic liver disease related to hepatitis B or C viral infection, or alcoholic or non-alcoholic fatty liver disease/steatohepatitis, in contrast to large duct type iCCA that is often related to hepatolithiasis and liver fluke infection. Cholangiolocarcinoma is a variant of small duct type iCCA composed of naïve-looking cuboidal cells forming cords or ductule-like structures, and shows better prognosis than the conventional small duct type. Fibrous tumor stroma, one of the characteristic features of iCCA, contains activated fibroblasts intermixed with innate and adaptive immune cells. The types of stroma (mature versus immature) are related to tumor behavior and prognosis. Low tumor-infiltrating lymphocyte density, *KRAS* alteration, and chromosomal instability are related to immune-suppressive tumor microenvironments with resistance to programmed death 1/ programmed death ligand 1 blockade. Data from recent large-scale exome analyses have revealed the heterogeneity in the molecular profiles of iCCA, showing that small duct type iCCA exhibit frequent *BAP1*, *IDH1/2* hotspot mutations and *FGFR2* fusion, in contrast to frequent mutations in *KRAS*, *TP53*, and *SMAD4* observed in large duct type iCCA. Multi-omics analyses have proposed several molecular classifications of iCCA, including inflammation class and proliferation class. The inflammation class is enriched in inflammatory signaling pathways and expression of cytokines, while the proliferation class has activated oncogenic growth signaling pathways. Diverse pathologic features of iCCA and its associated multi-omics characteristics are currently under active investigation, thereby providing insights into precision therapeutics for patients with iCCA. This review provides the latest knowledge on the histopathologic classification of iCCA and its associated molecular features, ranging from tumor microenvironment to genomic and transcriptomic research.

Keywords: intrahepatic cholangiocarcinoma, pathology, small duct, large duct, tumor microenvironment, genomics, transcriptomics

INTRODUCTION

Cholangiocarcinomas (CCAs) include intrahepatic CCA (iCCA), perihilar CCA, and distal CCA (1). Anatomically, iCCA, often called as "peripheral CCA," is defined as a tumor located in the periphery of the second-order bile ducts, ranging from segmental bile ducts to smaller branches of the intrahepatic biliary tree. Perihilar CCA, also known as Klatskin tumor, is defined as a tumor that arises at the junction where the right and left hepatic ducts meet, with the insertion site of the cystic duct as its distal limit. CCAs involving more of the distal area, such as the common bile duct, is defined as distal CCA. This review mainly focuses on iCCA.

Recent evaluation indicates that iCCA comprises approximately 10–15% of primary liver malignancies (2, 3), and its incidence worldwide has increased over the past decades (4). However, changes in the nomenclature, classification, and the disease coding system of CCA have hampered the accurate estimation of the incidence of iCCA (5). Countries with the highest incidence include South Korea (2.8 per 100,000 people/year), where *Clonorchis sinensis* infection was prevalent in the past, and Thailand (2.2 per 100,000 people/year), which still is an endemic area for infections due to *Opisthorchis viverrini* (4, 6, 7). In other countries where parasites are not endemic, the incidence of iCCA is low, usually below or around 1 per 100,000 people/year. Moreover, there are proposed risk factors such as choledochal cyst, primary sclerosing cholangitis, chronic B or C viral hepatitis, and non-alcoholic fatty liver disease caused by obesity or metabolic syndromes. However, a significant proportion of patients with iCCA have no known risk factors (4, 8). Since these patients rarely present symptoms in the early stage, they are often diagnosed with advanced disease with a dismal prognosis and 5-year overall survival rate of approximately 10% even in developed countries (9–11).

Intrahepatic cholangiocarcinoma is an epithelial neoplasm with biliary differentiation, and usually presents with abundant fibrous tumor stroma containing cancer-associated fibroblasts (CAFs), innate and adaptive immune cells, etc. Recently, iCCAs have been classified into two subtypes namely, small duct type and large duct type (3, 12). Furthermore, the molecular characteristics of iCCA are under active investigation owing to technological advances in nucleotide sequencing and the availability of massive data sources on cancer, such as The Cancer Genome Atlas (TCGA) and cBio Cancer Genomics Portal (13, 14). The combination of histopathological and multi-omics data have provided novel insights into understanding the molecular pathology and thereby, developing therapeutic options for iCCA.

This review aims to provide the latest knowledge on the histopathologic classification of iCCA based on the fifth edition of the World Health Organization (WHO) classification of digestive system tumors. In addition, we discuss the associated molecular features based on tumor microenvironment, genomic and transcriptomic research results presented so far.

PATHOLOGICAL FEATURES OF INTRAHEPATIC CHOLANGIOCARCINOMA

Intrahepatic cholangiocarcinoma is an adenocarcinoma arising in the intrahepatic biliary tree. Fibrous tumor stroma is one of the characteristic features of iCCA, and the fibrous stroma is various in amount and distribution. The tumor center is usually more fibrotic than the tumor periphery, showing proliferating tumor cells invading into the surrounding liver. Lymphovascular and perineural invasion are often detected even at an early stage.

Gross Features of Intrahepatic Cholangiocarcinoma

Macroscopically, iCCAs can be classified into three types: mass-forming, periductal infiltrating, and intraductal growing. Based on gross appearance, the mass-forming type is most common, and often exhibits mixed features (**Figure 1**) (15). The mass-forming type shows a definite round tumor mass with invasive border. The cut surface is usually white, pale tan or yellowish in color with firm consistency due to fibrous tumor stroma. The periductal infiltrating type shows a growth pattern that extends along the bile duct, exhibiting a whitish fibrotic and thickened bile duct wall. The intraductal growing type grows into the lumen of the bile duct, forming single or multiple soft papillary masses attached to the bile duct wall. The tumor mass and resultant obstruction often dilate the bile duct and make the tumor symptomatic. Since most of the intraductal growing type iCCA cases are now being considered as malignant transformations of intraductal papillary neoplasm of the bile duct (IPNB), in the latest fifth edition of WHO classification, gross morphologic types of iCCA include mass forming, periductal infiltrating and mixed type of these two (3, 16).

Abbreviations: CCA, cholangiocarcinoma; iCCA, intrahepatic cholangiocarcinoma; CAFs, cancer-associated fibroblasts; TCGA, The Cancer Genome Atlas; WHO, World Health Organization; MUC, mucin; CRP, c-reactive protein; EBER, Epstein–Barr virus-encoded small RNA; CKs, cytokeratins; FGB, fibrinopeptide B; CLC, cholangiolocarcinoma; HCC, hepatocellular carcinoma; DPM, ductal plate malformation; IPNB, intraductal papillary neoplasm of the bile duct; BilIN, biliary intraepithelial neoplasia; IPMN, intraductal papillary mucinous neoplasm; TAMs, tumor-associated macrophages.

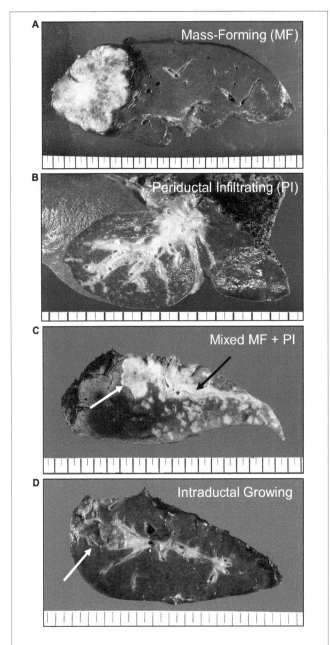

FIGURE 1 | Macroscopic types of intrahepatic cholangiocarcinoma.
(A) Mass-forming (MF) type showing a whitish tan tumor mass invading
adjacent liver parenchyma. **(B)** Periductal infiltrating (PI) type showing a
whitish periductal tumor growth along the bile duct branches. **(C)** Mixed type
of MF and PI showing a solid tumor of MF type (white arrow) and a periductal
growth of PI type (black arrow). **(D)** Intraductal growing type showing a friable
tumor mass in the dilated bile duct (white arrow). This type of tumor is
re-classified as intraductal papillary neoplasm of bile duct.

Classification of Small Duct Type and Large Duct Type

Conventional iCCA can be further classified into two
histopathological types according to the level or size of the
affected duct. Recently, small duct type and large duct type
iCCA have been introduced in the WHO classification (3).

Small duct type iCCA, which has been reported as a peripheral,
ductular, and cholangiolar type, accounts for 36–84% of iCCA
(12, 17–19). Small duct type iCCA shows small-sized tubular
growth of cuboidal or low-columnar tumor epithelial cells. There
is little or no mucin production, and occasional areas of growth
exhibit a pattern resembling ductular reaction with slit-like
glandular lumen (**Figures 2A,B**). Background liver of small duct
type iCCA often shows chronic liver disease related to B viral
hepatitis, C viral hepatitis, alcoholic hepatitis, and non-alcoholic
steatohepatitis (12, 17, 20).

Large duct type iCCA, which has been reported as bile duct
type or perihilar type, arises in large intrahepatic bile ducts and
comprises 8–60% of iCCA cases (12, 17–19). Large duct type
iCCA is composed of mucin-producing columnar cells forming
irregular shaped-and-sized tubules or gland-like structures. This
type usually shows a highly invasive growth pattern accompanied
by a desmoplastic reaction (**Figures 2D,E**) (3). Pathological
examination of the background liver of large duct type iCCA
often reveals chronic bile duct injury due to hepatolithiasis,
parasitic infection in bile ducts, or primary sclerosing cholangitis
(8, 20).

Furthermore, histopathological features of small duct type and
large duct type iCCA are related to their gross appearance. The
periductal infiltrative type of iCCA is exclusively large duct type,
whereas the mass-forming type is more heterogeneous, including
small duct and large duct types (17, 21). Mass-forming type iCCA
with small duct type histology showed better prognosis than other
types (17).

Putative Cells of Origin
Small duct type iCCA occurs in smaller intrahepatic bile ducts
compared to large duct type. Canals of Hering, which are
histological structures that link hepatic canaliculi and the biliary
tree, cuboidal cholangiocytes of bile ductules, and interlobular
bile ducts are considered as the putative cells of origin (22,
23). In contrast, large duct type iCCA might be derived from
columnar biliary epithelium producing mucin or peribiliary
glands around them (8, 20). However, the cellular origin of iCCA
is still controversial, since various lineage tracing animal studies
showed mixed results indicating hepatic stem or progenitor cells,
cholangiocytes or hepatocytes as the cells of origin of iCCA (24,
25). Further research is required to conclusively define the origin
of small duct and large duct type iCCAs.

Immunohistochemical Markers for Small Duct Type and Large Duct Type Intrahepatic Cholangiocarcinoma
Examination of a panel of immunohistochemical (IHC) markers
is useful to differentiate small duct type and large duct type.
In large duct type iCCAs, high expression of mucin (MUC)
core protein 5AC, MUC6, and S100 calcium-binding protein P
(S100P) has been reported (26, 27), whereas neural cell adhesion
molecule (NCAM, also known as CD56) and N-cadherin have
been found to be highly expressed in the small duct type. NCAM
and N-cadherin are normally expressed in cholangioles (28,
29). Intra- and/or extracellular mucin, detected by mucicarmine
or Alcian blue staining, is abundant in the large duct type

in contrast to its scarcity or absence in the small duct type. Examining a panel of these markers, including S100P, N-cadherin, NCAM, and Alcian blue, has been reported to be more effective in differentiating small duct and large duct types (12). Additionally, c-reactive protein (CRP) was recently found to be an effective marker for the diagnosis of small duct type iCCA (30) (**Figures 2C,F**). Biliary cytokeratins (CKs) such as CK7 and CK19 are useful for confirming biliary differentiation or biliary origin. However, their ability to differentiate between small duct type and large duct type iCCA is limited (31, 32).

Histopathological features of hematoxylin and eosin-stained slides usually provide insight to distinguish small duct and large duct type iCCA. In addition, application of immunohistochemical (IHC) markers (S100P, NCAM, and N-cadherin) and special stain for mucin is useful to support the diagnosis of iCCA subtypes, especially when the tissue is limited in biopsies.

Comparison of Prognosis and Treatment Response Between Small Duct Type and Large Duct Type Intrahepatic Cholangiocarcinoma

The prognosis of small duct type iCCA is generally favorable compared to that of large duct type iCCA (12, 17, 33, 34). Accordingly, inflammation-related markers [CRP and fibrinopeptide B (FGB)] and proliferation-related markers [extracellular signal-regulated kinases (ERK) 1/2 and Ki-67] are highly expressed in small duct type iCCA and large duct type iCCA, respectively (17). It has also been reported that the response to conventional chemotherapy is better with small duct type than with large duct type iCCA (35).

Differential Diagnosis of Intrahepatic Cholangiocarcinoma in a Biopsied Tissue

For liver primary tumors, diagnosis of iCCA requires differentiation from combined hepatocellular-cholangiocarcinoma (cHCC-CC), since both components of cHCC-CC may not clearly present due to the limitations of the biopsied tissue. Application of IHC markers for hepatocellular carcinoma (HCC) is helpful to identify portions of hepatocytic differentiation. Hepatocyte paraffin-1 (Hep Par 1) and arginase-1 (ARG1) are highly sensitive and specific (both exceeding 80%) markers, and addition of glypican-3 (GPC) is shown to be useful for the diagnosis of poorly differentiated areas of hepatocytic differentiation with sensitivity over 80% (36).

Since an iCCA is histopathologically an adenocarcinoma, it is necessary to differentiate it from metastatic adenocarcinoma from other organs. Application of the following IHC markers is helpful. Caudal-type homeobox 2 (CDX2) is a widely used marker for the diagnosis of metastatic colorectal adenocarcinoma with sensitivity over 90%. Since its specificity is relatively low (70%) (37), combination with CK7 and CK20, which are usually negative and positive in colorectal adenocarcinoma, respectively, is recommended (32). Adenocarcinoma of the lung and ductal carcinoma of the breast, which can be differentiated by IHC staining with antibodies of thyroid transcription factor-1 (TTF-1; 75% sensitivity and specificity) (38, 39) and GATA binding protein 3 (GATA-3; over 90% sensitivity and specificity),

respectively (38, 40, 41). Paired box 8 (PAX8) is a sensitive marker for ovarian and endometrial carcinomas, as well as for renal cell carcinomas with sensitivity approaching 90% (40). Metastatic prostate adenocarcinoma is usually positive for the antibodies against prostate specific antigen (PSA) and prostate specific acid phosphatase (PSAP), with sensitivity and specificity exceeding 95% (40, 42). However, in cases of metastatic adenocarcinomas originating from organs adjacent to the liver including gallbladder, pancreas, and stomach, etc., it is difficult to differentiate iCCA from these tumors, due to the lack of specific IHC marker. Some potentially promising markers have been introduced, and filamin A was reported to show high positivity (63%) by immunohistochemistry on iCCA (43). Recently, an *in situ* hybridization assay for albumin RNA was reported to show 90% sensitivity and 100% specificity for iCCA, particularly for the differentiation of small duct type iCCA and metastatic tumors (44–46).

Variants of Intrahepatic Cholangiocarcinoma
Cholangiolocarcinoma

Cholangiolocarcinoma (CLC) is a variant of iCCA that belongs to the small duct type. It is defined as an iCCA with more than 80% of the tumor area showing cholangiolocellular differentiation without hepatocellular differentiation. The prefix "cholangiolo" implies histopathological similarity to the cholangiole or canals of Hering (47). CLCs show small cuboidal cells forming cords or tubular structures with antler-like growth resembling the ductular reaction of non-tumorous liver (48). Often, the lumina of tumor cords are inconspicuous, the atypia or pleomorphism of tumor epithelial cells is minimal, and regularly spaced intervening stroma is also a characteristic feature (**Figure 3A**).

CLC is thought to arise at the bile ductule, containing hepatic stem or progenitor cells, and canals of Hering. It was previously classified as a subtype of combined hepatocellular-cholangiocarcinoma (49), however, molecular profiling studies favor the classification of CLC as part of iCCA (50). According to the current WHO classification, CLC without components of HCC or intermediate carcinoma is an iCCA and is not considered as combined hepatocellular-cholangiocarcinoma.

CLC is distinguished from conventional small duct type iCCAs based on its excellent outcome, which shows significantly higher overall and disease-free survival (49, 51). Even iCCAs with cholangiolocellular differentiation (> 10% of the tumor area) were found to have a better prognosis than those without (17, 52). A transcriptomic profiling study reported that iCCA with cholangiolocellular differentiation correlated with inflammation class, while iCCA without cholangiolocellular differentiation correlated with proliferation class (the molecular classification is discussed in more detail later in the genomic-transcriptomic profiles section) (52, 53).

Intrahepatic Cholangiocarcinoma With Ductal Plate Malformation Pattern

Ductal plate malformation (DPM) refers to a developmental anomaly characterized by pathologically existing embryonic bile duct structures ("ductal plates"). The percentage of iCCAs

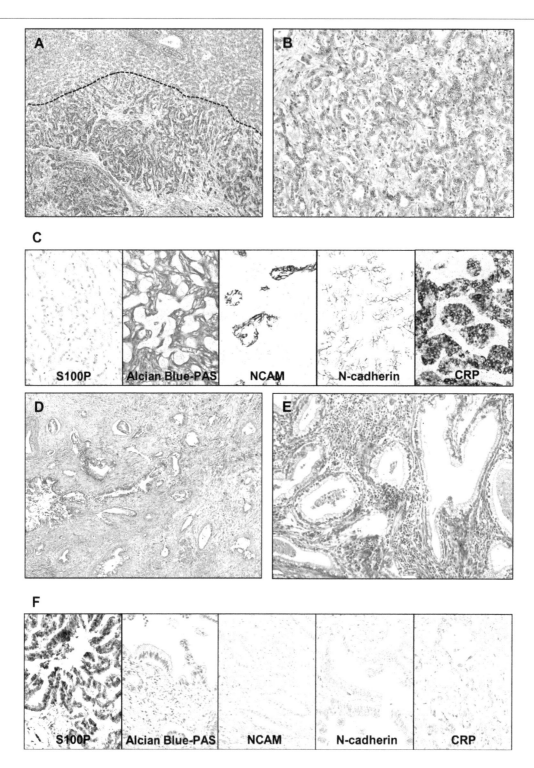

FIGURE 2 | Representative microscopic images of small duct type and large duct type intrahepatic cholangiocarcinoma (iCCA). **(A–C)** Small duct type iCCA. **(A)** A low-power view showing uniform-shaped tumor glands replacing hepatocellular trabeculae at the border (indicated by dashed line). **(B)** A higher magnification image showing the growth of cuboidal cells forming cords and small glandular structures, without intra- or extracellular mucin. **(C)** Microscopic images of special and immunohistochemical panel staining for small duct type iCCA; positive expression of NCAM, N-cadherin and CRP, negative expression of S100P, and absence of mucin in the Alcian blue staining is characteristic. **(D–F)** Large duct type iCCA. **(D)** A low magnification image shows infiltrative growth of adenocarcinoma with rich fibrous stroma. **(E)** A higher magnification image showing columnar cells with intracellular mucin forming irregular glandular spaces. **(F)** Microscopic images of special and immunohistochemical panel staining for large duct type iCCA; positive expression of S100P, presence of mucin in the Alcian blue staining, and negative expression of NCAM, N-cadherin, and CRP is characteristic. Original magnification: 40× for **(A,D)**, 100× for **(B,E)**, 200× for **(C,F)**. S100P, S100 calcium-binding protein P; NCAM, neural cell adhesion molecule; CRP, c-reactive protein; PAS, periodic acid–Schiff.

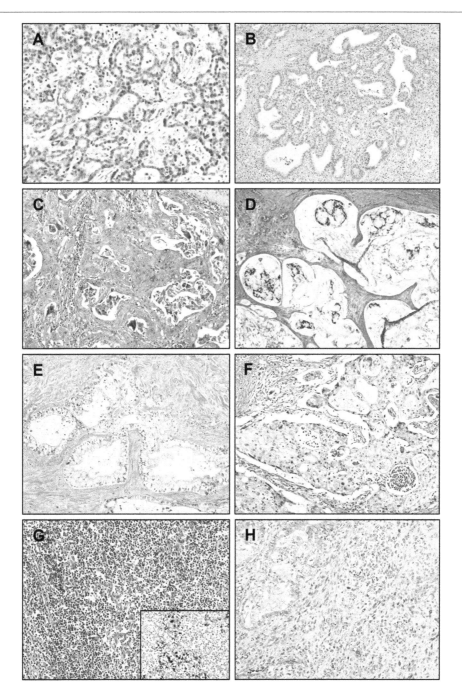

FIGURE 3 | Variants of intrahepatic cholangiocarcinoma (iCCA). **(A)** Cholangiolocarcinoma. Bland-looking small cuboidal tumor epithelial cells are forming cords or ductules, with antler-like branching pattern. **(B)** iCCA with ductal plate malformation pattern. Cuboidal tumor cells are forming irregularly dilated and coalesced spaces, resembling developmental anomaly of ductal plate. **(C)** Adenosquamous carcinoma showing both of gland-forming portion and portions with squamous differentiation. **(D)** Mucinous carcinoma. Mucin-producing tumor cell clusters are floating in mucin pools. **(E)** Clear cell carcinoma. Tumor cells have large clear cytoplasm with eccentric nuclei. **(F)** Mucoepidermoid carcinoma showing squamoid tumor cells intermixed with mucin-producing cells. **(G)** Lymphoepithelioma-like carcinoma showing marked lymphocytic infiltration into tumor epithelial component. Tumor epithelial cells are positive for Epstein–Barr virus (EBV), detected by *in situ* hybridization of EBV-encoded small RNA (inset). **(H)** Sarcomatous iCCA showing mainly pleomorphic spindle cells, with adenocarcinoma components in the upper left corner. Original magnification: 100×.

that are diagnosed as iCCAs with DPM pattern is very small, approximately 2.9% of cases in a cohort of 175 resected iCCAs (54). Histopathologically, the tumor epithelial cell lining is usually benign-looking cuboidal cells without mucin production, and they form glandular structures that are elongated, tortuous, and coalesced, mimicking ductal plates (**Figure 3B**) (55). Genetic alterations in iCCA with DPM pattern include point mutations in *FGFR2*, *PTPRT*, *ARID1A*, and *CDKN2A*, and fusion of *FGFR2* (54, 56). Patient survival seems better than that of conventional small duct type iCCAs (54).

Adenosquamous Carcinoma/Squamous Carcinoma

Adenosquamous carcinoma of the liver has both squamous epithelial and glandular components (**Figure 3C**), and its incidence is rare (57). Squamous carcinoma, showing squamous differentiation in the entire tumor is extremely rare. This type of variant iCCA is reported to be correlated with chronic cholangitis caused by liver flukes or hepatolithiasis (58). The prognosis of adenosquamous carcinoma of the liver is usually poor, with a median survival of approximately 6 months (57).

Mucinous Carcinoma/Signet Ring Cell Carcinoma

Mucinous carcinoma is a variant that belongs to large duct type iCCA. It contains an overwhelming amount of extracellular mucin in the luminal space of tumor glands, usually over 50% of the total tumor volume by convention (59), often causing tumor epithelial cells to float in the mucin pool (**Figure 3D**). This type of tumor usually occurs due to the malignant transformation of the IPNB. Signet ring cell carcinoma occasionally presents as a mucinous carcinoma with varying distribution; however, pure signet ring cell carcinoma of the liver is extremely rare. The absence of ovarian-like stroma differentiates this variant of iCCA from mucinous cystic neoplasm (60).

Clear Cell Carcinoma

Clear cell carcinoma is characterized by bulky cytoplasmic clearing and eccentrically located nuclei in most tumor epithelial cells with glandular and trabecular growth patterns (**Figure 3E**) (58, 61). Primary clear cell carcinoma of the liver can be differentiated from HCC with clear cell change, metastatic clear cell carcinoma of the kidney, and metastasis from other gastrointestinal tract tumors by IHC staining for hepatocyte paraffin 1 (HepPar-1), CD10, and CK20, respectively (62).

Mucoepidermoid Carcinoma

Primary mucoepidermoid carcinoma of the liver shows features similar to those in other organs, including the salivary glands. It reveals a more intimate mixture of epidermoid or squamous and mucin-secreting elements, compared to adenosquamous carcinoma where mucin-secreting cells and foci of squamous differentiation exist separately (**Figure 3F**) (63). There have been only a few reports, and most of them have shown a poor prognosis (64).

Lymphoepithelioma-Like Carcinoma

Lymphoepithelioma-like carcinoma is characterized by dense lymphoid stroma around the tumor epithelial cells, often forming lymphoid follicles. Tumor epithelial cells show an undifferentiated or gland-forming pattern, rarely with well-differentiated or bland-looking glands (**Figure 3G**). Almost all cases are Epstein–Barr virus-encoded small RNA (EBER) positive and usually have favorable outcomes (65, 66).

Sarcomatous Intrahepatic Cholangiocarcinoma

Sarcomatous iCCA usually shows mixed features of conventional iCCA and undifferentiated components of cells with spindle or rhabdoid features (**Figure 3H**). When a conventional iCCA component is not present, a definite diagnosis is difficult, since the sarcomatoid component is often negative for epithelial markers by IHC staining (67). Sarcomatous iCCA usually has a worse prognosis than conventional iCCAs (68).

Precursor Lesions
Biliary Intraepithelial Neoplasia

Biliary intraepithelial neoplasia (BilIN), a precursor lesion of CCA, occurs at the epithelium of intra- and extrahepatic bile ducts and in the peribiliary glands. Large duct type iCCA, but not small duct type, is often accompanied by BilIN (17, 21). BilIN is virtually invisible upon gross examination, although it may be associated with subtle changes such as mucosal thickening. Microscopically, BilIN consists of flat or micropapillary (less than 3 mm in height) epithelial lesions that are graded as low-grade or high-grade (carcinoma *in situ*) based on the highest degree of cytoarchitectural atypia (69, 70). This two-tiered classification replaces the former three-tiered classification, wherein the former BilIN-1 and BilIN-2 are now classified as low-grade, and the former BilIN-3 is now classified as high-grade.

Low-grade BilIN shows mild cytoarchitectural atypia, including flat pseudopapillary and/or micropapillary growth pattern, nuclear stratification, hyperchromatic nuclei, and increased nuclear-cytoplasmic ratio; however, nuclear polarity is preserved. High-grade BilIN is characterized by moderate to severe cytoarchitectural atypia, including more complex patterns, complete loss of polarity, marked nuclear atypia, and frequent mitosis. While IHC staining for p53 is usually negative in low-grade BilIN, it is often overexpressed in high-grade BilIN (71). The expression of p16 is relatively preserved in low-grade BilIN and decreased in high-grade BilIN (72). A notable mutation in BilIN lesions is alterations in *KRAS*, which is reported to be approximately 30% (73) (**Figures 4A,B**).

Differentiating BilIN from reactive epithelial atypia may be difficult, especially in biopsy samples. Reactive atypia shows overlapping attenuated basophilic cells with nuclei having fine and diffuse chromatin. The nucleoli are small or conspicuous. Mitotic activity may be prominent. Reactive epithelial atypia usually shows a gradual transition from uninvolved epithelium, in contrast to the abrupt change usually seen in BilIN. The IHC detection of S100P was shown to be useful, being mostly negative in reactive epithelial atypia. However, its expression increased sequentially from low-grade BilIN to high-grade BilIN and subsequently in iCCA (74).

Intraductal Papillary Neoplasm of the Bile Duct

Intraductal papillary neoplasm of the bile duct (IPNB) is defined as a grossly visible premalignant neoplasm showing intraductal papillary or villous growth of biliary-type epithelium (70). It is considered to be a counterpart of a similar tumor arising in the pancreas, the so-called intraductal papillary mucinous neoplasm (IPMN). IPNB is divided into low-grade and high-grade based on the highest degree of cytoarchitectural atypia.

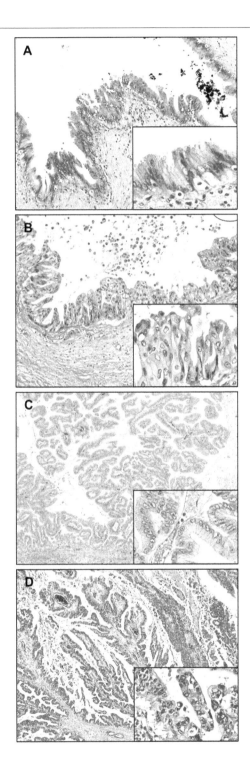

FIGURE 4 | Precursor lesions of intrahepatic cholangiocarcinoma. **(A,B)** Biliary intraepithelial neoplasia (BilIN). **(A)** Low-grade BilIN composed of columnar cells with intact nuclear polarity and minimal atypia. **(B)** High-grade BilIN showing stratification of cells with marked nuclear atypia and loss of polarity. **(C,D)** Intraductal papillary neoplasm of the bile ducts (IPNB). **(C)** Low-grade IPNB showing a papillary growth of columnar biliary type epithelial cells with mild pleomorphism and preserved nuclear polarity. **(D)** High-grade IPNB showing irregular papillary projections, composed of highly pleomorphic and stratified cells with increased nuclear-cytoplasmic ratio. Original magnification: 100× for **(A,B)**, 40× for **(C,D)**, 200× for inset images.

When invasive carcinoma develops in this lesion, it is diagnosed as IPNB with associated invasive carcinoma. High-grade IPNBs are often associated with stromal invasive carcinoma, usually consisting of tubular adenocarcinoma and occasionally mucinous carcinoma (75).

Grossly, IPNBs appear as polypoid masses with dilatation of the bile ducts. These are usually isolated papillary lesions, whereas some IPNBs appear as multiple contiguous papillary or polypoid lesions. Some IPNBs are characterized by mucus hypersecretion, forming mucin-containing fusiform dilatation or cysts, similar to those observed in IPMNs (76). Microscopically, IPNBs form papillary structures with fine fibrovascular cores (**Figures 4C,D**). Four histological subtypes are generally accepted based on cytological appearance and immunophenotype, namely, – pancreatobiliary, intestinal, gastric, and oncocytic. Immunohistochemically, MUC1 is mostly expressed in the pancreatobiliary type. Gastric type usually express MUC5AC and MUC6, and the intestinal type frequently express MUC2. CK20 is positive in the intestinal type, but not in the gastric and oncocytic types (70, 77). The presence of two or more histopathological types is common in IPNB, therefore these tumors are diagnosed based on the most prevalent histopathological type. The pancreatobiliary type is most common, with higher prevalence in western countries than in Asia. In contrast, intestinal type is more common in Asian populations than in western populations, while oncocytic and gastric types are least frequent (78). Although the clinical implications of histopathologic subtypes are still controversial, the pancreatobiliary type is reported to be linked with a higher frequency of associated invasive carcinoma, frequent lymph node metastasis, and recurrence (77).

A recent consensus has proposed a different classification for IPNBs of type 1 and type 2 (79, 80). Type 1 IPNB shows more homogeneous appearance than type 2 IPNB, and is composed of regular villous, papillary, or tubular structures usually with low-grade dysplasia, but may present with high-grade dysplasia with foci of low-grade dysplasia. Mucin overproduction is frequently observed, whereas stromal invasion is uncommon. This is most commonly found in intrahepatic bile ducts. Histological similarity with IPMN of the pancreas is also characteristic. Type 2 IPNB exhibits heterogenous appearance composed of irregular and complicated villous, papillary or tubular structures. This is usually composed of high-grade dysplasia, and foci of low-grade dysplasia are absent or minimal. Invasive carcinoma is more frequently associated with type 2 IPNB than type 1 IPNB. Mucin overproduction is not common. Type 2 IPNB arises throughout the biliary tree, including intrahepatic and extrahepatic bile ducts.

The mutational profile studies on IPNB have reported that diverse cancer driver mutations are frequently observed, including *KRAS*, *TP53*, *STK11*, *CTNNB1*, *APC*, *SMAD4*, and *GNAS*. Type 1 IPNBs show higher mutation rates of *KRAS*, *GNAS*, and *RNF43*, whereas type 2 IPNBs have higher *TP53* and *SMAD4* mutation rates (81, 82).

Although IPNBs present papillary morphology, sometimes tubular growth pattern of epithelial components with less mucin production is predominantly observed, similar to intraductal tubulopapillary neoplasm (ITPN) of the pancreas (83). Such cases have been described as intraductal tubular neoplasms or ITPNs. Recently, ITPN has been reported to show more frequent intrahepatic occurrence in contrast to IPNB, which favors both intra- and extrahepatic locations. Furthermore, IPNB and ITPN differ in their genomic and epigenomic profiles. Recently, IPNB has been reported to share mutational profiles with extrahepatic CCA, including mutations in *TP53*, *SMAD4*, and *KRAS* and deletions on chromosomes 9q, 17p, and 18q. However, ITPN shows low overall mutational burden, and distinct DNA methylation pattern that clustered together with iCCA rather than extrahepatic CCA, suggesting that IPNB and ITPN are distinct entities (84).

TUMOR MICROENVIRONMENT OF INTRAHEPATIC CHOLANGIOCARCINOMA

One of the characteristics of iCCA is the abundance of fibrous stroma (85). The amount of fibrous stroma has been reported to be associated with poor prognosis (86). Furthermore, so-called "scirrhous type" iCCA, which is defined as iCCA having scirrhous area (where the amount of fibrous stromal component is at least equal to the area of epithelial component) more than 70% of the largest cut surface, has been reported to show worse prognosis than conventional iCCAs (87). More recently, the characteristics of immature and mature fibrous tumor stroma have been reported to be related to tumor behavior (88, 89). Immature stroma is composed of myxoid stroma with randomly oriented short keloid-like collagen bundles. In contrast, mature stroma shows multilayered mature collagen fibers (**Figure 5**). Accordingly, iCCAs with immature stroma have been reported to show poorer prognosis compared to iCCAs with mature stroma (88, 89).

Activated CAFs, one of the major components of the tumor microenvironment, have been demonstrated to facilitate tumor growth and progression, and promote immunosuppression in tumors (90). CAFs are thought to be recruited from hepatic stellate cells, portal fibroblasts, or circulating mesenchymal cells, but the exact source is currently unknown (91). Transforming growth factor β (TGF-β) and platelet-derived growth factor D (PDGF-D) secreted by tumor epithelial cells recruit CAFs. Recruited CAFs not only promote desmoplastic reaction by collagen and matrix metalloproteinases, but also cause tumor epithelial cells to proliferate, invade, and resist antitumor mechanisms by secreting growth factors such as PDGF-B and epidermal growth factors (92, 93). Patients with iCCA with a high proportion of activated CAFs were reported to have a shorter survival rate than patients with low CAF proportion (94).

Immune cells, including tumor-associated macrophages (TAMs) and tumor-infiltrating lymphocytes, are also main components of the tumor microenvironment. The hepatic macrophage population consists of activated macrophages derived from Kupffer cells or bone marrow-derived macrophages (95), and activated macrophages can be classified as M1- (classical) and M2 (alternative)-polarized types (96). The M2 phenotype forms the majority of TAM population in iCCA, having anti-inflammatory and pro-tumor functions mediated by

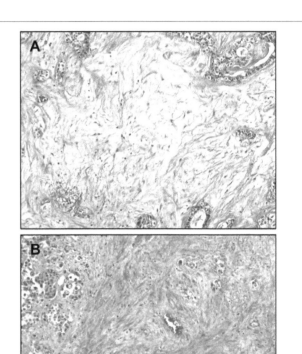

FIGURE 5 | Stromal features of intrahepatic cholangiocarcinoma. **(A)** Immature stroma showing pale basophilic myxoid appearance. Activated fibroblasts are the main components of the stroma. Collagen fibers are incomplete and thin. **(B)** Mature stroma showing thick collagen bundles, making its eosinophilic color. Original magnification: 100×.

the secretion of anti-inflammatory cytokines, including IL-4, IL-10, IL-13, and TGF-β (97). These cells also promote intratumoral angiogenesis, which is vital for tumor survival and metastasis (85, 98). A high proportion of M2 TAMs in iCCA is correlated with increased invasiveness of tumor cells and poor disease-free survival (97, 99). In contrast, M1 TAMs have been reported to exert pro-inflammatory functions, including secretion of pro-inflammatory cytokines such as TNF-α, interleukin (IL)-6, and IL-1β (99).

Tumor-infiltrating lymphocytes include B cells (CD20+), helper T cells (CD4+), cytotoxic T cells (CD8+), and regulatory T cells (Tregs, FOXP3+). The major proportion of tumor-infiltrating lymphocytes comprises T cells rather than B cells (100). The distribution and proportion of CD4+ and CD8+ T cells varies among iCCAs, and increased population of these cells is correlated with better prognosis (8, 85). In addition, iCCAs with B cell infiltration have been reported to be associated with better survival than iCCAs without B cells (101). Treg cells are a subset of CD4+ T cells that suppress innate and adaptive immune responses mainly by secreting IL-10 and TGF-β, which are known to promote tumor progression by inhibiting antitumor immune response. Regarding iCCA, while there are a few studies on the clinical aspects of the presence of Treg cells, there is no sufficient evidence to draw a conclusion. Therefore, additional investigation is required (101–103).

With the advent of immune checkpoint blockade therapeutics, the expression status of cell surface proteins with immune escape mechanisms is currently under active investigation. Cytotoxic T-lymphocyte antigen-4 (CTLA-4), expressed on the surface of Treg cells, suppresses cytotoxic T cell activity by binding to CD80 of antigen-presenting cells (85). High CTLA-4 expression has been reported to be related to worse relapse-free survival of patients with CCA, raising the possibility of effective immunotherapy targeting CTLA-4 (104). Programmed death 1 (PD-1), expressed on T cells, and its ligand programmed death ligand 1 (PD-L1), on tumor epithelial cells, are other major immune checkpoints of interest. Binding of PD-L1 to PD-1 diminishes the immunological function of cytotoxic T cells. Approximately 9–30% of iCCA has been reported to be PD-L1 positive as observed by IHC staining (105–107). Recently, our group reported that KRAS alteration and chromosomal instability were associated with resistance to PD-1/PD-L1 blockade immunotherapy, whereas high intratumoral tumor-infiltrating lymphocyte density was associated with a favorable immunotherapy response in patients with CCA (35). Many clinical trials for iCCA using immune checkpoint inhibitors are ongoing based on the expression status of markers, including PD-1, PD-L1, and CTLA-4, with expectations of promising results in the near future (108).

MULTI-OMICS FEATURES OF INTRAHEPATIC CHOLANGIOCARCINOMA

Germline and Somatic Mutational Profile of Intrahepatic Cholangiocarcinoma
Germline Predisposition

There are a few germline predispositions for cancers, including proto-oncogenes and tumor suppressor genes, either by inheritance from parents or *de novo* mutation at the zygote level. Approximately 8–12% of iCCAs have been reported to have known pathogenic or possibly deleterious germline mutations, and the most commonly found germline-mutated genes are BRCA1 and BRCA2, which are associated with DNA repair mechanism and hereditary cancer syndromes (109–112) (**Table 1**). Other germline variants linked with iCCA include APC, an antagonist of the Wnt signaling pathway, BAP1, which mediates deubiquitination, and mismatch repair mechanism-related genes, namely MLH1 and MSH2 (109, 111, 113). However, evidence regarding the association between known hereditary cancer syndromes and iCCA is currently not fully established and requires further investigation.

Somatic Short Mutations, Structural Variations, and Copy Number Aberrations

Among somatic mutations identified in iCCA, the most well-known and frequent variants are at exons 5–8 of TP53 and

TABLE 1 | Summary of germline mutations reported in intrahepatic cholangiocarcinoma.

Gene	Frequency of occurrence (%)	References
BRCA1	1–3	(109–111)
BRCA2	1–3	(109–111)
MLH1	2	(109)
MSH2	2	(109)
MUTYH	2	(111)
BAP1	1	(111)
PMS2	1	(111)
APC	1	(111)

hotspots at codons 12/13 of KRAS, which are involved in cell cycle arrest/DNA repair and mitogen-activated protein kinase (MAPK) signaling pathway, respectively (114–116). Other MAPK pathway genes such as NRAS and BRAF are also frequently mutated in iCCA (117). Owing to the advancement and wide use of massive parallel sequencing techniques, many other driver gene mutations have been discovered in the last decade. Single-nucleotide variants of chromatin remodeling-related genes such as ARID1A, BAP1, and PBRM1 have been reported with frequencies ranging from 6 to over 30% (115, 118–120). Moreover, mutations in IDH1/2, which acts as an epigenetic regulator, are most frequently observed, with an average incidence of approximately 15% (115, 121–124). Other somatic short mutations include Akt signaling pathway-associated genes such as PTEN, PIK3CA, and PIK3C2A, and SMAD4, a TGF-β signaling pathway gene (115, 118, 125, 126).

The most frequently found structural variation in iCCA is FGFR gene fusion, notably FGFR2, which has been reported in 6–14% of iCCAs (127, 128). The most common fusion partner is BICC1; however, several other genes were also found, including AHCYL1 and PPHLN1 (128–130). Driver gene amplification was found in ERBB2 (2–12%), MDM2 (0–13%), EGFR (1–16%), and CCND1 (10–13%). Deletion of 9p21.3, or the locus including genes CDKN2A and CDKN2B is found in 10–20% of iCCA (13, 126, 127, 131).

Microsatellite instability-high cases are usually determined by three methods namely, observing the size change in more than three out of five marker loci by polymerase chain reaction, IHC for mismatch repair proteins including, MLH1, MSH2, MSH6, and PMS2, or estimation of tumor mutation burden by NGS. Such cases are known to be rare (around 1%) in iCCA (126, 132–134). The mutational characteristics of iCCA are summarized in **Table 2**.

Genetic alterations are also correlated with pathological features. Hotspot mutations in KRAS have been reported in periductal infiltrating type, but not in mass-forming type (135). Histopathologically, small duct type has been reported to have more frequent BAP1 and IDH1/2 hotspot mutations and FGFR2 fusion, and lower incidence of KRAS mutation than large duct type (12, 26, 51, 122, 136, 137). On the contrary, large duct type is known to have frequent mutations in TP53, KRAS and some

TABLE 2 | Major somatic variants and reported incidence in intrahepatic cholangiocarcinoma.

	Groups	Gene or locus	Frequency of occurrence (range, %)	References
Small nucleotide variants	DNA repair	TP53	2.5–39.3	(13, 35, 115, 120, 123, 125, 126, 131)
	Chromatin remodeling	ARID1A	7–36	(13, 35, 115, 120, 123, 126, 131)
		BAP1	6–16	(13, 35, 116, 121, 123, 126, 131)
		PBRM1	9–14.3	(13, 35, 116, 119, 121, 123, 126, 131)
	MAPK signaling pathway	KRAS	2–30.3	(13, 35, 115, 121, 123, 125, 126, 131)
		NRAS	3–9.3	(13, 115, 117, 119, 125, 126, 131)
		BRAF	3–5	(13, 35, 117, 125, 126, 131)
	Epigenetic regulator	IDH1	5–36	(13, 35, 115, 126, 131)
		IDH2	3.7–36	(13, 115, 117, 119, 121, 126, 131)
	TGF-β signaling pathway	SMAD4	0–9	(13, 35, 115, 126, 131)
	Akt signaling Pathway	PTEN	0.6–11	(13, 115, 117, 125, 126, 131)
		PIK3CA	3–7	(13, 35, 115, 117, 119, 120, 125, 126, 131)
		PIK3C2A	0–7.1	(117)
Structural variation	Translocation	FGFR2	6–14	(13, 127, 128, 131)
	Amplification	CCND1	10–13	(13, 35, 131)
		EGFR	1–16	(126, 131)
		ERBB2	2–12	(35, 126, 131)
		MDM2	0–13	(131)
	Deletion	9p21.3 (CDKN2A/B)	10–20	(126, 131)
Microsatellite instability			~1	(126, 131, 133)

TGF-β pathway genes, including *SMAD4*, *TGFBR2*, *FBXW7*, and *MYC* (35).

From an etiological point of view, liver fluke *O. viverrini* infection-related iCCA had a higher *TP53* mutation rate, while *BAP1* and *IDH1/2* mutations were more frequently found in non-fluke-related cases (131, 138). *TP53* mutation was also found to be significantly correlated with hepatitis B virus (HBV) infection (127, 139). Regarding patient outcome, worse overall survival of patients with mutated *TP53*, *KRAS*, and *TERT* or deleted *CDKN2A* has been reported (126).

Genomic-Transcriptomic Profiles: Molecular Classification of Intrahepatic Cholangiocarcinoma

Several multi-omics approaches have been reported in the past decade, and several molecular classifications of iCCA have been presented (**Table 3**).

Inflammation/Proliferation Class

Integrated gene expression and mutational analyses performed by Sia et al. revealed two classes (inflammation and proliferation) of iCCA (53). The inflammation class accounted for approximately 40% of iCCA, and it was characterized by activation of immune response-related pathways, including dendritic cell signature and cytokines such as IL-4 and IL-10. The proliferation class showed activation of several oncogenic pathways including receptor tyrosine kinase pathway genes, such as *EGF*, *RAS*, *AKT*, *MET*, and other growth factor genes. Patient outcomes were worse in the proliferation class than in the inflammation class.

Prognosis-Based Classes

Transcriptomic profiling of iCCA and perihilar CCA by Andersen et al. revealed two prognostic groups (C1 and C2) with 5-year survival rate. The group with poor prognosis (C2) indicated increased activation of *VEGF/ERBB*, *CTNNB1/MYC*, and *TNF* signaling network and *KRAS* mutation, whereas these characteristics were not seen in the group with good prognosis (C1) (140). Recently, the gene expression pattern of iCCAs with cholangiolocellular differentiation trait, having favorable prognosis, was reported to be similar to that of C1, and has a signature including upregulated expression of inflammation-related genes and downregulated expression of proliferation-related genes based on Gene Ontology terms (52, 141).

Tumor Microenvironment-Based Classes

A recent study on the classification of iCCA according to its tumor microenvironment presented four subtypes based on gene signature analysis: "immunogenic," which shows high innate and adaptive immune cell infiltration, "myeloid-rich," which has strong macrophage and myeloid signatures, "mesenchymal," with strong activated fibroblast signature, and "immune-desert," which is characterized by lowest expression of all signatures (142). The immunogenic subtype had the best outcome, whereas the mesenchymal subtype had the worst outcome, in agreement with the prognostic features of the tumor microenvironment of iCCA discussed previously.

Other Classifications

Multi-omics data from TCGA project revealed that *IDH1/2*- and *PBRM1*-mutant subgroups showed upregulation of

TABLE 3 | Notable classification of intrahepatic cholangiocarcinoma from multi-omics studies.

Base of classification	Number of cases	Molecular classification and characteristics	References

Inflammation versus proliferation signature	149	• Inflammation class
		  - Enriched in immune response-related pathways
		  - Overexpression of *IL-4* and *IL-10* (Th2 marker)
		  - Favorable prognosis
		• Proliferation class
		  - Enriched in oncogenic pathways including RTK and angiogenic pathways, increased expression of *EGF*, *RAS*, *AKT*, *MET*, and growth factors
		  - Worse outcome compared to inflammation class
			Sia et al. (53)

Prognosis	104*	• Cluster 1 (group with good prognosis)
		  - No *KRAS* mutation
		  - Absence or weak expression of *HER2* and *MET*
		• Cluster 2 (group with poor prognosis)
		  - Enriched *VEGF/ERBB*, *CTNNB1/MYC*, and TNF pathway and *KRAS* mutation
			Andersen et al. (140)

Tumor microenvironment	78	• Immune desert subtype
		  - Minimal expression of all TME signatures
		• Immunogenic subtype
		  - High innate and adaptive immune cell presence
		  - Strong activation of fibroblasts and inflammatory and immune checkpoint pathways
		  - Best outcome
		• Myeloid-rich subtype
		  - Strong monocyte-derived myeloid cell signatures
		  - Low lymphoid signatures
		• Mesenchymal subtype
		  - Strong active fibroblast signatures
		  - Worst outcome
			Job et al. (142)

TCGA project	32	• *IDH*-mutant cluster
		  - *IDH1/2* mutation
		  - Enriched mitochondrial gene expression
		  - Loss of function of *ARID1A* and *PBRM1*
		• *CCND1* amplification cluster
		  - Highly methylated
		  - *BAP1/FGFR* cluster
		• *BAP1* mutation or *FGFR2* fusion
		• Survival difference is not significant between clusters
			Farshidfar et al. (13)

Etiologic factor-associated	69	• Cluster 1
		  - Liver fluke-related
		  - *ARID1A*, *BRCA1/2*, and *TP53* mutations
		  - *ERBB2* amplification
		  - CpG island hypermethylation
		• Cluster 2
		  - Partly liver-fluke-related
		  - *TP53* mutation
		  - High expression of *CTNNB1*, *WNT5B* and *AKT1*
		• Cluster 3
		  - High CNA burden
		  - Enriched immune-related pathways
		• Cluster 4
		  - Associated with viral hepatitis
		  - *BAP1* or *IDH1/2* mutation
		  - High expression of *FGFR* family proteins
		  - CpG shore hypermethylation
		  - Favorable prognosis
			Jusakul et al. (131)

*Whether only intrahepatic cholangiocarcinoma was included is not certain.
CNA, copy number aberration; HCC, hepatocellular carcinoma; IL, interleukin; RTK, receptor tyrosine kinase; TCGA-CHOL, The Cancer Genome Atlas-Cholangiocarcinoma Consortium; TME, tumor microenvironment.

mitochondrial genes and downregulation of chromatin-modifying genes such as *ARID1A* and *ARID1B* due to hypermethylation of the promoter CpG region, while cases with *FGFR2* fusion showed downregulation of mitochondrial genes (13). Furthermore, another study has proposed a classification based on the correlation of multi-omics features with etiologic

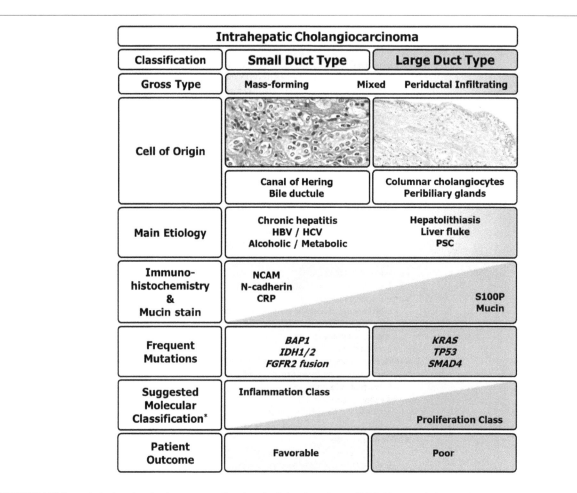

FIGURE 6 | Clinico-pathologic and molecular summary of intrahepatic cholangiocarcinoma (iCCA). Macro and microscopic, immunohistochemical, mutational, and clinical overview of iCCA. HBV, hepatitis B virus; HCV, hepatitis C virus; PSC, primary sclerosing cholangitis; S100P, S100 calcium-binding protein P; NCAM, neural cell adhesion molecule; CRP, c-reactive protein. *Based on the classification by Sia et al. (53).

background, showing that liver fluke-associated clusters 1 and 2, which harbor *TP53* mutation and *ERBB2* amplification in common, can be differentiated based on hypermethylated CpG island (for cluster 1). Furthermore, liver fluke-negative clusters 3 and 4 can be subdivided based on immune-related pathway enrichment (for cluster 3), and *IDH1/2* mutations, *FGFR2* fusion, and hypermethylated CpG promoter shores associated with viral hepatitis (for cluster 4) (131).

Moleculo-Pathological Correlation

The two major pathological types, small duct type and large duct type iCCA differ in their molecular characteristics. Small duct type iCCAs frequently have *BAP1*, *IDH1/2*, and *FGFR* mutations, while large duct type iCCAs more commonly show *KRAS*, *TP53*, and *SMAD4* mutations. Interestingly, iCCA with cholangiolocellular differentiation trait, which belongs to the small duct type, has been reported to be correlated with inflammation class and group with good prognosis (C1) (52, 53, 140). The pathological, clinical, and molecular characteristics of iCCA based on currently available evidence are summarized in **Figure 6**.

Perspectives on Targeted Therapies

Large-scale genomic analyses have identified target molecules for chemotherapy of patients with iCCA. Thus far, use of fibroblast growth factor receptor (FGFR) inhibitors and isocitrate dehydrogenase (IDH) 1 and 2 inhibitors are promising strategies against iCCA (130, 143).

Fibroblast growth factor receptor family proteins are localized on the cell membrane and transfer extracellular growth signals through intracellular tyrosine kinase domains. Pemigatinib, an oral inhibitor of FGFR1-3, has been approved by the United States Food and Drug Administration (FDA) for the treatment of patients with refractory advanced CCA with *FGFR2* fusion (130).

Isocitrate dehydrogenase 1 and 2 proteins are essential components of the tricarboxylic acid cycle, that normally generate NADPH *via* conversion of isocitrate into α-ketoglutarate. Mutant IDH1/2 proteins accelerate this process, resulting in excess production of the byproduct, 2-hydroxyglutarate, which acts as an oncometabolite by interfering with histone and DNA methylation regulation (143). A recent phase 3 clinical trial of the IDH1 inhibitor ivosidenib in patients with advanced iCCA has shown promising results in increasing overall survival, and the FDA has approved its use in previously treated *IDH1*-mutated iCCA patients (143, 144).

Even though there is hope for these approved target agents, application is limited to those who harbor specific mutations, and antitumor efficacy is limited by intratumoral heterogeneity and drug resistance. Other targeted protein inhibitor molecules are in active clinical trials, including other inhibitors of FGFR family; multi-kinase inhibitors that act on epidermal growth factor receptor, vascular endothelial growth factor receptor and platelet-derived growth factor receptor; specific tyrosine kinase inhibitors targeting HER2, BRAF inhibitors, and immune checkpoint inhibitors (145, 146). To detect a variety of potential actionable mutations, the European Society for Medical Oncology has recommended routine use of NGS in patients with advanced cholangiocarcinoma (147).

CONCLUSION

Intrahepatic cholangiocarcinoma is a very heterogenous malignancy with respect to histomorphology and molecular

perspectives. The tumor microenvironment of iCCA also varies significantly depending on the type of immune cell infiltration and tumor stromal characteristics. Histopathological classification of small duct and large duct types shows differences in etiology, molecular features, and clinical outcomes. Analyses of NGS and multi-omics studies have suggested molecular classifications of iCCA and identified *FGFR2* fusion and *IDH1/2* mutations as indications for targeted drugs. Further studies are needed for better pathological-molecular correlation and marker development for targeted therapy as well as immunotherapy to improve the treatment efficacy of patients with iCCA.

AUTHOR CONTRIBUTIONS

TC and YP contributed to the conception and design of this manuscript. TC performed the literature search, data analysis, and wrote the first draft of the manuscript. YP critically revised the manuscript. Both authors approved the submitted version.

REFERENCES

1. Nagorney DM, Pawlik TM, Chun YS, Ebata T, Vauthey J-N. Perihilar bile ducts. 8th ed. In: Edge SB, American Joint Committee on Cancer editors. *AJCC Cancer Staging Manual*. New York, NY: Springer (2017).

2. Massarweh NN, El-Serag HB. Epidemiology of Hepatocellular carcinoma and intrahepatic cholangiocarcinoma. *Cancer Control*. (2017) 24:1073274817729245. doi: 10.1177/1073274817729245

3. Nakanuma Y, Klimstra DS, Komuta M, Zen Y. Intrahepatic cholangiocarcinoma. 5th ed. In: WHO Classification of Tumours Editorial Board editor. *Digestive System Tumours*. Lyon: International Agency for Research on Cancer (2019).

4. Florio AA, Ferlay J, Znaor A, Ruggieri D, Alvarez CS, Laversanne M, et al. Global incidence of and trends in intrahepatic and extrahepatic cholangiocarcinoma from 1993 to 2012. *Cancer*. (2020) 126:2666–78. doi: 10.1002/cncr.32803

5. Khan SA, Tavolari S, Brandi G. Cholangiocarcinoma: epidemiology and risk factors. *Liver Int*. (2019) 39:19–31. doi: 10.1111/liv.14095

6. Jeong Y-I, Shin H-E, Lee S-E, Cheun H-I, Ju J-W, Kim J-Y, et al. Prevalence of *Clonorchis sinensis* Infection among residents along 5 major rivers in the republic of Korea. *Korean J Parasitol*. (2016) 54:215–9. doi: 10.3347/kjp.2016.54.2.215

7. Kitphati R, Watanawong O, Wongsaroj T, Nithikathkul C. National program of opisthorchiasis in Thailand; situation and policy strategy. *Int J Geoinf*. (2021) 17:61–8. doi: 10.52939/ijg.v17i2.1759

8. Banales JM, Marin JJG, Lamarca A, Rodrigues PM, Khan SA, Roberts LR, et al. Cholangiocarcinoma 2020: the next horizon in mechanisms and management. *Nat Rev Gastroenterol Hepatol*. (2020) 17:557–88. doi: 10.1038/s41575-020-0310-z

9. Buettner S, van Vugt JL, Jn IJ, Groot Koerkamp B. Intrahepatic cholangiocarcinoma: current perspectives. *OncoTargets Ther*. (2017) 10:1131–42. doi: 10.2147/ott.S93629

10. Yu T-H, Chen X, Zhang X-H, Zhang E-C, Sun C-X. Clinicopathological characteristics and prognostic factors for intrahepatic cholangiocarcinoma:

a population-based study. *Sci Rep*. (2021) 11:3990. doi: 10.1038/s41598-021-83149-5

11. Lee Y-T, Wang JJ, Luu M, Noureddin M, Nissen NN, Patel TC, et al. Comparison of clinical features and outcomes between intrahepatic cholangiocarcinoma and hepatocellular carcinoma in the United States. *Hepatology*. (2021) 74:2622–32. doi: 10.1002/hep.32007

12. Hayashi A, Misumi K, Shibahara J, Arita J, Sakamoto Y, Hasegawa K, et al. Distinct clinicopathologic and genetic features of 2 histologic subtypes of intrahepatic cholangiocarcinoma. *Am J Surg Pathol*. (2016) 40:1021–30. doi: 10.1097/pas.0000000000000670

13. Farshidfar F, Zheng S, Gingras MC, Newton Y, Shih J, Robertson AG, et al. Integrative genomic analysis of cholangiocarcinoma identifies distinct IDH-mutant molecular profiles. *Cell Rep*. (2017) 18:2780–94. doi: 10.1016/j.celrep.2017.02.033

14. Cerami E, Gao J, Dogrusoz U, Gross BE, Sumer SO, Aksoy BA, et al. The cBio cancer genomics portal: an open platform for exploring multidimensional cancer genomics data. *J Cancer Discov*. (2012) 2:401–4. doi: 10.1158/2159-8290.CD-12-0095

15. Yamasaki S. Intrahepatic cholangiocarcinoma: macroscopic type and stage classification. *J Hepatobiliary Pancreat Surg*. (2003) 10:288–91. doi: 10.1007/s00534-002-0732-8

16. Nakanuma Y, Miyata T, Uchida T. Latest advances in the pathological understanding of cholangiocarcinomas. *Expert Rev Gastroenterol Hepatol*. (2016) 10:113–27. doi: 10.1586/17474124.2016.1104246

17. Chung T, Rhee H, Nahm JH, Jeon Y, Yoo JE, Kim Y-J, et al. Clinicopathological characteristics of intrahepatic cholangiocarcinoma according to gross morphologic type: cholangiolocellular differentiation traits and inflammation- and proliferation-phenotypes. *HPB*. (2020) 22:864–73. doi: 10.1016/j.hpb.2019.10.009

18. Kim Y, Lee K, Jeong S, Wen X, Cho NY, Kang GH. DLEC1 methylation is associated with a better clinical outcome in patients with intrahepatic cholangiocarcinoma of the small duct subtype. *Virchows Arch*. (2019) 475:49–58. doi: 10.1007/s00428-018-02511-7

19. Sigel CS, Drill E, Zhou Y, Basturk O, Askan G, Pak LM, et al. Intrahepatic cholangiocarcinomas have histologically and immunophenotypically distinct

small and large duct patterns. *Am J Surg Pathol.* (2018) 42:1334–45. doi: 10.1097/pas.0000000000001118

20. Aishima S, Oda Y. Pathogenesis and classification of intrahepatic cholangiocarcinoma: different characters of perihilar large duct type versus peripheral small duct type. *J Hepatobiliary Pancreat Sci.* (2015) 22:94–100. doi: 10.1002/jhbp.154

21. Akita M, Sofue K, Fujikura K, Otani K, Itoh T, Ajiki T, et al. Histological and molecular characterization of intrahepatic bile duct cancers suggests an expanded definition of perihilar cholangiocarcinoma. *HPB (Oxford).* (2019) 21:226–34. doi: 10.1016/j.hpb.2018.07.021

22. Komuta M, Govaere O, Vandecaveye V, Akiba J, Van Steenbergen W, Verslype C, et al. Histological diversity in cholangiocellular carcinoma reflects the different cholangiocyte phenotypes. *Hepatology.* (2012) 55:1876–88. doi: 10.1002/hep.25595

23. Theise ND, Saxena R, Portmann BC, Thung SN, Yee H, Chiriboga L, et al. The canals of Hering and hepatic stem cells in humans. *Hepatology.* (1999) 30:1425–33. doi: 10.1002/hep.510300614

24. Guest RV, Boulter L, Kendall TJ, Minnis-Lyons SE, Walker R, Wigmore SJ, et al. Cell lineage tracing reveals a biliary origin of intrahepatic cholangiocarcinoma. *J Cancer Res.* (2014) 74:1005–10. doi: 10.1158/0008-5472.CAN-13-1911

25. Moeini A, Haber PK, Sia D. Cell of origin in biliary tract cancers and clinical implications. *JHEP Rep.* (2021) 3:100226. doi: 10.1016/j.jhepr.2021.100226

26. Tsai JH, Huang WC, Kuo KT, Yuan RH, Chen YL, Jeng YM. S100P immunostaining identifies a subset of peripheral-type intrahepatic cholangiocarcinomas with morphological and molecular features similar to those of perihilar and extrahepatic cholangiocarcinomas. *Histopathology.* (2012) 61:1106–16. doi: 10.1111/j.1365-2559.2012.04316.x

27. Aishima S, Kuroda Y, Nishihara Y, Taguchi K, Taketomi A, Maehara Y, et al. Gastric mucin phenotype defines tumour progression and prognosis of intrahepatic cholangiocarcinoma: gastric foveolar type is associated with aggressive tumour behaviour. *Histopathology.* (2006) 49:35–44. doi: 10.1111/j.1365-2559.2006.02414.x

28. Yu TH, Yuan RH, Chen YL, Yang WC, Hsu HC, Jeng YM. Viral hepatitis is associated with intrahepatic cholangiocarcinoma with cholangiolar differentiation and N-cadherin expression. *Mod Pathol.* (2011) 24:810–9. doi: 10.1038/modpathol.2011.41

29. Kozaka K, Sasaki M, Fujii T, Harada K, Zen Y, Sato Y, et al. A subgroup of intrahepatic cholangiocarcinoma with an infiltrating replacement growth pattern and a resemblance to reactive proliferating bile ductules: 'bile ductular carcinoma'. *Histopathology.* (2007) 51:390–400. doi: 10.1111/j.1365-2559.2007.02735.x

30. Akita M, Sawada R, Komatsu M, Suleman N, Itoh T, Ajiki T, et al. An immunostaining panel of C-reactive protein, N-cadherin, and S100 calcium binding protein P is useful for intrahepatic cholangiocarcinoma subtyping. *Hum Pathol.* (2021) 109:45–52. doi: 10.1016/j.humpath.2020.12.005

31. Vijgen S, Terris B, Rubbia-Brandt L. Pathology of intrahepatic cholangiocarcinoma. *Hepatobiliary Surg Nutr.* (2017) 6:22–34. doi: 10.21037/hbsn.2016.11.04

32. Park JH, Kim JH. Pathologic differential diagnosis of metastatic carcinoma in the liver. *Clin Mol Hepatol.* (2019) 25:12–20. doi: 10.3350/cmh.2018.0067

33. Misumi K, Hayashi A, Shibahara J, Arita J, Sakamoto Y, Hasegawa K, et al. Intrahepatic cholangiocarcinoma frequently shows loss of BAP1 and PBRM1 expression, and demonstrates specific clinicopathological and genetic characteristics with BAP1 loss. *Histopathology.* (2017) 70:766–74. doi: 10.1111/his.13127

34. Jeon Y, Kwon SM, Rhee H, Yoo JE, Chung T, Woo HG, et al. Molecular and radiopathologic spectrum between HCC and intrahepatic cholangiocarcinoma. *Hepatology* (2022). doi: 10.1002/hep.32397. [Epub ahead of print].

35. Yoon JG, Kim MH, Jang M, Kim H, Hwang HK, Kang CM, et al. Molecular characterization of biliary tract cancer predicts chemotherapy and PD-1/PD-L1 blockade responses. *Hepatology.* (2021) 74:1914–31. doi: 10.1002/hep.31862

36. Choi W-T, Ramachandran R, Kakar S. Immunohistochemical approach for the diagnosis of a liver mass on small biopsy specimens. *Hum Pathol.* (2017) 63:1–13. doi: 10.1016/j.humpath.2016.12.025

37. Werling RW, Yaziji H, Bacchi CE, Gown AM. CDX2, a Highly sensitive and specific marker of adenocarcinomas of intestinal origin: an immunohistochemical survey of 476 primary and metastatic carcinomas. *Am J Surg Pathol.* (2003) 27:303–10. doi: 10.1097/00000478-200303000-00003

38. Stenhouse G, Fyfe N, King G, Chapman A, Kerr KM. Thyroid transcription factor 1 in pulmonary adenocarcinoma. *J Clin Pathol.* (2004) 57:383–7. doi: 10.1136/jcp.2003.007138

39. Surrey LF, Frank R, Zhang PJ, Furth EE. TTF-1 and Napsin-A are expressed in a subset of cholangiocarcinomas arising from the gallbladder and hepatic ducts: continued caveats for utilization of immunohistochemistry panels. *Am J Surg Pathol.* (2014) 38:224–7. doi: 10.1097/pas.0000000000000138

40. Selves J, Long-Mira E, Mathieu M-C, Rochaix P, Ilié M. Immunohistochemistry for diagnosis of metastatic carcinomas of unknown primary site. *Cancers (Basel).* (2018) 10:108. doi: 10.3390/cancers10040108

41. Miettinen M, McCue PA, Sarlomo-Rikala M, Rys J, Czapiewski P, Wazny K, et al. GATA3: a multispecific but potentially useful marker in surgical pathology: a systematic analysis of 2500 epithelial and nonepithelial tumors. *Am J Surg Pathol.* (2014) 38:13–22. doi: 10.1097/PAS.0b013e3182a0218f

42. Varma M, Morgan M, Jasani B, Tamboli P, Amin MB. Polyclonal anti-PSA is more sensitive but less specific than monoclonal anti-PSA: implications for diagnostic prostatic pathology. *Am J Clin Pathol.* (2002) 118:202–7. doi: 10.1309/BGWQ-P26T-7TR6-VGT3

43. Guedj N, Zhan Q, Perigny M, Rautou PE, Degos F, Belghiti J, et al. Comparative protein expression profiles of hilar and peripheral hepatic cholangiocarcinomas. *J Hepatol.* (2009) 51:93–101. doi: 10.1016/j.jhep.2009.03.017

44. Shahid M, Mubeen A, Tse J, Kakar S, Bateman AC, Borger D, et al. Branched chain in situ hybridization for albumin as a marker of hepatocellular differentiation: evaluation of manual and automated in situ hybridization platforms. *Am J Surg Pathol.* (2015) 39:25–34. doi: 10.1097/PAS.0000000000000343

45. Ferrone CR, Ting DT, Shahid M, Konstantinidis IT, Sabbatino F, Goyal L, et al. The ability to diagnose intrahepatic cholangiocarcinoma definitively using novel branched DNA-enhanced albumin RNA in situ hybridization technology. *Ann Surg Oncol.* (2016) 23:290–6. doi: 10.1245/s10434-014-4247-8

46. Collins K, Newcomb PH, Cartun RW, Ligato S. Utility and limitations of albumin mRNA in situ hybridization detection in the diagnosis of hepatobiliary lesions and metastatic carcinoma to the liver. *Appl Immunohistochem Mol Morphol.* (2021) 29:180–7. doi: 10.1097/pai.0000000000000885

47. Banales JM, Huebert RC, Karlsen T, Strazzabosco M, LaRusso NF, Gores GJ. Cholangiocyte pathobiology. *Nat Rev Gastroenterol Hepatol.* (2019) 16:269–81. doi: 10.1038/s41575-019-0125-y

48. Steiner PE, Higginson J. Cholangiolocellular carcinoma of the liver. *Cancer.* (1959) 12:753–9. doi: 10.1002/1097-0142(195907/08)12:4<753::aid-cncr2820120420>3.0.co;2-l

49. Komuta M, Spee B, Vander Borght S, De Vos R, Verslype C, Aerts R, et al. Clinicopathological study on cholangiolocellular carcinoma suggesting hepatic progenitor cell origin. *Hepatology.* (2008) 47:1544–56. doi: 10.1002/hep.22238

50. Moeini A, Sia D, Zhang Z, Camprecios G, Stueck A, Dong H, et al. Mixed hepatocellular cholangiocarcinoma tumors: cholangiolocellular carcinoma is a distinct molecular entity. *J Hepatol.* (2017) 66:952–61. doi: 10.1016/j.jhep.2017.01.010

51. Liau JY, Tsai JH, Yuan RH, Chang CN, Lee HJ, Jeng YM. Morphological subclassification of intrahepatic cholangiocarcinoma: etiological, clinicopathological, and molecular features. *Mod Pathol.* (2014) 27:1163–73. doi: 10.1038/modpathol.2013.241

52. Rhee H, Ko JE, Chung T, Jee BA, Kwon SM, Nahm JH, et al. Transcriptomic and histopathological analysis of cholangiolocellular differentiation trait in intrahepatic cholangiocarcinoma. *Liver Int.* (2018) 38:113–24. doi: 10.1111/liv.13492

53. Sia D, Hoshida Y, Villanueva A, Roayaie S, Ferrer J, Tabak B, et al. Integrative molecular analysis of intrahepatic cholangiocarcinoma reveals 2 classes that have different outcomes. *Gastroenterology.* (2013) 144:829–40. doi: 10.1053/j.gastro.2013.01.001

54. Chung T, Rhee H, Shim HS, Yoo JE, Choi GH, Kim H, et al. Genetic, clinicopathological, and radiological features of intrahepatic cholangiocarcinoma with ductal plate malformation pattern. *Gut Liver.* (2021). doi: 10.5009/gnl210174

55. Nakanuma Y, Sato Y, Ikeda H, Harada K, Kobayashi M, Sano K, et al. Intrahepatic cholangiocarcinoma with predominant "ductal plate malformation" pattern: a new subtype. *Am J Surg Pathol.* (2012) 36:1629–35. doi: 10.1097/PAS.0b013e31826e0249

56. Sasaki M, Sato Y, Nakanuma Y. Cholangiolocellular carcinoma with "ductal plate malformation" pattern may be characterized by ARID1A genetic alterations. *Am J Surg Pathol.* (2019) 43:352–60. doi: 10.1097/pas.0000000000001201

57. Gou Q, Fu S, Xie Y, Zhang M, Shen Y. Treatment and survival patterns of primary adenosquamous carcinoma of the liver: a retrospective analysis. *Front Oncol.* (2021) 11:621594. doi: 10.3389/fonc.2021.621594

58. Nakanuma Y, Sato Y, Harada K, Sasaki M, Xu J, Ikeda H. Pathological classification of intrahepatic cholangiocarcinoma based on a new concept. *World J Hepatol.* (2010) 2:419–27. doi: 10.4254/wjh.v2.i12.419

59. Chi Z, Bhalla A, Saeed O, Cheng L, Curless K, Wang HL, et al. Mucinous intrahepatic cholangiocarcinoma: a distinct variant. *Hum Pathol.* (2018) 78:131–7. doi: 10.1016/j.humpath.2018.04.010

60. Sumiyoshi T, Shima Y, Okabayashi T, Ishikawa A, Matsumoto M, Iwata J, et al. Mucinous cholangiocarcinoma: clinicopathological features of the rarest type of cholangiocarcinoma. *Ann Gastroenterol Surg.* (2017) 1:114–21. doi: 10.1002/ags3.12016

61. Haas S, Gütgemann I, Wolff M, Fischer HP. Intrahepatic clear cell cholangiocarcinoma: immunohistochemical aspects in a very rare type of cholangiocarcinoma. *Am J Surg Pathol.* (2007) 31:902–6. doi: 10.1097/PAS.0b013e31802c0c8a

62. Yamamoto T, Abe T, Oshita A, Yonehara S, Katamura Y, Matsumoto N, et al. Intrahepatic cholangiocarcinoma with clear cell type following laparoscopic curative surgery. *Surg Case Rep.* (2020) 6:264. doi: 10.1186/s40792-020-01041-2

63. Guo XQ, Li B, Li Y, Tian XY, Li Z. Unusual mucoepidermoid carcinoma of the liver misdiagnosed as squamous cell carcinoma by intraoperative histological examination. *Diagn Pathol.* (2014) 9:24. doi: 10.1186/1746-1596-9-24

64. Arakawa Y, Shimada M, Ikegami T, Kubo T, Imura S, Morine Y, et al. Mucoepidermoid carcinoma of the liver: report of a rare case and review of the literature. *Hepatol Res.* (2008) 38:736–42. doi: 10.1111/j.1872-034X.2008.00335.x

65. Tsai J-H, Liau J-Y, Lee C-H, Jeng Y-M. Lymphoepithelioma-like intrahepatic cholangiocarcinoma is a distinct entity with frequent pTERT/TP53 mutations and comprises 2 subgroups based on epstein-barr virus infection. *Am J Surg Pathol.* (2021) 45:1409–18. doi: 10.1097/PAS.0000000000001716

66. Khandakar B, Liu J-R, Thung S, Li Y, Rhee H, Kagen AC, et al. Lymphoepithelioma-like neoplasm of the biliary tract with 'probable low malignant potential'. *Histopathology.* (2022) 80:720–8. doi: 10.1111/his.14580

67. Malhotra S, Wood J, Mansy T, Singh R, Zaitoun A, Madhusudan S. Intrahepatic sarcomatoid cholangiocarcinoma. *J Oncol.* (2010) 2010:701476. doi: 10.1155/2010/701476

68. Matsukuma KE, Yeh MM. Update on the pathology of liver neoplasms. *Ann Diagn Pathol.* (2019) 38:126–37. doi: 10.1016/j.anndiagpath.2018.10.005

69. Geramizadeh B. Precursor lesions of cholangiocarcinoma: a clinicopathologic review. *Clin Pathol.* (2020) 13:2632010X20925045. doi: 10.1177/2632010x20925045

70. Who Classification of Tumours Editorial Board. *Digestive System Tumours.* 5th ed. Lyon: International Agency for Research on Cancer (2019).

71. Nakanishi Y, Zen Y, Kondo S, Itoh T, Itatsu K, Nakanuma Y. Expression of cell cycle-related molecules in biliary premalignant lesions: biliary intraepithelial neoplasia and biliary intraductal papillary neoplasm. *Hum Pathol.* (2008) 39:1153–61. doi: 10.1016/j.humpath.2007.11.018

72. Ettel M, Eze O, Xu R. Clinical and biological significance of precursor lesions of intrahepatic cholangiocarcinoma. *World J Hepatol.* (2015) 7:2563–70. doi: 10.4254/wjh.v7.i25.2563

73. Hsu M, Sasaki M, Igarashi S, Sato Y, Nakanuma Y. KRAS and GNAS mutations and p53 overexpression in biliary intraepithelial neoplasia and intrahepatic cholangiocarcinomas. *Cancer.* (2013) 119:1669–74. doi: 10.1002/cncr.27955

74. Aishima S, Fujita N, Mano Y, Kubo Y, Tanaka Y, Taketomi A, et al. Different roles of S100P overexpression in intrahepatic cholangiocarcinoma: carcinogenesis of perihilar type and aggressive behavior of peripheral type. *Am J Surg Pathol.* (2011) 35:590–8. doi: 10.1097/PAS.0b013e31820ffdf1

75. Nakanuma Y, Kakuda Y, Uesaka K, Miyata T, Yamamoto Y, Fukumura Y, et al. Characterization of intraductal papillary neoplasm of bile duct with respect to histopathologic similarities to pancreatic intraductal papillary mucinous neoplasm. *Hum Pathol.* (2016) 51:103–13. doi: 10.1016/j.humpath.2015.12.022

76. Rocha FG, Lee H, Katabi N, DeMatteo RP, Fong Y, D'Angelica MI, et al. Intraductal papillary neoplasm of the bile duct: a biliary equivalent to intraductal papillary mucinous neoplasm of the pancreas? *Hepatology.* (2012) 56:1352–60. doi: 10.1002/hep.25786

77. Kim KM, Lee JK, Shin JU, Lee KH, Lee KT, Sung J-Y, et al. Clinicopathologic features of intraductal papillary neoplasm of the bile duct according to histologic subtype. *Am J Gastroenterol.* (2012) 107:118–25. doi: 10.1038/ajg.2011.316

78. Schlitter AM, Born D, Bettstetter M, Specht K, Kim-Fuchs C, Riener M-O, et al. Intraductal papillary neoplasms of the bile duct: stepwise progression to carcinoma involves common molecular pathways. *Mod Pathol.* (2014) 27:73–86. doi: 10.1038/modpathol.2013.112

79. Nakanuma Y, Uesaka K, Kakuda Y, Sugino T, Kubota K, Furukawa T, et al. Intraductal papillary neoplasm of bile duct: updated clinicopathological characteristics and molecular and genetic alterations. *J Clin Med.* (2020) 9:3991. doi: 10.3390/jcm9123991

80. Nakanuma Y, Uesaka K, Okamura Y, Terada T, Fukumura Y, Kakuda Y, et al. Reappraisal of pathological features of intraductal papillary neoplasm of bile duct with respect to the type 1 and 2 subclassifications. *Hum Pathol.* (2021) 111:21–35. doi: 10.1016/j.humpath.2021.01.002

81. Yang CY, Huang WJ, Tsai JH, Cheng A, Chen CC, Hsu HP, et al. Targeted next-generation sequencing identifies distinct clinicopathologic and molecular entities of intraductal papillary neoplasms of the bile duct. *Mod Pathol.* (2019) 32:1637–45. doi: 10.1038/s41379-019-0306-9

82. Aoki Y, Mizuma M, Hata T, Aoki T, Omori Y, Ono Y, et al. Intraductal papillary neoplasms of the bile duct consist of two distinct types specifically associated with clinicopathological features and molecular phenotypes. *J Pathol.* (2020) 251:38–48. doi: 10.1002/path.5398

83. Schlitter AM, Jang K-T, Klöppel G, Saka B, Hong S-M, Choi H, et al. Intraductal tubulopapillary neoplasms of the bile ducts: clinicopathologic, immunohistochemical, and molecular analysis of 20 cases. *Mod Pathol.* (2015) 28:1249–64. doi: 10.1038/modpathol.2015.61

84. Goeppert B, Stichel D, Toth R, Fritzsche S, Loeffler MA, Schlitter AM, et al. Integrative analysis reveals early and distinct genetic and epigenetic changes in intraductal papillary and tubulopapillary cholangiocarcinogenesis. *Gut.* (2022) 71:391–401. doi: 10.1136/gutjnl-2020-322983

85. Fabris L, Sato K, Alpini G, Strazzabosco M. The tumor microenvironment in cholangiocarcinoma progression. *Hepatology.* (2021) 73:75–85. doi: 10.1002/hep.31410

86. Jing C-Y, Fu Y-P, Huang J-L, Zhang M-X, Yi Y, Gan W, et al. Prognostic nomogram based on histological characteristics of fibrotic tumor stroma in patients who underwent curative resection for intrahepatic cholangiocarcinoma. *Oncologist.* (2018) 23:1482–93. doi: 10.1634/theoncologist.2017-0439

87. Kajiyama K, Maeda T, Takenaka K, Sugimachi K, Tsuneyoshi M. The significance of stromal desmoplasia in intrahepatic cholangiocarcinoma: a special reference of 'scirrhous-type' and 'nonscirrhous-type'. *Growth.* (1999) 23:892. doi: 10.1097/00000478-199908000-00006

88. Zhang X-F, Dong M, Pan Y-H, Chen J-N, Huang X-Q, Jin Y, et al. Expression pattern of cancer-associated fibroblast and its clinical relevance in intrahepatic cholangiocarcinoma. *Hum Pathol.* (2017) 65:92–100. doi: 10.1016/j.humpath.2017.04.014

89. Kojima S, Hisaka T, Midorikawa R, Naito Y, Akiba J, Tanigawa M, et al. Prognostic impact of desmoplastic reaction evaluation for intrahepatic cholangiocarcinoma. *Anticancer Res.* (2020) 40:4749–54. doi: 10.21873/anticanres.14476

90. De Jaeghere EA, Denys HG, De Wever O. Fibroblasts fuel immune escape in the tumor microenvironment. *Trends Cancer.* (2019) 5:704–23. doi: 10.1016/j.trecan.2019.09.009

91. Okabe H, Beppu T, Hayashi H, Ishiko T, Masuda T, Otao R, et al. Hepatic stellate cells accelerate the malignant behavior of cholangiocarcinoma cells. *Ann Surg Oncol.* (2011) 18:1175–84. doi: 10.1245/s10434-010-1391-7

92. Clapéron A, Mergey M, Aoudjehane L, Ho-Bouldoires THN, Wendum D, Prignon A, et al. Hepatic myofibroblasts promote the progression of human cholangiocarcinoma through activation of epidermal growth factor receptor. *Hepatology.* (2013) 58:2001–11. doi: 10.1002/hep.26585

93. Fingas CD, Bronk SF, Werneburg NW, Mott JL, Guicciardi ME, Cazanave SC, et al. Myofibroblast-derived PDGF-BB promotes hedgehog survival signaling in cholangiocarcinoma cells. *Hepatology.* (2011) 54:2076–88. doi: 10.1002/hep.24588

94. Chuaysri C, Thuwajit P, Paupairoj A, Chau-In S, Suthiphongchai T, Thuwajit C. Alpha-smooth muscle actin-positive fibroblasts promote biliary cell proliferation and correlate with poor survival in cholangiocarcinoma. *Oncol Rep.* (2009) 21:957–69. doi: 10.3892/or_00000309

95. Shan Z, Ju C. Hepatic macrophages in liver injury. *Front Immunol.* (2020) 11:322. doi: 10.3389/fimmu.2020.00322

96. Sato K, Hall C, Glaser S, Francis H, Meng F, Alpini G. Pathogenesis of Kupffer cells in cholestatic liver injury. *Am J Pathol.* (2016) 186:2238–47. doi: 10.1016/j.ajpath.2016.06.003

97. Yuan H, Lin Z, Liu Y, Jiang Y, Liu K, Tu M, et al. Intrahepatic cholangiocarcinoma induced M2-polarized tumor-associated macrophages facilitate tumor growth and invasiveness. *Cancer Cell Int.* (2020) 20:586. doi: 10.1186/s12935-020-01687-w

98. Høgdall D, Lewinska M, Andersen JB. Desmoplastic tumor microenvironment and immunotherapy in cholangiocarcinoma. *Trends Cancer.* (2018) 4:239–55. doi: 10.1016/j.trecan.2018.01.007

99. Hasita H, Komohara Y, Okabe H, Masuda T, Ohnishi K, Lei XF, et al. Significance of alternatively activated macrophages in patients with intrahepatic cholangiocarcinoma. *Cancer Sci.* (2010) 101:1913–9. doi: 10.1111/j.1349-7006.2010.01614.x

100. Kasper HU, Drebber U, Stippel DL, Dienes HP, Gillessen A. Liver tumor infiltrating lymphocytes: comparison of hepatocellular and cholangiolar carcinoma. *World J Gastroenterol.* (2009) 15:5053–7. doi: 10.3748/wjg.15.5053

101. Goeppert B, Frauenschuh L, Zucknick M, Stenzinger A, Andrulis M, Klauschen F, et al. Prognostic impact of tumour-infiltrating immune cells on biliary tract cancer. *Br J Cancer.* (2013) 109:2665–74. doi: 10.1038/bjc.2013.610

102. Yugawa K, Itoh S, Yoshizumi T, Iseda N, Tomiyama T, Toshima T, et al. Prognostic impact of tumor microvessels in intrahepatic cholangiocarcinoma: association with tumor-infiltrating lymphocytes. *Mod Pathol.* (2021) 34:798–807. doi: 10.1038/s41379-020-00702-9

103. Kim H-D, Kim JH, Ryu Y-M, Kim D, Lee S, Shin J, et al. Spatial distribution and prognostic implications of tumor-infiltrating FoxP3- CD4+ T cells in biliary tract cancer. *Cancer Res Treat.* (2021) 53:162–71. doi: 10.4143/crt.2020.704

104. Ghidini M, Cascione L, Carotenuto P, Lampis A, Trevisani F, Previdi MC, et al. Characterisation of the immune-related transcriptome in resected biliary tract cancers. *Eur J Cancer.* (2017) 86:158–65. doi: 10.1016/j.ejca.2017.09.005

105. Fontugne J, Augustin J, Pujals A, Compagnon P, Rousseau B, Luciani A, et al. PD-L1 expression in perihilar and intrahepatic cholangiocarcinoma. *Oncotarget.* (2017) 8:24644–51. doi: 10.18632/oncotarget.15602

106. Wu H, Wei Y, Jian M, Lu H, Song Q, Hao L, et al. Clinicopathological and prognostic significance of immunoscore and PD-L1 in intrahepatic cholangiocarcinoma. *OncoTargets Ther.* (2021) 14:39–51. doi: 10.2147/ott.S288982

107. Sabbatino F, Villani V, Yearley JH, Deshpande V, Cai L, Konstantinidis IT, et al. PD-L1 and HLA class I antigen expression and clinical course of the disease in intrahepatic cholangiocarcinoma. *J Clin Cancer Res.* (2016) 22:470–8. doi: 10.1158/1078-0432.CCR-15-0715

108. Rizzo A, Ricci AD, Brandi G. PD-L1, TMB, MSI, and other predictors of response to immune checkpoint inhibitors in biliary tract cancer. *Cancers (Basel).* (2021) 13:558. doi: 10.3390/cancers13030558

109. Wardell CP, Fujita M, Yamada T, Simbolo M, Fassan M, Karlic R, et al. Genomic characterization of biliary tract cancers identifies driver genes and predisposing mutations. *J Hepatol.* (2018) 68:959–69. doi: 10.1016/j.jhep.2018.01.009

110. Terashima T, Umemoto K, Takahashi H, Hosoi H, Takai E, Kondo S, et al. Germline mutations in cancer-predisposition genes in patients with biliary tract cancer. *Oncotarget.* (2019) 10:5949–57. doi: 10.18632/oncotarget.27224

111. Maynard H, Stadler ZK, Berger MF, Solit DB, Ly M, Lowery MA, et al. Germline alterations in patients with biliary tract cancers: a spectrum of significant and previously underappreciated findings. *Cancer.* (2020) 126:1995–2002. doi: 10.1002/cncr.32740

112. Golan T, Raitses-Gurevich M, Kelley RK, Bocobo AG, Borgida A, Shroff RT, et al. Overall survival and clinical characteristics of BRCA-associated cholangiocarcinoma: a multicenter retrospective study. *Oncologist.* (2017) 22:804–10. doi: 10.1634/theoncologist.2016-0415

113. Brandi G, Deserti M, Palloni A, Turchetti D, Zuntini R, Pedica F, et al. Intrahepatic cholangiocarcinoma development in a patient with a novel BAP1 germline mutation and low exposure to asbestos. *Cancer Genet.* (2020) 24:57–62. doi: 10.1016/j.cancergen.2020.10.001

114. Kiba T, Tsuda H, Hirohashi S, Inoue S, Sugimura T, Pairojkul C. Mutations of the p53 tumor suppressor gene and the ras gene family in intrahepatic cholangiocellular carcinomas in Japan and Thailand. *Mol Carcinog.* (1993) 8:312–8. doi: 10.1002/mc.2940080415

115. Ross JS, Wang K, Gay L, Al-Rohil R, Rand JV, Jones DM, et al. New routes to targeted therapy of intrahepatic cholangiocarcinomas revealed by next-generation sequencing. *Oncologist.* (2014) 19:235–42. doi: 10.1634/theoncologist.2013-0352

116. Chaisaingmongkol J, Budhu A, Dang H, Rabibhadana S, Pupacdi B, Kwon SM, et al. Common molecular subtypes among asian hepatocellular carcinoma and cholangiocarcinoma. *Cancer Cell.* (2017) 32:57–70.e3. doi: 10.1016/j.ccell.2017.05.009

117. Simbolo M, Fassan M, Ruzzenente A, Mafficini A, Wood LD, Corbo V, et al. Multigene mutational profiling of cholangiocarcinomas identifies actionable molecular subgroups. *Oncotarget.* (2014) 5:2839–52. doi: 10.18632/oncotarget.1943

118. Churi CR, Shroff R, Wang Y, Rashid A, Kang HC, Weatherly J, et al. Mutation profiling in cholangiocarcinoma: prognostic and therapeutic implications. *PLoS One.* (2014) 9:e115383. doi: 10.1371/journal.pone.0115383

119. Jiao Y, Pawlik TM, Anders RA, Selaru FM, Streppel MM, Lucas DJ, et al. Exome sequencing identifies frequent inactivating mutations in BAP1, ARID1A and PBRM1 in intrahepatic cholangiocarcinomas. *Nat Genet.* (2013) 45:1470–3. doi: 10.1038/ng.2813

120. Nakamura H, Arai Y, Totoki Y, Shirota T, Elzawahry A, Kato M, et al. Genomic spectra of biliary tract cancer. *Nat Genet.* (2015) 47:1003–10. doi: 10.1038/ng.3375

121. Fujimoto A, Furuta M, Shiraishi Y, Gotoh K, Kawakami Y, Arihiro K, et al. Whole-genome mutational landscape of liver cancers displaying biliary phenotype reveals hepatitis impact and molecular diversity. *Nat Commun.* (2015) 6:6120. doi: 10.1038/ncomms7120

122. Wang T, Drill E, Vakiani E, Pak LM, Boerner T, Askan G, et al. Distinct histomorphological features are associated with IDH1 mutation in intrahepatic cholangiocarcinoma. *Hum Pathol.* (2019) 91:19–25. doi: 10.1016/j.humpath.2019.05.002

123. Jolissaint JS, Soares KC, Seier KP, Kundra R, Gönen M, Shin PJ, et al. Intrahepatic cholangiocarcinoma with lymph node metastasis: treatment-related outcomes and the role of tumor genomics in patient selection. *Clin Cancer Res.* (2021) 27:4101–8. doi: 10.1158/1078-0432.CCR-21-0412

124. Kipp BR, Voss JS, Kerr SE, Barr Fritcher EG, Graham RP, Zhang L, et al. Isocitrate dehydrogenase 1 and 2 mutations in cholangiocarcinoma. *Hum Pathol.* (2012) 43:1552–8. doi: 10.1016/j.humpath.2011.12.007

125. Zhu AX, Borger DR, Kim Y, Cosgrove D, Ejaz A, Alexandrescu S, et al. Genomic profiling of intrahepatic cholangiocarcinoma: refining prognosis and identifying therapeutic targets. *Ann Surg Oncol.* (2014) 21:3827–34. doi: 10.1245/s10434-014-3828-x

126. Boerner T, Drill E, Pak LM, Nguyen B, Sigel CS, Doussot A, et al. Genetic determinants of outcome in intrahepatic cholangiocarcinoma. *Hepatology.* (2021) 74:1429–44. doi: 10.1002/hep.31829

127. Nepal C, O'Rourke CJ, Oliveira DVNP, Taranta A, Shema S, Gautam P, et al. Genomic perturbations reveal distinct regulatory networks in intrahepatic

cholangiocarcinoma. *Hepatology*. (2018) 68:949–63. doi: 10.1002/hep. 29764

128. Lowery MA, Ptashkin R, Jordan E, Berger MF, Zehir A, Capanu M, et al. Comprehensive molecular profiling of intrahepatic and extrahepatic cholangiocarcinomas: potential targets for intervention. *Clin Cancer Res*. (2018) 24:4154–61. doi: 10.1158/1078-0432.CCR-18-0078

129. Borad MJ, Champion MD, Egan JB, Liang WS, Fonseca R, Bryce AH, et al. Integrated genomic characterization reveals novel, therapeutically relevant drug targets in FGFR and EGFR pathways in sporadic intrahepatic cholangiocarcinoma. *PLoS Genet*. (2014) 10:e1004135. doi: 10.1371/journal. pgen.1004135

130. Goyal L, Kongpetch S, Crolley VE, Bridgewater J. Targeting FGFR inhibition in cholangiocarcinoma. *Cancer Treat Rev*. (2021) 95:102170. doi: 10.1016/j. ctrv.2021.102170

131. Jusakul A, Cutcutache I, Yong CH, Lim JQ, Huang MN, Padmanabhan N, et al. Whole-genome and epigenomic landscapes of etiologically distinct subtypes of cholangiocarcinoma. *Cancer Discov*. (2017) 7:1116–35. doi: 10. 1158/2159-8290.CD-17-0368

132. Winkelmann R, Schneider M, Hartmann S, Schnitzbauer AA, Zeuzem S, Peveling-Oberhag J, et al. Microsatellite instability occurs rarely in patients with cholangiocarcinoma: a retrospective study from a German tertiary care hospital. *Int J Mol Sci*. (2018) 19:1421. doi: 10.3390/ijms19051421

133. Goeppert B, Roessler S, Renner M, Singer S, Mehrabi A, Vogel MN, et al. Mismatch repair deficiency is a rare but putative therapeutically relevant finding in non-liver fluke associated cholangiocarcinoma. *Br J Cancer*. (2019) 120:109–14. doi: 10.1038/s41416-018-0199-2

134. Li K, Luo H, Huang L, Luo H, Zhu X. Microsatellite instability: a review of what the oncologist should know. *Cancer Cell Int*. (2020) 20:16. doi: 10.1186/s12935-019-1091-8

135. Ohashi K, Nakajima Y, Kanehiro H, Tsutsumi M, Taki J, Aomatsu Y, et al. Ki-ras mutations and p53 protein expressions in intrahepatic cholangiocarcinomas: relation to gross tumor morphology. *Gastroenterology*. (1995) 109:1612–7. doi: 10.1016/0016-5085(95)90650-9

136. Goeppert B, Toth R, Singer S, Albrecht T, Lipka DB, Lutsik P, et al. Integrative analysis defines distinct prognostic subgroups of intrahepatic cholangiocarcinoma. *Hepatology*. (2019) 69:2091–106. doi: 10.1002/hep. 30493

137. Ma B, Meng H, Tian Y, Wang Y, Song T, Zhang T, et al. Distinct clinical and prognostic implication of IDH1/2 mutation and other most frequent mutations in large duct and small duct subtypes of intrahepatic cholangiocarcinoma. *BMC Cancer*. (2020) 20:318. doi: 10.1186/s12885-020-06804-6

138. Chan-on W, Nairismägi M-L, Ong CK, Lim WK, Dima S, Pairojkul C, et al. Exome sequencing identifies distinct mutational patterns in liver fluke–related and non-infection-related bile duct cancers. *Nat Genet*. (2013) 45:1474–8. doi: 10.1038/ng.2806

139. Zou S, Li J, Zhou H, Frech C, Jiang X, Chu JSC, et al. Mutational landscape of intrahepatic cholangiocarcinoma. *Nat Commun*. (2014) 5:5696. doi: 10.1038/ncomms6696

140. Andersen JB, Spee B, Blechacz BR, Avital I, Komuta M, Barbour A, et al. Genomic and genetic characterization of cholangiocarcinoma identifies therapeutic targets for tyrosine kinase inhibitors. *Gastroenterology*. (2012) 142:1021–31.e15. doi: 10.1053/j.gastro.2011.12.005

141. Ashburner M, Ball CA, Blake JA, Botstein D, Butler H, Cherry JM, et al. Gene ontology: tool for the unification of biology. *Nat Genet*. (2000) 25:25–9. doi: 10.1038/75556

142. Job S, Rapoud D, Dos Santos A, Gonzalez P, Desterke C, Pascal G, et al. Identification of four immune subtypes characterized by distinct composition and functions of tumor microenvironment in intrahepatic cholangiocarcinoma. *Hepatology*. (2020) 72:965–81. doi: 10.1002/hep. 31092

143. Rizzo A, Ricci AD, Brandi G. IDH inhibitors in advanced cholangiocarcinoma: another arrow in the quiver? *Cancer Treat Res Commun*. (2021) 27:100356. doi: 10.1016/j.ctarc.2021.100356

144. Zhu AX, Macarulla T, Javle MM, Kelley RK, Lubner SJ, Adeva J, et al. Final overall survival efficacy results of Ivosidenib for patients with advanced cholangiocarcinoma with IDH1 mutation: the phase 3 randomized clinical ClarIDHy trial. *JAMA Oncol*. (2021) 7:1669–77. doi: 10.1001/jamaoncol. 2021.3836

145. Acher AW, Paro A, Elfadaly A, Tsilimigras D, Pawlik TM. Intrahepatic cholangiocarcinoma: a summative review of biomarkers and targeted therapies. *Cancers (Basel)*. (2021) 13:5169. doi: 10.3390/cancers13205169

146. Mondaca S, Razavi P, Xu C, Offin M, Myers M, Scaltriti M, et al. Genomic characterization of ERBB2-driven biliary cancer and a case of response to Ado-Trastuzumab Emtansine. *JCO Precis Oncol*. (2019) 3:1–9. doi: 10.1200/po.19.00223

147. Mosele F, Remon J, Mateo J, Westphalen CB, Barlesi F, Lolkema MP, et al. Recommendations for the use of next-generation sequencing (NGS) for patients with metastatic cancers: a report from the ESMO precision medicine working group. *Ann Oncol*. (2020) 31:1491–505. doi: 10.1016/j.annonc.2020. 07.014

16

Investigation of Functional Synergism of CENPF and FOXM1 Identifies POLD1 as Downstream Target in Hepatocellular Carcinoma

Daniel Wai-Hung Ho†, Wai-Ling Macrina Lam†, Lo-Kong Chan† and Irene Oi-Lin Ng*

Department of Pathology and State Key Laboratory of Liver Research, University of Hong Kong, Hong Kong, Hong Kong SAR, China

*Correspondence:
Irene Oi-Lin Ng
iolng@hku.hk

†These authors have contributed equally to this work

Background: Lines of evidence implicate CENPF and FOXM1 may have novel co-operative roles in driving hepatocellular carcinoma (HCC).

Objective: We investigated the clinicopathological correlation, functional characterization, molecular mechanism and translational significance of CENPF and FOXM1.

Methods: We carried out integrative studies investigating functional synergism of CENPF and FOXM1 in HCC and its metastasis. Human HCC samples, HCC cell lines and mouse model were used in the studies. Stable knockdown, q-PCR, Western blotting, whole-transcriptomic sequencing (RNA-seq), as well as cell and mouse assays were performed.

Results: Upon clinicopathological correlation, we found that co-overexpression of CENPF and FOXM1 in human HCCs was associated with more aggressive tumor behavior including presence of venous invasion, tumor microsatellite formation, and absence of tumor encapsulation. Moreover, co-silencing FOXM1 and CENPF using shRNA approach in HCC cell lines resulted in significantly reduced cell proliferation. Furthermore, our RNA-seq and differential gene expression analysis delineated that CENPF and FOXM1 co-regulated a specific set of target genes in various metabolic processes and oncogenic signaling pathways. Among them, POLD1, which encodes the catalytic subunit of DNA polymerase δ, was ranked as the top downstream target co-regulated by CENPF and FOXM1. POLD1 expression was positively correlated with that of FOXM1 and CENPF in HCCs. In addition, POLD1 expression was significantly upregulated in HCC tumors. Functionally, *in vivo* orthotopic injection model showed that stable knockdown of POLD1 in HCC cells suppressed tumor incidence and tumorigenicity and had a trend of diminished lung metastasis.

Conclusion: Taken together, our data suggest that CENPF and FOXM1 could synergistically support hepatocarcinogenesis via the regulation of POLD1. CENPF and FOXM1 may represent new vulnerabilities to novel drug-based therapy in HCC.

Keywords: CENPF, FOXM1, POLD1, liver cancer, HCC, functional synergism

INTRODUCTION

Hepatocellular carcinoma (HCC) is one of the leading causes of cancer death worldwide (1, 2) and the second and third commonest cancer, respectively, in China and Hong Kong. Indeed, 55% of all new liver cancers worldwide each year occur in China including Hong Kong, due to a high prevalence of hepatitis B viral (HBV) infection (3, 4). It has a poor prognosis and only few effective treatment options are available. Despite years of efforts in studying the molecular mechanism of HCC carcinogenesis, current understanding on this lethal disease is still limited. In a recent study of our group (5), we have utilized whole-transcriptome sequencing technology to perform a differential gene expression (DGE) analysis using the dataset of 50 pairs (tumor and the corresponding non-tumorous liver tissue) of HCC cases from The Cancer Genome Atlas (TCGA). By comparing the gene expression in HCC tumors and their corresponding non-tumorous liver tissues, differentially expressed genes in HCC were identified. Among the 734 differentially expressed genes, CENPF and FOXM1 were listed as the first and third most upregulated genes respectively in HCC. Both FOXM1 and CENPF are crucial for cell-cycle progression, especially in the G2/M phase.

In a study on mitosis regulation and aging, CENPF was demonstrated to be a direct target of the cell cycle master regulator FOXM1 (6). Hence, it is traditionally believed that CENPF is a downstream target of FOXM1 and under the regulation by FOXM1. Interestingly, CENPF and FOXM1 were predicted to be master regulators of prostate cancer malignancy in a cross-species computational analysis by comparing interactomes of human and mice (7), and experimental validation demonstrated that they function synergistically to promote tumor growth by regulating prostate cancer-associated target gene expression profiles. Knockdown of CENPF and FOXM1 synergistically reduced the proliferation of cancer cells and tumor growth in cell-line-derived xenografts. It was further demonstrated that knockdown of CENPF expression reduced the binding of FOXM1 to its targets, suggesting CENPF is required for appropriate genomic binding by FOXM1. Additional data showed that they were co-localized in nucleus and their subcellular co-localization was mutually dependent.

Taken together, multiple lines of evidence imply CENPF and FOXM1 may have novel cooperative roles in regulating the expression of shared target genes. Hence, we postulate that they may have functional synergism in driving hepatocarcinogenesis.

MATERIALS AND METHODS

Quantitative Real-Time Polymerase Chain Reaction

RNA was extracted by Trizol (Thermo Fisher Scientific, Waltham, MA, United States) and cDNA was synthesized by a reverse transcription kit (Thermo Fisher Scientific, Waltham, MA, United States). Quantitative real-time polymerase chain reaction (qRT-PCR) was performed with target-specific TaqMan probes (Thermo Fisher Scientific, Waltham, MA, United States)

listed in **Supplementary Table 1**. The mRNA expression was normalized by the expression of the housekeeping gene *HPRT*.

Clinical Specimens and Clinicopathological Correlation Analysis

The primary HCC specimens and their corresponding non-tumorous liver tissues of randomly selected 118 human HCC cases were surgically resected from HCC patients in Queen Mary Hospital of Hong Kong between year 1991 and 2017. None of the patients had received therapies before hepatic tumor resection. Total RNA of these 118 pairs clinical specimens were isolated for subsequent qRT-PCR and clinicopathological correlation analysis using SPSS24.0 software, as previously described (8). We did not differentiate into micro- or macrovascular invasion. However, although the venous invasion included both microvascular and macrovascular invasion, mostly it was microvascular invasion. The tumor microsatellites were defined as microscopic or small tumor nodules less than 1 cm in diameter and in close proximity to the main tumor. Direct liver invasion was defined as invasion of the tumor cells into the non-tumorous liver parenchyma without separation by tumor capsule or fibrous layer (9). The use of clinical specimens was approved by the Institutional Review Board of the University of Hong Kong and the Hospital Authority.

Cell Lines and Culture Conditions

Hepatocellular carcinoma cell line Hep3B (HB-8064) was obtained from the American Type Culture Collection (ATCC) and HCC cell line Huh7 (JCRB0403) was obtained from JCRB Cell Bank. MHCC97L was a gift from Liver Cancer Institute, Fudan University. Hep3B cells were cultured in Minimum Essential Medium (MEM) supplemented with 1mM sodium pyruvate (NaPy). MHCC97L cells were cultured in Dulbecco's modified Eagle minimal high glucose essential medium (DMEM-HG) supplemented with 1mM NaPy. Huh7 cells were cultured in DMEM-HG media. All cell culture media mentioned above were further supplemented with 10% fetal bovine serum (FBS), 1% penicillin, and 1% streptomycin unless otherwise specified. Cell line cultures were maintained in 37°C and 5% CO_2 incubator.

Authentication of HCC cell lines used in this study was performed by short tandem repeat (STR) DNA Profiling in March 2018 and no cellular cross-contamination was detected. STR result for MHCC97L is provided in **Supplementary Figure 1**. Cell cultures were tested negative for Mycoplasma contamination. "Xenome," utilizing RNA-seq data, estimated a negligible 0.04–0.42% ($n = 3$) for MHCC97L, while 0.15–0.40% for clinical human NTL and HCC samples ($n = 6$) with mouse contamination, thus indicating our MHCC97L cells do not contain cells of murine origin (10). Furthermore, MHCC97L used in this study contains HBV integration in the TERT locus of the genome (8).

Stable Lentiviral-Based Short-Hairpin RNA Knockdown Cell Models

FOXM1, CENPF, and POLD1 were stably knocked down in MHCC97L HCC cells by the lentiviral-based short-hairpin

RNA (shRNA) approach as previously described (11, 12). The oligonucleotide sequences encoding non-targeted control (shNTCC) shRNA and shRNAs that specifically target FOXM1 (shFOXM1), CENPF (shCENPF), and POLD1 (shPOLD1) (Integrated DNA Technologies, Coralville, IA, United States) were summarized in **Supplementary Table 2**. The forward and reverse oligonucleotides were reannealed to generate shRNA cassettes and each of them was individually cloned into pLKO.1-Puro plasmid with puromycin resistance gene as selection marker. For lentiviral packaging, individual shRNA plasmid was co-transfected with the packaging mix into 293FT cells by lipofectamine 2000 transfection reagent (Invitrogen) at a plasmid to lipofectamine ratio (μg:μL) of 1:2. The viral supernatants were harvested 48 h post-transfection and used to transduce MHCC97L cells. About 1 μg/mL puromycin was applied to the viral-transduced cells for at least 4 days to select for stable knockdown clones. The knockdown efficiencies of FOXM1 and CENPF were examined by RT-qPCR and western blot.

Western Blot Analysis

Cells were lysed by 6X protein sample buffer (0.35 M Tris-HCl, pH 6.8, 30% glycerol, 20% SDS, 9.3% DTT and 0.05% bromophenol blue) and resolved by SDS-polyacrylamide gel electrophoresis. Immunoblots were incubated with primary antibody rabbit anti-human FOXM1 (D12D5) XP (Cell Signaling Technology, Danvers, MA, United States), rabbit anti-human CENPF (D6X4L) (Cell Signaling Technology, Danvers, MA, United States) and mouse anti-human β-actin (Sigma Aldrich, St. Louis, MO, United States) at 4 C overnight, followed by horseradish peroxidase-labeled anti-rabbit or anti-mouse secondary antibodies (Sigma Aldrich, St. Louis, MO, United States) at room temperature for 2 h. The chemiluminescence signal was detected with the ECL detection system (GE Healthcare, Lafayette, CO, United States).

Cell Proliferation Assay by Direct Cell Counting

About 2 $\times$ 10^4 cells of each cell line were seeded into each well of multiple 24-well culture plates in triplicates and incubated in a 37°C humidified incubator with 5% CO$_2$. Cell growth was assessed by determining the number of cells in each well every 24 h for 4 consecutive days. Direct cell counting was performed using COULTER COUNTER Z1 Cell and Particle Counter (Beckman Coulter).

Cell Growth Inhibition Assay by XTT Assay

Cell Proliferation II Kit (XTT) (Roche, Basel, Switzerland) was used to determine the percentage of cell growth inhibition according to the manufacturer's instructions.

Animal Studies

All animal studies were approved by the Animals (Control of Experiments) Ordinance of Hong Kong and the Committee on the Use of Live Animals in Teaching and Research (CULATR) of the University of Hong Kong (CULATR number: 3848-15), and strictly following the institutional regulations and guidelines. All animal studies were performed on 4 to 6 weeks old BALB/c-nu/nu (nude) athymic male mice, which were provided by the Centre for Comparative Medicine Research of the University of Hong Kong.

In vivo Orthotopic Liver Injection Model

POLD1 was knocked down in luciferase-labeled MHCC97L (MHCC97L-Luc) HCC cells by shRNA approach. The orthotopic liver injection was performed on 4 to 6 weeks old BALB/c-nu/nu (nude) athymic male mice to assess the metastatic potential of the injected HCC cells as previously described (13). About 1 $\times$ 10^6 of MHCC97L-luc stable cells were resuspended in 15 μL of Matrigel Basement Membrane Matrix (Corning) diluted with serum-free cell culture medium in a 1:1 ratio and then injected into the left lobe of the livers of mice by a 29-gauge needle (Hamilton, Reno, NV, United States). The abdominal wound was sutured after the injection. At 6-week post-injection, bioluminescence imaging of the xenografts was performed. Mice were anesthetized with Pentobarbital at 80 mg/kg, followed by injection of D-luciferin at 100 mg/kg (Perkin-Elmer, Waltham, MA, United States) into the tumor-bearing mice intraperitoneally. Bioluminescence images were acquired by IVIS Spectrum *in vivo* imaging system (Perkin-Elmer, Waltham, MA, United States) to measure the total flux of the bioluminescent signals emitted from the dissected liver tumor xenografts and the distant lung metastases.

Identification of FOXM1 and CENPF Co-regulated Genes by RNA-Sequencing

RNA-sequencing (RNA-seq) was performed to identify downstream target genes that were co-regulated by FOXM1 and CENPF. FOXM1 and CENPF were either individually silenced or co-silenced in Huh7, Hep3B and MHCC97L using small-interfering RNA (siRNA) approach and subjected to RNA-seq subsequently. Before transfection, 1.5 $\times$ 10^5 per well of cells were seeded onto a 6-well plate (for RNA extraction) and 3.5 $\times$ 10^5 per well of cells were seeded onto a 60-mm plate (for protein extraction) and were incubated in a 37°C humidified incubator with 5% CO$_2$ overnight. The siRNAs of the non-target control (NTC), FOXM1 and/or CENPF (Dharmacon, GE Healthcare, Lafayette, CO, United States) listed in **Supplementary Table 3** were transfected into the HCC cells with DharmaFECT 1 transfection reagent (Dharmacon, GE Healthcare, Lafayette, CO, United States). The cells were incubated for further 72 h and then subjected to RNA and protein extraction. Real-time PCR and western blot analysis were performed to confirm the knockdown efficiencies of FOXM1 and CENPF. Successful individual and co-knockdown cells were subjected to bioanalyzer analysis (Agilent) for RNA sample quality control followed by RNA-seq analysis (polyA and mRNA) at the Center for PanorOmic Sciences of the University of Hong Kong. The RNA-seq data has been deposited to NCBI SRA (PRJNA800214).

The DGE profiles of FOXM1 and/or CENPF knockdown HCC cell lines were analyzed by edgeR. Furthermore, additional filters were applied to confine the candidate gene list co-regulated

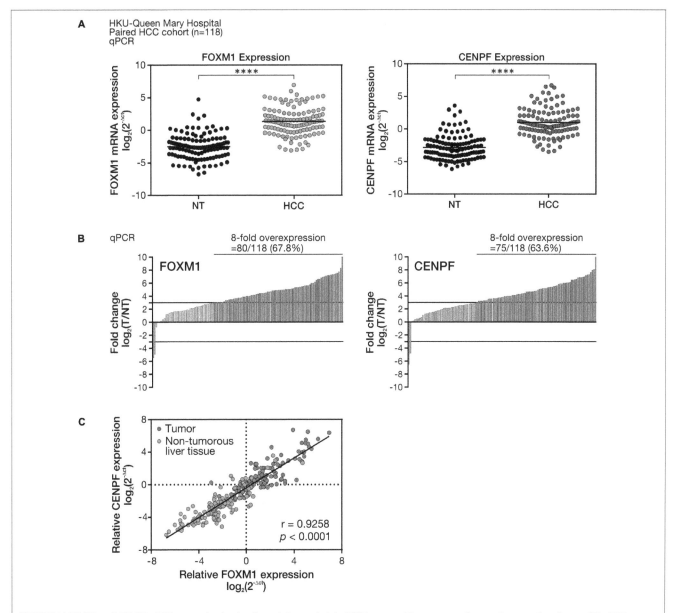

FIGURE 1 | FOXM1 and CENPF mRNA expression level and correlation analysis in HCC tumor and the corresponding non-tumorous liver tissues. **(A)** mRNA expression levels of FOXM1 and CENPF in 118 pairs of HCC and NT samples. mRNA expressions were normalized by housekeeping gene, *HPRT*. **(B)** Waterfall plot showing overall distribution of the fold change of FOXM1 and CENPF mRNA expression in 118 HCC clinical paired samples. **(C)** Pearson correlation analysis between FOXM1 and CENPF relative mRNA expression. Statistical significance was calculated by one-sample *t*-test (****$p < 0.001$).

by FOXM1 and CENPF based on four criteria: (i) they were differentially expressed with a *p*-value less than 0.05; (ii) with log CPM (counts per million) greater than 1; (iii) with an absolute log fold change greater than 1; and (iv) they were commonly differentially expressed in all 3 HCC cell lines with co-knockdown of FOXM1 and CENPF. Criteria (i)–(iii) applied to DGE analysis using both TCGA and our in-house whole-transcriptome sequencing of HCC clinical cases. To validate with DGE analysis results from the knockdown cell lines, correlation analysis between the candidate genes and FOXM1 and/or CENPF was performed using the TCGA and our in-house whole-transcriptome sequencing cohort of HCC clinical cases (14). The

activated and repressed candidate genes that were potentially co-regulated by FOXM1 and CENPF were also subjected to gene set enrichment analysis (15).

RESULTS

Expression and Clinical Relevance of FOXM1 and CENPF in Human HCCs

To validate FOXM1 and CENPF expression in our cohort of HCC patients, we examined the abundance of mRNA expression of FOXM1 and CENPF in 118 randomly selected pairs of HCC

TABLE 1 | Clinicopathological correlation analysis of FOXM1 and CENPF.

Clinical parameters		FOXM1 expression(T/NT)			CENPF expression(T/NT)			FOXM1 and CENPF expression (T/NT)		
		≥8-Fold	<8-Fold	*p*-Value	≥8-Fold	<8-Fold	*p*-Value	≥8-Fold	<8-Fold	*p*-Value
Gender	Male	63	28	0.348	60	31	0.223	54	37	0.446
	Female	17	10		15	12		15	12	
Venous invasion	Yes	48	19	0.204	49	18	**0.011***	45	22	**0.022***
	No	32	19		26	25		24	27	
Tumor encapsulation	Yes	23	15	0.146	20	18	0.057	18	20	0.059
	No	57	22		55	24		51	28	
Tumor microsatellite formation	Yes	48	16	**0.045***	47	17	**0.010***	44	20	**0.009***
	No	31	22		27	26		24	29	
Direct liver invasion	Yes	32	10	0.123	29	13	0.254	27	15	0.225
	No	44	25		42	27		38	31	
Tumor size	>5 cm	53	22	0.221	50	25	0.204	46	29	0.228
	≤5 cm	26	16		24	18		22	20	
Cirrhosis	Yes	35	23	0.066	36	22	0.445	31	27	0.183
	No	45	15		39	21		38	22	
Chronic liver disease	Yes	73	37	0.205	68	42	0.140	62	48	0.084
	No	7	1		7	1		7	1	
Cellular differentiation (Edmonson's grading)	I–II	34	18	0.403	33	19	0.560	31	21	0.459
	III–IV	45	20		41	24		37	28	
Tumor stage	I/II	25	16	0.195	22	19	0.093	21	20	0.195
	III/IV	53	22		51	24		46	29	

Clinicopathological correlation analysis between the indicated clinical parameters and the individual and co-expression of FOXM1 and CENPF in human HCC (n = 118) at an 8-fold difference cut-off. Statistical analyses were done by SPSS software 24.0. Asterisks (*) indicate statistically significant (p < 0.05). T; HCC tumorous tissue; NT; corresponding non-tumorous liver tissue. P values are shown in bold to emphasize they are < 0.05.

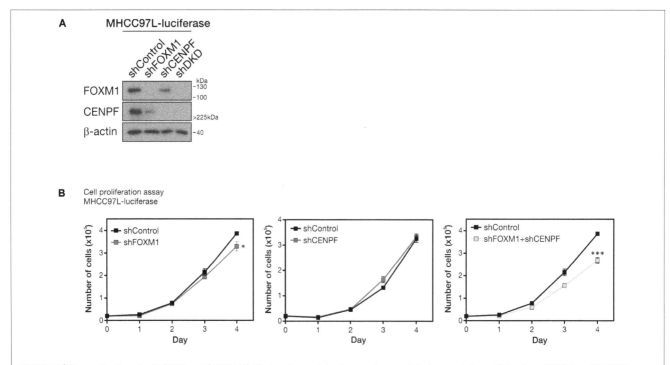

FIGURE 2 | Pro-proliferative role of FOXM1 and CENPF. **(A)** Western blot analysis showing single and double knockdown efficiencies of FOXM1 and CENPF in MHCC97L-Luc cells. **(B)** Representative cell proliferation assay showing the growth curves of HCC cells with single and co-knockdown of FOXM1 and CENPF for four consecutive days. Statistical significance was calculated by one-sample *t*-test (*p < 0.05; ***p < 0.001). shDKD, shRNA double knockdown of FOXM1 and CENPF cells.

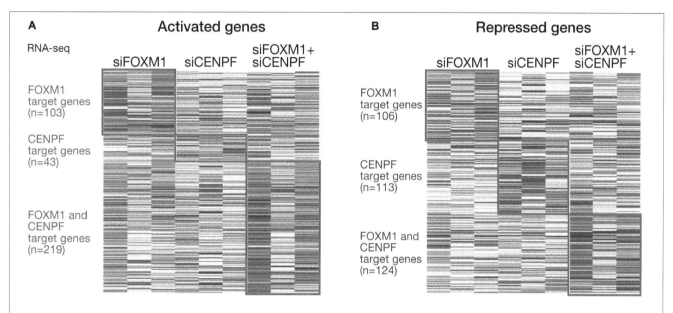

FIGURE 3 | Heatmaps of the differentially expressed genes in HCC cells with knockdown of FOXM1 and CENPF. **(A)** Orange color indicates genes that were activated upon silencing of FOXM1 and/or CENPF. 103 genes were upregulated upon FOXM1 knockdown. About 43 genes were upregulated upon CENPF knockdown. 219 genes were upregulated upon FOXM1 and CENPF co-knockdown. **(B)** Blue color indicates genes that were repressed upon silencing of FOXM1 and/or CENPF. About 106 genes were downregulated upon FOXM1 knockdown. 113 genes were downregulated upon CENPF knockdown. About 124 genes were downregulated upon FOXM1 and CENPF co-knockdown.

clinical samples (tumor, HCC, and corresponding non-tumorous liver tissues, NT) by real-time RT-PCR analysis. By comparing the mRNA expression levels between the HCC and NT samples, both FOXM1 and CENPF were shown to be significantly upregulated (****$p < 0.0001$), respectively (**Figure 1A**). The overall distribution of FOXM1 and CENPF expression in our cohort was displayed in the waterfall plot (**Figure 1B**). Using a cut-off at 8-fold difference between HCC and NT, 80 of the 118 HCC cases (67.8%) showed an overexpression of FOXM1, and 75 of the 118 HCC cases (63.6%) showed an overexpression of CENPF, whereas only 2 HCC cases (1.69%) had under-expression of either FOXM1 or CENPF. Interestingly, when we compared the relative expression of FOXM1 and CENPF in HCC and NT, respectively, we observed that they were positively correlated with each other ($r = 0.9258$, $p < 0.0001$), and substantially higher expressions in the tumor samples (**Figure 1C**).

To examine the clinical relevance of FOXM1 and CENPF, either in terms of their expression alone or co-expression, clinicopathological correlation analysis was performed. Using a threshold of 8-fold difference between T and NT, we showed that the overexpression of FOXM1 was positively correlated with the presence of tumor microsatellite formation ($p = 0.045$), whereas the overexpression of CENPF was positively correlated with the presence of venous invasion ($p = 0.011$) and the presence of tumor microsatellite ($p = 0.010$). Remarkably, co-overexpression of FOXM1 and CENPF were positively correlated with the presence of venous invasion ($p = 0.022$) and the presence of tumor microsatellite formation ($p = 0.009$), while the absence of tumor encapsulation ($p = 0.059$) was also suggested but did not reach statistical significance (**Table 1**).

FOXM1 and CENPF Were Critical for Cell Proliferation

FOXM1 and CENPF were individually silenced and co-silenced in MHCC97L-Luc HCC cell line by shRNA approach. We confirmed the successful knockdown by Western blot analysis (**Figure 2A**). To investigate the role of FOXM1 and CENPF in cell proliferation *in vitro*, the established stable knockdown cell lines were analyzed by anchorage-dependent cell proliferation assay. Co-knockdown of FOXM1 and CENPF cells showed the most significantly reduced proliferation rate ($p < 0.05$) (**Figure 2B**).

Identification of Commonly Regulated Genes by FOXM1 and CENPF Using RNA-Seq

To investigate the potential synergistic underlying mechanism of FOXM1 and CENPF in HCC, we have established single and co-knockdown FOXM1 and CENPF cell lines using small-interfering RNA (siRNA) transient knockdown approach for subsequent RNA-seq. siRNA knockdown cell lines were established in Huh7, Hep3B and MHCC97L HCC cells. The knockdown efficiencies were confirmed by real-time RT-PCR and western blot analysis (**Supplementary Figure 2**). Among all, siFOXM1-6, siCENPF-10 and siFOXM1-6/siCENPF-10 exhibited strongest knockdown efficiencies consistently in all 3 HCC cell lines. Thus, they were used for RNA-seq, together with the siRNA control cells.

We analyzed the expression profiles from the HCC cell lines in which they were individually silenced or co-silenced by DGE analysis. From the DGE analysis across all 3 sets of knockdown cell lines, we have identified 209 genes that

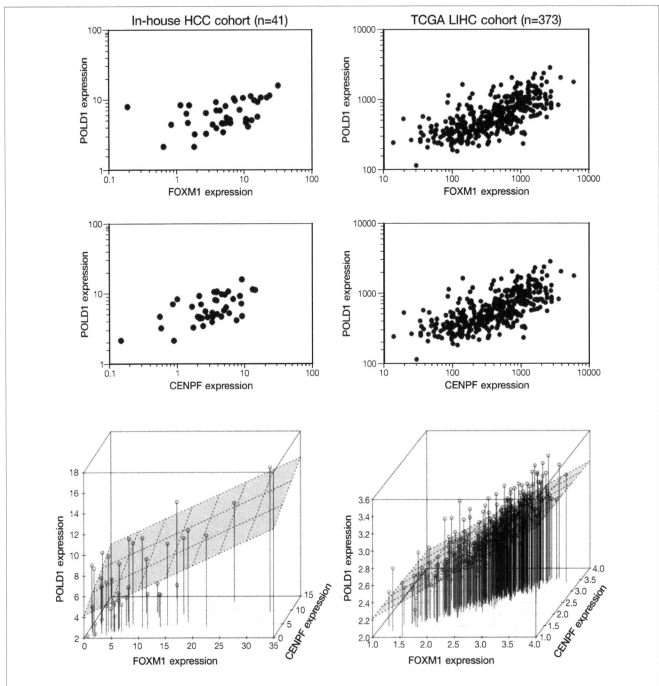

FIGURE 4 | POLD1 was positively correlated with FOXM1 and CENPF. Correlation analysis among the list of repressed candidate genes using our in-house RNA-seq dataset and the TCGA RNA-seq dataset. Both analyses indicated POLD1 was significantly correlated to both FOXM1 and CENPF ($p < 0.05$). Three-dimensional plot showed the correlation between the expressions of FOXM1, CENPF and POLD1 in both datasets.

were regulated by FOXM1, with 103 being activated and 106 being repressed upon FOXM1 knockdown; 156 genes that were regulated by CENPF, with 43 being activated and 113 being repressed upon CENPF knockdown; and 343 genes that were co-regulated by FOXM1 and CENPF, with 219 being activated and 124 being repressed upon co-knockdown of FOXM1 and CENPF (**Figure 3**). Among 343 candidate genes that were potentially being co-regulated by FOXM1 and CENPF, we further filtered

out 29 genes that were activated and 4 genes that were repressed upon co-knockdown of FOXM1 and CENPF in HCC cells (**Supplementary Figure 3**).

To elucidate the molecular pathways underlying the synergistic interaction of FOXM1 and CENPF, we subjected the list of activated and repressed candidate genes for gene set enrichment analysis using two databases, including Gene Ontology (biological process) and Reactome Pathway. We found

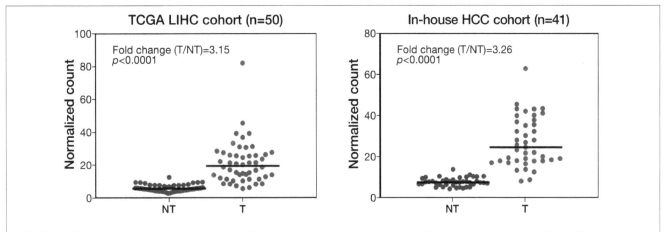

FIGURE 5 | POLD1 was significantly upregulated in human HCC. Differential gene expression analysis of POLD1 in the Cancer Genome Atlas (TCGA) RNA-seq dataset of 50 pairs of human HCC and our in-house RNA-seq dataset of 41 matched pairs of human HCC.

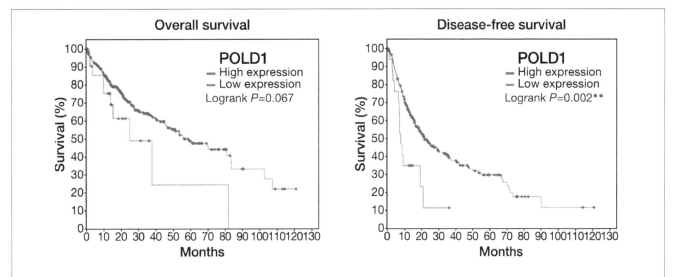

FIGURE 6 | Upregulation of POLD1 in HCC tumors was associated with poorer prognosis in TCGA dataset. Kaplan-Meier curves displayed the overall survival and disease free survival rates of HCC patients with higher POLD1 expression relative to those with lower expression. Higher POLD1 expression was based on a threshold of 2 for the mRNA expression z-scores relative to diploid samples.

that the differentially expressed genes were mainly enriched in biological pathways associated with various metabolic processes and biological signaling pathways. Notably, these genes were also enriched in several signaling pathways that are associated with tumorigenesis, including insulin growth factor (IGF) and platelet-derived growth factor (PDGF) signaling pathways (**Supplementary Figure 4**).

Among the 4 repressed gene candidates (**Supplementary Figure 3**), correlation analysis was performed using our in-house RNA-seq and the TCGA dataset. We found that *POLD1* (DNA Polymerase Delta 1) is positively correlated with both FOXM1 and CENPF, respectively and concurrently, in both RNA-seq datasets (**Figure 4**). In addition, *POLD1* expression was significantly upregulated in HCC tumor when compared with the corresponding liver tissue in TCGA RNA-seq dataset (fold change = 3.15, $p < 0.0001$) and in our in-house RNA-seq dataset (fold change = 3.26,

$p < 0.0001$) (**Figure 5**). Furthermore, we found that HCC patients with higher expression of *POLD1* had shorter overall survival and disease-free survival rates from the TCGA data analysis (**Figure 6**).

Effect of Knockdown of POLD1 in Tumorigenicity and Lung Metastasis in HCC

We knockdown *POLD1* (shPOLD1) in MHCC97L HCC cells by shRNA approach and performed *in vivo* liver orthotopic injection assay to assess the functional role of *POLD1* in liver tumorigenicity and lung metastasis. We showed that shPOLD1 strongly reduced tumor incidence. The tumor sizes (measured by total flux signal) were significantly reduced in mice injected with shPOLD1 HCC cells. We also observed a trend of diminished lung metastasis upon knockdown

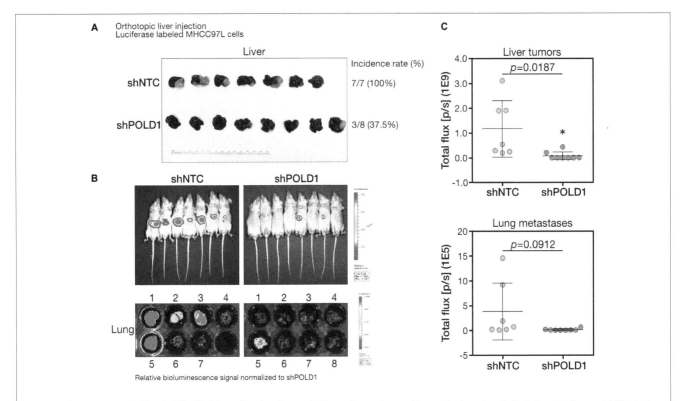

FIGURE 7 | Knockdown of POLD1 in MHCC97L-luc cells reduced tumor incidence, tumor sizes and lung metastases in orthotopic liver injection model. The *in vivo* functional role of POLD1 knockdown was evaluated as compared to the non-target control (NTC). Comparison was based on **(A)** tumorigenicity and **(B,C)** tumor size and lung metastasis.

of POLD1, but the difference could not reach statistical significance (**Figure 7**).

DISCUSSION

Development of HCC is a multistep process results from accumulation of mutational events in cancer driver genes. The alterations in driver genes promote oncogenic functions, such as proliferation, survival, cell motility and immune evasion. Moreover, accumulation of genetic and epigenetic alterations could contribute to tumor initiation, progression, metastasis and resistance to therapy (16). The malignant phenotype of cancer entails the dysregulation of cell cycle machinery, which serves as a convergence point for cellular transformation (17).

In this study, we demonstrated the significant roles of FOXM1 and CENPF in hepatocarcinogenesis. First, we found the co-overexpression of FOXM1 and CENPF in HCC was associated with aggressive tumor behavior, including the presence of venous invasion, tumor microsatellite formation, and the absence of tumor encapsulation by clinicopathological correlation analysis. Second, we demonstrated that FOXM1 and CENPF are important for cell growth. Third, our RNA-seq study further delineated that FOXM1 and CENPF co-regulated a set of genes that play essential roles in various metabolic processes and oncogenic signaling pathways. Among all differentially expressed genes between the wild-type HCC cells and FOXM1 and/or

CENPF knockdown cell lines, *POLD1*, which encodes for the catalytic subunit of DNA polymerase δ, was ranked as the top downstream target co-regulated by FOXM1 and CENPF.

In addition to the delineation of underlying mechanism of FOXM1 and CENPF in HCC, we have also been able to demonstrate their therapeutic implications in HCC using *in vitro* models. Despite the efficacy of existing molecularly targeted drugs, e.g., sorafenib and regorafenib, there is still an unmet medical need for patients with advanced HCC. With the successful advent of immune checkpoint inhibitors (ICIs), the combo of atezolizumab and bevacizumab has become the standard of care. However, although early clinical outcomes are impressive, a significant proportion of patients do not respond to this regimen. Uncontrolled cell growth is one of the characteristics of cancer, which entails aberrant activities of cell cycle proteins. Upregulation of FOXM1 and CENPF were shown to be crucial for the deregulated cell proliferation in HCC in this study. HCC may be uniquely dependent on FOXM1 and CENPF for cell growth; thus, we speculated that targeting these two cell cycle regulators offer considerable potentials in treating HCC. Thiostrepton is a potential inhibitor of FOXM1 (18, 19) while zoledronic acid is a potential inhibitor of CENPF (20–22). Indeed, we observed thiostrepton and zoledronic acid inhibited HCC cells selectively, as compared to the normal liver cells (**Supplementary Figure 5**). Further studies are awaited to confirm their potential usage in HCC treatment. It would also be interesting to test these inhibitors in the presence of ICI treatment, for instance in immunocompetent mouse models.

Taken together, our study provided new insight into the underlying synergistic mechanism of FOXM1 and CENPF via the regulation of POLD1, which plays a significant role in HCC progression. Moreover, FOXM1 and CENPF also represent new vulnerabilities to novel drug-based therapy in HCC.

AUTHOR CONTRIBUTIONS

DH and IN: study concept and design. DH, W-LL, L-KC, and IN: acquisition of data, analysis and interpretation of data, and drafting of the manuscript. IN: acquisition of clinical samples. All authors reviewed and approved the final draft of the manuscript.

FUNDING

The study was supported by the National Natural Science Foundation of China (81872222), Health and Medical Research Fund (03142836 and 07182546), General Research Fund (17100021 and 17117019), Hong Kong Research Grants Council Theme-based Research Scheme (T12-704/16-R), and Innovation and Technology Commission grant for State Key Laboratory of Liver Research. IN is Loke Yew Professor in Pathology.

ACKNOWLEDGMENTS

We thank the Center for PanorOmic Sciences of The University of Hong Kong for the RNA-seq service.

SUPPLEMENTARY MATERIAL

Supplementary Figure 1 | Short tandem repeat (STR) DNA profiling of MHCC97L.

Supplementary Figure 2 | Transient knockdown efficiencies of FOXM1 and CENPF in Huh7, Hep3B and MHCC97L. **(A)** mRNA expression and **(B)** protein expression of FOXM1 and CENPF upon siRNA transfection.

Supplementary Figure 3 | Candidate genes that were co-regulated by FOXM1 and CENPF. Additional filters (differential expression with $p < 0.05$; logCPM > 1; and | logFC| > 1) were used to narrow down the list of candidate genes. Among all, there were 29 genes being activated and 4 being repressed upon co-silencing of FOXM1 and CENPF across Huh7, Hep3B and MHCC97L.

Supplementary Figure 4 | Gene set enrichment analysis of the candidate genes co-regulated by FOXM1 and CENPF. The analysis was performed using Gene Ontology (GO) biological processes and Reactome Pathway.

Supplementary Figure 5 | Half-maximal inhibitory concentration (IC_{50}) of thiostrepton and zoledronic acid in HCC cell and non-tumorigenic liver cells. The percent growth inhibition curve showed the response of the Huh7 HCC cell line and two non-tumorigenic liver cell lines, including MIHA and LO2, to thiostrepton or zoledronic acid treatments at varying dosage. Thio, thiostrepton; ZOL, zoledronic acid.

REFERENCES

1. Sung H, Ferlay J, Siegel RL, Laversanne M, Soerjomataram I, Jemal A, et al. Global cancer statistics 2020: globocan estimates of incidence and mortality worldwide for 36 cancers in 185 countries. *CA Cancer J Clin*. (2021) 71:209–49. doi: 10.3322/caac.21660

2. Llovet JM, Kelley RK, Villanueva A, Singal AG, Pikarsky E, Roayaie S, et al. Hepatocellular carcinoma. *Nat Rev Dis Primers*. (2021) 7:6. doi: 10.1038/s41572-020-00240-3

3. Ho DW, Lo RC, Chan LK, Ng IO. Molecular pathogenesis of hepatocellular carcinoma. *Liver Cancer*. (2016) 5:290–302. doi: 10.1159/000449340

4. Ho DW, Lyu X, Ng IO. Viral integration detection strategies and a technical update on virus-clip. *Biocell*. (2021) 45:1495—-500. doi: 10.32604/biocell.2021.017227

5. Ho DW, Kai AK, Ng IO. TCGA whole-transcriptome sequencing data reveals significantly dysregulated genes and signaling pathways in hepatocellular carcinoma. *Front Med*. (2015) 9:322–30. doi: 10.1007/s11684-015-0408-9

6. Laoukili J, Kooistra MR, Bras A, Kauw J, Kerkhoven RM, Morrison A, et al. FoxM1 is required for execution of the mitotic programme and chromosome stability. *Nat Cell Biol*. (2005) 7:126–36. doi: 10.1038/ncb1217

7. Aytes A, Mitrofanova A, Lefebvre C, Alvarez MJ, Castillo-Martin M, Zheng T, et al. Cross-species regulatory network analysis identifies a synergistic interaction between FOXM1 and CENPF that drives prostate cancer malignancy. *Cancer Cell*. (2014) 25:638–51. doi: 10.1016/j.ccr.2014.03.017

8. Sze KM, Ho DW, Chiu YT, Tsui YM, Chan LK, Lee JM, et al. Hepatitis B virus-telomerase reverse transcriptase promoter integration harnesses host ELF4, resulting in telomerase reverse transcriptase gene transcription in hepatocellular carcinoma. *Hepatology*. (2021) 73:23–40. doi: 10.1002/hep.31231

9. Ng IO, Lai EC, Ng MM, Fan ST. Tumor encapsulation in hepatocellular carcinoma. A pathologic study of 189 cases. *Cancer*. (1992) 70:45–9. doi: 10.1002/1097-0142(19920701)70:1<45::aid-cncr2820700108>3.0.co;2-7

10. Conway T, Wazny J, Bromage A, Tymms M, Sooraj D, Williams ED, et al. Xenome–a tool for classifying reads from xenograft samples. *Bioinformatics*.

(2012) 28:i172–8. doi: 10.1093/bioinformatics/bts236

11. Ho DWH, Chan LK, Chiu YT, Xu IMJ, Poon RTP, Cheung TT, et al. TSC1/2 mutations define a molecular subset of HCC with aggressive behaviour and treatment implication. *Gut*. (2017) 66:1496–506. doi: 10.1136/gutjnl-2016-312734

12. Ho DW, Tsui YM, Sze KM, Chan LK, Cheung TT, Lee E, et al. Single-cell transcriptomics reveals the landscape of intra-tumoral heterogeneity and stemness-related subpopulations in liver cancer. *Cancer Lett*. (2019) 459:176–85. doi: 10.1016/j.canlet.2019.06.002

13. Ma W, Ho DW, Sze KM, Tsui YM, Chan LK, Lee JM, et al. APOBEC3B promotes hepatocarcinogenesis and metastasis through novel deaminase-independent activity. *Mol Carcinog*. (2019) 58:643–53. doi: 10.1002/mc.22956

14. Ho DW, Tsui YM, Chan LK, Sze KM, Zhang X, Cheu JW, et al. Single-cell RNA sequencing shows the immunosuppressive landscape and tumor heterogeneity of HBV-associated hepatocellular carcinoma. *Nat Commun*. (2021) 12:3684. doi: 10.1038/s41467-021-24010-1

15. Ho DW, Ng IO. uGPA: unified gene pathway analyzer package for high-throughput genome-wide screening data provides mechanistic overview on human diseases. *Clin Chim Acta*. (2015) 441:105–8.

16. Llovet JM, Zucman-Rossi J, Pikarsky E, Sangro B, Schwartz M, Sherman M, et al. Hepatocellular carcinoma. *Nat Rev Dis Primers*. (2016) 2:16018. doi: 10.1038/nrdp.2016.18

17. Williams GH, Stoeber K. The cell cycle and cancer. *J Pathol*. (2012) 226:352–64.

18. Hegde NS, Sanders DA, Rodriguez R, Balasubramanian S. The transcription factor FOXM1 is a cellular target of the natural product thiostrepton. *Nat Chem*. (2011) 3:725–31. doi: 10.1038/nchem.1114

19. Kwok JM, Myatt SS, Marson CM, Coombes RC, Constantinidou D, Lam EW. Thiostrepton selectively targets breast cancer cells through inhibition of forkhead box M1 expression. *Mol Cancer Ther*. (2008) 7:2022–32. doi: 10.1158/1535-7163.MCT-08-0188

20. Brown HK, Ottewell PD, Coleman RE, Holen I. The kinetochore protein Cenp-F is a potential novel target for zoledronic acid in breast cancer

cells. *J Cell Mol Med.* (2011) 15:501–13. doi: 10.1111/j.1582-4934.2009.0 0995.x

21. Mi YJ, Gao J, Xie JD, Cao JY, Cui SX, Gao HJ, et al. Prognostic relevance and therapeutic implications of centromere protein F expression in patients with esophageal squamous cell carcinoma. *Dis Esophagus.* (2013) 26:636–43. doi: 10.1111/dote.12002

22. Cao JY, Liu L, Chen SP, Zhang X, Mi YJ, Liu ZG, et al. Prognostic significance and therapeutic implications of centromere protein F expression in human nasopharyngeal carcinoma. *Mol Cancer.* (2010) 9:237. doi: 10.1186/1476-4598-9-237

17

Histopathological Evidence of Occipital Involvement in Male Androgenetic Alopecia

Saranya Khunkhet [1,2†], Kumutnart Chanprapaph [1†], Suthinee Rutnin [1†] and Poonkiat Suchonwanit [1*†]

[1] Division of Dermatology, Department of Medicine, Faculty of Medicine, Ramathibodi Hospital, Mahidol University, Bangkok, Thailand, [2] Skin Center, Srinakharinwirot University, Bangkok, Thailand

*Correspondence:
Poonkiat Suchonwanit
poonkiat@hotmail.com

†ORCID:
Saranya Khunkhet
orcid.org/0000-0001-9968-4243
Kumutnart Chanprapaph
orcid.org/0000-0001-7931-3816
Suthinee Rutnin
orcid.org/0000-0001-8268-8790
Poonkiat Suchonwanit
orcid.org/0000-0001-9723-0563

Background: The occipital region of the scalp is generally accepted as an unaffected area of androgenetic alopecia (AGA) for both genders. However, evidence of AGA involving the occipital scalp has been demonstrated in women; meanwhile, it is unclear whether occipital involvement also occurs in men.

Objective: We aimed to determine if there is occipital involvement in men with AGA.

Methods: This case-control study compared hair counts of scalp biopsy specimens from the occipital region of 82 men with Hamilton-Norwood III-VII and 82 unaffected men.

Results: The mean ages of men with AGA and controls were 40.1 ± 8.9 and 38.6 ± 10.5 years, respectively ($P = 0.291$). A significant decrease in total hair follicles, terminal hair follicles, follicular units and terminal to vellus (T:V) ratio, along with a significant increase in follicular stelae was indicated in the AGA group compared to controls (all $P < 0.05$). Subgroup analyses revealed that average counts of total hair follicles, terminal hair follicles and T:V ratios were also significantly lower in males with Hamilton-Norwood VI and VII than in controls (all $P < 0.05$). There were no correlations between increasing age and hair count parameters, but a significant negative association was found between total follicle numbers and disease duration ($r = -0.23$, $P = 0.02$).

Conclusions: AGA can involve the occipital area of male patients with advanced disease. Therefore, the occiput of particular cases should not be used to determine reference data for normal scalp hair, and preoperative measurements of miniaturized hairs in the donor site are strongly recommended in all persons undergoing hair transplantation.

Keywords: pattern hair loss, transverse section, hair count, donor site, hair transplantation, miniaturization

INTRODUCTION

The most common cause of hair loss in both men and women is androgenetic alopecia (AGA), also known as pattern hair loss, and is characterized by gradual hair thinning within a specific distribution on the scalp in genetically susceptible individuals (1). Male patients typically present with hairline recession in the frontotemporal areas as well as balding of the vertex and mid-scalp whereas female patients usually manifest as diffuse hair thinning over the central scalp with a preserved frontal hairline (2). Androgens are apparently implicated in the pathogenesis of male

AGA; by contrast, the role of androgens in women is much less established (3, 4). Although the etiologies between men and women are not identical, they share similar features which include a miniaturization of hair follicles and a progressive shortening of anagen duration (1, 5).

The diagnosis of AGA is usually straightforward and based upon characteristic clinical findings; however, scalp biopsies, in particular transverse sections, may be required to achieve a definite diagnosis in uncertain cases. The main histopathological features of AGA are as follows: (i) decreased terminal hair follicles and increased vellus hair follicles resulting in a reduced ratio of terminal to vellus (T:V) follicles of <4:1; (ii) a slightly increased telogen count, standardly accounting for 15–20%; (iii) the presence of follicular stelae below miniaturized hair follicles; and (iv) normal follicular density, apart from long-standing and advanced stages, which reveal an actual decrease in total hair follicles (6, 7).

The occipital region of the scalp has been widely accepted as an uninvolved area of AGA for both sexes, under the concept that affected persons have androgen-sensitive and androgen-insensitive scalp regions. This principle has led to the subsequent introduction of donor dominance theory and hair transplantation as a treatment option. Nonetheless, in our practice, we have observed hair thinning extending toward the occipital scalp in some advanced AGA, with more frequent observations among female patients. This may be partly due to the fact that androgen-independent mechanisms also play a role in many women. Moreover, it was highlighted in the field of hair restoration surgery that hair miniaturization can occur in the back and sides of the scalp (the donor sites), which will negatively influence transplant outcomes (8).

Occipital involvement has been demonstrated in female patients with AGA. Previous phototrichogram studies comparing hair characteristics in the occipital area between female AGA and normal controls showed highly consistent results (9–12). Statistically significant decreases in hair density and thickness relative to controls were confirmed in subjects with Ludwig II and III. Additionally, Ekmekci et al. conducted hair counts in biopsy specimens from the mid-scalp and occipital areas of forty female subjects with Ludwig I and II. A quarter of the subjects possessed occipital findings compatible with AGA (T:V ratios of <4:1), and almost 40% of the subjects had findings of suspected AGA in the occipital scalp (T:V ratios ranged from 4:1 to 7:1) (13).

On the contrary, occipital involvement in male AGA has not been proved. The results of phototrichogram studies, performed on the occipital region of men with AGA and normal men, have also been inconsistent. One study showed no significant differences in all hair parameters (14). Another study found statistically significant decreases in hair density and hair diameter in male subjects with the U type of the Basic and Specific classification, corresponding to Hamilton-Norwood VI and VII (15). The aim of our study was to determine whether occipital involvement existed in male patients with AGA.

MATERIALS AND METHODS

Study Design and Participants

This study was approved by the Mahidol University Institutional Review Board for Ethics in Human Research (MURA2020/165) and was conducted in accordance with the principles of the Declaration of Helsinki and in compliance with the International Conference on Harmonization-Good Clinical Practice and local regulatory requirements. Informed consent was obtained from the study participants or their families, as appropriate. All male patients with biopsy-proven AGA, who underwent paired 4 mm punch biopsies from both affected frontal/vertex and clinically normal occipital regions of the scalp for transverse sectioning from 2014 to 2019, were enrolled into this case-control study. Patient demographics and clinical data were collected. Principal exclusion criteria included incomplete medical records and the presence of other hair and scalp disorders. Additional exclusion criteria were documented systemic diseases related to hair loss, the use of medications or energy-based devices which can affect hair growth within 6 months and a history of hair transplantation.

As being considered the most reliable method, histological examination of transverse sections from scalp biopsy specimens was chosen to confirm androgenetic changes. Regarding the biopsy protocol in patients with AGA at our institution, the biopsy landmark on the occipital scalp was the external occipital protuberance of the skull. Paired biopsy specimens from the balding and non-balding occipital scalp were horizontally sectioned using the techniques described by Whiting DA (6). Tissue slides of the biopsy specimen from the occipital scalp in each study subject were reviewed. Two cases were excluded as we were unable to obtain the slides and three cases were excluded on account of tangential cuts, which complicated histologic interpretation. A total of 82 cases remained for analysis.

Control Subjects

The control group consisted of 82 male adult decedents who required an autopsy for legal documentation at our institution. These decedents had no type of hair loss and received a 4 mm punch biopsy on the normal occipital scalp, following our AGA biopsy protocol, for transverse sectioning within 8 h of death to avoid autolysis, after receiving written informed consent from the bereaved relatives. Controls were randomly selected from a pool of male deceased subjects in our previous studies on hair counts from scalp biopsy specimens in the Thai population (16, 17), with an equal number of cases and controls. The biopsy specimens of controls were processed using a protocol identical to those of the study cases. The exclusion criteria used were also indistinguishable.

Assessments

Histology slides of specimens from the occipital scalp of both case and control subjects were re-examined by a blinded dermatopathologist. All follicular structures were identified at various anatomical levels from the epidermis to subcutis. The numbers of total, terminal, and vellus hair follicles, along with the number of follicular units, were recorded. Anagen and telogen hair follicles, as well as follicular stelae were also counted. Catagen hair follicles were included in the group of telogen hair follicles. Half of the intermediate hair follicles were assigned to terminal hair follicles with the other half to vellus hair follicles. Differences in hair parameters between groups were subsequently analyzed.

Statistical Analyses

The minimum sample size for estimation of population mean with a 10% margin of error was 26, calculated using data from the previous study assessing values of hair counts per 4 mm diameter punch biopsy from the occipital scalp of Koreans, demonstrating that the mean number of total hair follicles in male subjects was 15.3 ± 3.9 (18).

Comparisons between study and control groups were performed using the Student's t-test, the Mann-Whitney U test, or the Chi-squared test as appropriate. For further analyses among study subgroups based on disease severity was conducted using the analysis of variance, the Kruskal-Wallis test, or the Chi-squared test. When the overall comparison $P < 0.05$, pairwise

comparisons of subgroups were performed using the Turkey's honest significance difference test, the Mann-Whitney U test, or the Chi-squared test as appropriate. The impact of advancing age on hair changes was determined using the Pearson correlation coefficient. A $P < 0.05$ was considered significant, and all statistical analyses were performed with SPSS software (PASW version 18.0; SPSS Inc., Chicago, IL).

RESULTS

Comparisons of Hair Count Parameters Between AGA and Control Groups

Hair counts from the clinically normal occipital scalp of patients with AGA, compared to controls, are shown in **Table 1**. The mean age of 82 patients with AGA was 40.1 ± 8.9 years whereas the mean age of 82 control subjects was 38.6 ± 10.5 years. The age difference between groups was not statistically significant ($P = 0.291$), representing only 18 months; therefore, an age adjustment was not applied. The mean number of total hair follicles in AGA subjects was 17.6 ± 4.2 (95% confidence interval [CI]: 16.68–18.52), showing a significantly lower number compared with controls (mean: 19.1 ± 6.1, 95% CI: 18.56–21.24, $P = 0.005$). Average counts of terminal hair follicles and follicular units were also significantly lower in patients with AGA than in controls ($P = 0.001$ and 0.002, respectively). In addition, there was a significant decrease in T:V ratio and a significant increase in follicular stelae in the AGA group ($P = 0.001$ and 0.035, respectively).

Subgroup Analyses of Subjects With AGA

The summary of hair counts in the control and AGA subgroups based on disease severity are exhibited in **Table 2**. As for the severity of AGA according to Hamilton-Norwood classification, 14 (17%), 18 (22%), 15 (18%), 19 (23%), and 16 (20%) patients were grades III, IV, V, VI, and VII, respectively. The overall comparisons among subgroups revealed statistically significant differences in total hair follicles, terminal hair follicles,

TABLE 1 | Hair counts per 4 mm diameter punch biopsy from the occipital scalp of male patients with androgenetic alopecia and controls.

	Controls	AGA	P-value
Number of cases	82	82	
Age, y, mean (SD)	38.6 (10.5)	40.1 (8.9)	0.291
Total hair follicles, mean (SD)	19.9 (6.1)	17.6 (4.2)	0.005*
Terminal hair follicles, mean (SD)	17.9 (4.2)	15.9 (3.8)	0.001*
Vellus hair follicles, median (range)	2 (0–7)	3 (0–14)	0.359
Follicular units, mean (SD)	9.3 (1.9)	8.4 (1.8)	0.002*
Follicular stelae, median (range)	1 (0–4)	3 (0–12)	0.035*
Terminal:vellus ratio	8.9:1	7.4:1	0.001*
Anagen:telogen ratio	92.2:7.8	87.6:12.4	0.889

AGA, androgenetic alopecia; SD, standard deviation; y, year.
*Statistically significant.

TABLE 2 | Hair counts in the occipital scalp of controls and patient subgroups with different disease severity of androgenetic alopecia.

	Controls	Hamilton-Norwood stages of AGA subjects					P-value
		III	IV	V	VI	VII	
Number of cases	82	14	18	15	19	16	
Age, y, mean (SD)	38.6 (10.5)	40.5 (11.4)	38.2 (12.4)	44.6 (10.2)	38.8 (8.4)	49.5 (7.4)	0.079
Disease duration, y, mean (SD)	–	3.6 (0.8)	5.2 (1.5)	6.5 (2.2)	6.9 (1.9)	8.3 (2.3)	0.001*
Total HFs, mean (SD)	19.9 (6.1)	18.6 (4.9)	19.1 (5.2)	17.8 (5.1)	15.3 (5.4)	14.2 (4.4)	0.002*
Terminal HFs, mean (SD)	17.9 (4.2)	17.9 (4.8)	18.3 (4.9)	16.1 (5.2)	13.1 (4.2)	11.9 (3.9)	0.002*
Vellus HFs, median (range)	2 (0–7)	2 (0–5)	2 (0–8)	3 (0–10)	3 (0–11)	4 (0–14)	0.146
Follicular units, mean (SD)	9.3 (1.9)	8.7 (1.9)	8.8 (2.1)	8.5 (1.6)	7.9 (1.4)	8.1 (2.5)	0.035*
Stelae, median (range)	1 (0–4)	1 (0–4)	1 (0–6)	2 (0–8)	2 (0–7)	3 (0–12)	0.294
Terminal:vellus ratio	8.9:1	8.6:1	8.8:1	7.9:1	6.8:1	5.3:1	0.001*
Anagen:telogen ratio	92.2:7.8	90.7:9.3	91.2:8.8	88.6:11.4	85.4:14.6	83.2:16.8	0.294

AGA, androgenetic alopecia; HF, hair follicle; SD, standard deviation; y, year.
*Statistically significant.

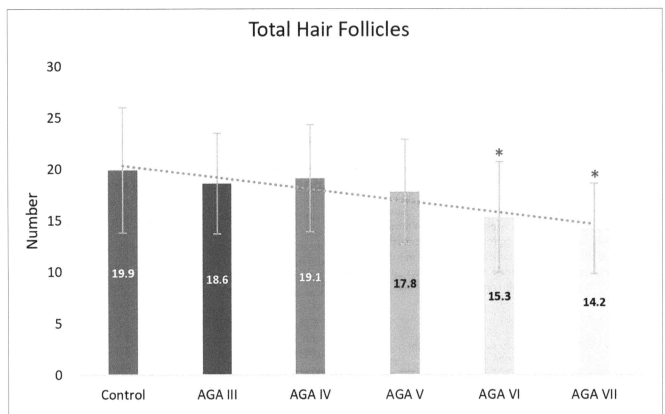

FIGURE 1 | Total hair follicles between controls and patient subgroups with different disease severity of androgenetic alopecia **(AGA)**. *$P < 0.05$ when compared to the control group.

follicular units and T:V ratios ($P = 0.002$, 0.002, 0.035 and 0.001, respectively).

Subgroup analyses showed no significant differences in age between groups; nevertheless, pairwise comparisons displayed significant decreases in the average numbers of total and terminal hair follicles, as well as T:V ratios, in patients with AGA grades VI and VII, when compared to the control group (all $P < 0.05$) (**Figures 1–3**). There were no significant associations between increasing age and changes in any of the hair parameters; however, a significant negative association between total follicle numbers and disease duration was found (r = −0.23, $P = 0.02$).

DISCUSSION

We assessed the histopathological changes in the occipital scalp of men with AGA compared with the normal occipital scalp of unaffected men and found a significant reduction in total hair follicles, terminal hair follicles and T:V ratio, along with a significant increase of follicular stelae in the occipital scalp of male subjects with AGA. Furthermore, AGA patients had a somewhat wider range of vellus follicle numbers than unaffected men, even though a significant difference in statistics was not achieved among median values. These results parallel the findings from previous histopathological studies analyzing biopsy specimens from the frontal or vertex area of men with

AGA compared to the same scalp sites of normal controls (6, 19, 20).

Based on subgroup comparisons, the more advanced the AGA, the more pronounced the changes in hair parameters, but statistically significant differences from controls were established only in subgroups with advanced disease (Hamilton-Norwood VI-VII). These findings are consonant with two previous comparative studies using phototrichogram analysis on the occipital scalp between male AGA and normal controls. The study showing no significant differences solely recruited subjects with mild to moderate severity (Hamilton-Norwood I–V) (14), whereas the other study revealed a significant change of hair density and diameter in patients with the U type, the most severe type of the Basic and Specific classification, compatible with Hamilton-Norwood VI–VII (15).

Androgenetic changes in the occipital region appear dissimilar to changes in the frontal and vertex regions. An approximate 25% reduction of total follicle numbers in patients with Hamilton-Norwood VI–VII was noticed while the average T:V ratios in these patients were 6.8:1 and 5.3:1, reduced from a normal ratio of 8.9:1 in controls. A noticeable depletion of total hair follicles can be observed in conjunction with an unsubstantial degree of hair miniaturization. In contrast to changes in the frontal and vertex regions, an actual reduction of total follicle numbers is particularly recognized

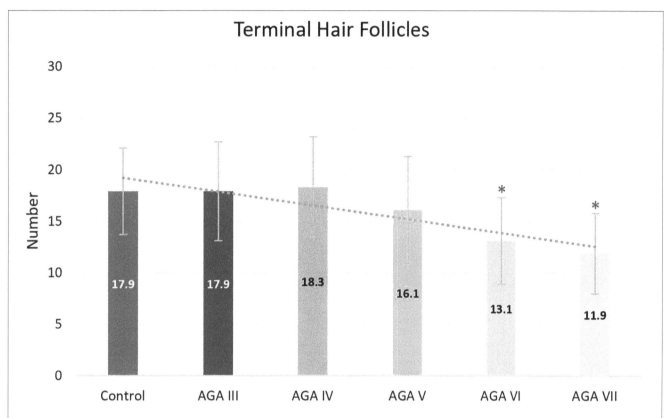

FIGURE 2 | Terminal hair follicles between controls and patient subgroups with different disease severity of androgenetic alopecia **(AGA)**. *$P < 0.05$ when compared to the control group.

at advanced stages of disease, when a reversal of terminal to vellus hair follicles seems to be obvious (6, 19). Hence, these feature deviations may imply unique characteristics of the occipital scalp in the process of AGA. We hypothesize that occipital hair follicles comprise two populations: one small component influenced by AGA and the unaffected majority. Therefore, clinical changes of AGA in the occipital scalp can be detected only in very advanced disease when the small population experiences pronounced androgenetic changes, including follicular dropout. Meanwhile, the impact on the T:V ratio remains minimal as a large number of normal hair follicles from the unaffected population are included in the ratio calculation.

Distinct anatomical structures and properties related to androgens are suspected to be mainly responsible for site-specific alterations in the occipital scalp of individuals with AGA (21, 22). Accumulating evidence suggests that hair follicles in the occipital area might elicit less androgen-regulated cellular responses than hair follicles in the other scalp areas (22, 23). Frontal hair follicles contained a significantly higher level of androgen receptors and 5α-reductase enzymes, known for converting testosterone into a more potent androgen called dihydrotestosterone, compared to occipital hair follicles for both genders (24–27). Scalp biopsies also demonstrated a greater amount of aromatase, the enzyme accountable for lowering androgen levels by turning into estrogens, within the occipital

rather than the frontal hair follicles in both men and women (21, 24, 28). Moreover, distinctive characteristics of the occipital scalp are perhaps due to its unique embryological origin. In regard to structural development of the head in vertebrates, a large portion is of neural crest origin while some posterior parts of the head, including the occipital region, are derived from the mesoderm (29).

As no correlation was established in this study between increasing age and total follicle numbers, the follicular dropout that occurred among the men with AGA seems not to result from senescent alopecia. These male patients also displayed an increase of miniaturized hairs and telogen counts, which are not features of age-related alopecia (30–34). On the other hand, a negative correlation between total follicle numbers and disease duration was indicated, showing a coherence with histopathological features of AGA in the original sites where follicular dropout can be observed in long-standing disease (7, 35).

The limitation of this study includes the limited ethnic population. Physical properties of hair, such as hair shapes and density, differ between ethnicities. Our findings might not be generalized to other racial and ethnic groups. Further well-designed prospective studies with diverse racial subjects are required to confirm the present findings.

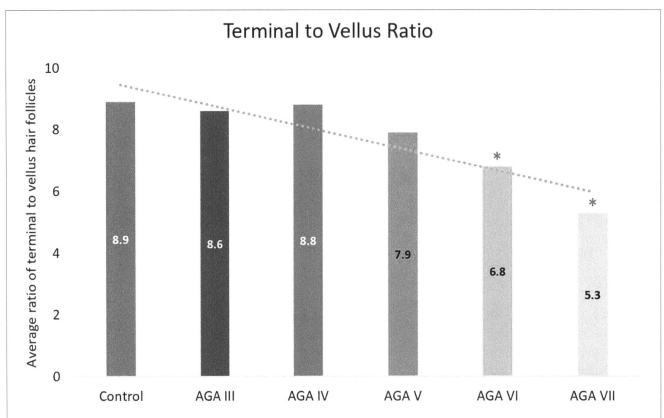

FIGURE 3 | Terminal to vellus hair ratio between controls and patient subgroups with different disease severity of androgenetic alopecia **(AGA)**. *$P < 0.05$ when compared to the control group.

CONCLUSION

Three main issues and recommendations are derived from this study. First, AGA extendedly involves the occipital area in male patients with advanced disease. Second, androgenetic changes can occur even in the clinically normal occipital scalp; therefore, the occiput of individuals with AGA, especially in advanced stages, should not be used to determine reference data for normal scalp hair. Third, preoperative measurements of miniaturized hairs present in the donor site are strongly recommended in all persons undergoing hair transplantation due to their impact on the success of surgery.

AUTHOR CONTRIBUTIONS

PS and KC: conceptualization and writing—review and editing. PS and SR: methodology and validation. PS, KC, and SK: formal analysis. PS and SK: investigation and data curation. SK and KC: writing—original draft preparation. All authors have read and agreed to the published version of the manuscript.

REFERENCES

1. Meephansan J, Thummakriengkrai J, Ponnikorn S, Yingmema W, Deenonpoe R, Suchonwanit P. Efficacy of topical tofacitinib in promoting hair growth in non-scarring alopecia: possible mechanism via VEGF induction. *Arch Dermatol Res.* (2017) 309:729–38. doi: 10.1007/s00403-017-

2. Leerunyakul K, Suchonwanit P. Asian hair: a review of structures, properties, and distinctive disorders. *Clin Cosmet Investig Dermatol.* (2020) 13:309–18. doi: 10.2147/CCID.S247390

3. Suchonwanit P, Iamsumang W, Rojhirunsakool S. Efficacy of topical combination of 0.25% finasteride and 3% minoxidil versus 3% minoxidil solution in female pattern hair loss: a randomized, double-blind, controlled study. *Am J Clin Dermatol.* (2019) 20:147–53. doi: 10.1007/s40257-018-0387-0

4. Lamsumang W, Leerunyakul K, Suchonwanit P. Finasteride and its potential for the treatment of female pattern hair loss: evidence to date. *Drug Des Devel Ther.* (2020) 14:951–9. doi: 10.2147/DDDT.S240615

5. Suchonwanit P, Rojhirunsakool S, Khunkhet S. A randomized, investigator-blinded, controlled, split-scalp study of the efficacy and safety of a 1550-nm fractional erbium-glass laser, used in combination with topical 5% minoxidil versus 5% minoxidil alone, for the treatment of androgenetic alopecia. *Lasers Med Sci.* (2019) 34:1857–64. doi: 10.1007/s10103-019-02783-8

6. Whiting DA. Diagnostic and predictive value of horizontal sections of scalp biopsy specimens in male pattern androgenetic alopecia. *J Am Acad Dermatol.* (1993) 28(Pt. 1):755–63. doi: 10.1016/0190-9622(93)70106-4

7. Olsen EA, Messenger AG, Shapiro J, Bergfeld WF, Hordinsky MK, Roberts JL, et al. Evaluation and treatment of male and female pattern hair loss. *J Am Acad Dermatol.* (2005) 52:301–11. doi: 10.1016/j.jaad.2004.04.008

8. Bernstein R, Rassman W. Densitometry and video-microscopy. *Hair Transplant Forum Int.* (2007) 17:49–51. doi: 10.33589/17.2.0041

9. Ekmekci TR, Koslu A. Phototrichogram findings in women with androgenetic alopecia. *Skin Res Technol.* (2006) 12:309–12. doi: 10.1111/j.0909-752X.2006.00196.x

10. Kang H, Kang TW, Lee SD, Park YM, Kim HO, Kim SY. The changing patterns of hair density and thickness in South Korean women with hair loss: clinical office-based phototrichogram analysis. *Int J Dermatol.* (2009) 48:14–21. doi: 10.1111/j.1365-4632.2009.03795.x

11. Mai W, Sun Y, Liu X, Lin D, Lu D. Characteristic findings by phototrichogram in southern Chinese women with female pattern hair loss. *Skin Res Technol.* (2019) 25:447–55. doi: 10.1111/srt.12672

12. Rojhirunsakool S, Suchonwanit P. Parietal scalp is another affected area in female pattern hair loss: an analysis of hair density and hair diameter. *Clin Cosmet Investig Dermatol.* (2018) 11:7–12. doi: 10.2147/CCID.S153768

13. Ekmekci TR, Sakiz D, Koslu A. Occipital involvement in female pattern hair loss: histopathological evidences. *J Eur Acad Dermatol Venereol.* (2010) 24:299–301. doi: 10.1111/j.1468-3083.2009.03411.x

14. Leroy T, Van Neste D. Contrast enhanced phototrichogram pinpoints scalp hair changes in androgen sensitive areas of male androgenetic alopecia. *Skin Res Technol.* (2002) 8:106–11. doi: 10.1034/j.1600-0846.2002.00329.x

15. Kim JY, Kim MH, Hong SP, Park BC. Characteristics of nonbalding scalp zones of androgenetic alopecia in East Asians. *Clin Exp Dermatol.* (2015) 40:279–85. doi: 10.1111/ced.12554

16. Visessiri Y, Pakornphadungsit K, Leerunyakul K, Rutnin S, Srisont S, Suchonwanit P. The study of hair follicle counts from scalp histopathology in the Thai population. *Int J Dermatol.* (2020) 59:978–81. doi: 10.1111/ijd.14989

17. Rutnin S, Chanprapaph K, Pakornphadungsit K, Leerunyakul K, Visessiri Y, Srisont S, et al. Variation of hair follicle counts among different scalp areas: a quantitative histopathological study. *Skin Appendage Disord.* (2021) 1–7. doi: 10.1159/000518434. [Epub ahead of print].

18. Lee HJ, Ha SJ, Lee JH, Kim JW, Kim HO, Whiting DA. Hair counts from scalp biopsy specimens in Asians. *J Am Acad Dermatol.* (2002) 46:218–21. doi: 10.1067/mjd.2002.119558

19. Aslani FS, Dastgheib L, Banihashemi BM. Hair counts in scalp biopsy of males and females with androgenetic alopecia compared with normal subjects. *J Cutan Pathol.* (2009) 36:734–9. doi: 10.1111/j.1600-0560.2008.01149.x

20. El-Domyati M, Attia S, Saleh F, Abdel-Wahab H. Androgenetic alopecia in males: a histopathological and ultrastructural study. *J Cosmet Dermatol.* (2009) 8:83–91. doi: 10.1111/j.1473-2165.2009.00439.x

21. Suchonwanit P, Triyangkulsri K, Ploydaeng M, Leerunyakul K. Assessing biophysical and physiological profiles of scalp seborrheic dermatitis in the Thai population. *Biomed Res Int.* (2019) 2019:5128376. doi: 10.1155/2019/5128376

22. Chanprapaph K, Sutharaphan T, Suchonwanit P. Scalp biophysical characteristics in males with androgenetic alopecia: a comparative study with healthy controls. *Clin Interv Aging.* (2021) 16:781–7. doi: 10.2147/CIA.S310178

23. Suchonwanit P, McMichael AJ. Alopecia in association with malignancy: a review. *Am J Clin Dermatol.* (2018) 19:853–65. doi: 10.1007/s40257-018-0378-1

24. Sawaya ME, Price VH. Different levels of 5alpha-reductase type I and II, aromatase, and androgen receptor in hair follicles of women and men with androgenetic alopecia. *J Invest Dermatol.* (1997) 109:296–300. doi: 10.1111/1523-1747.ep12335779

25. Suchonwanit P, Iamsumang W, Leerunyakul K. Topical finasteride for the treatment of male androgenetic alopecia and female pattern hair loss: a review of the current literature. *J Dermatolog Treat.* (2020) 1–6. doi: 10.1080/09546634.2020.1782324. [Epub ahead of print].

26. Hibberts NA, Howell AE, Randall VA. Balding hair follicle dermal papilla cells contain higher levels of androgen receptors than those from non-balding scalp. *J Endocrinol.* (1998) 156:59–65. doi: 10.1677/joe.0.1560059

27. Chanprapaph K, Mahasaksiri T, Kositkuljorn C, Leerunyakul K, Suchonwanit P. Prevalence and risk factors associated with the occurrence of autoimmune diseases in patients with Alopecia Areata. *J Inflamm Res.* (2021) 14:4881–91. doi: 10.2147/JIR.S331579

28. Suchonwanit P, Triamchaisri S, Wittayakornrerk S, Rattanakaemakorn P. Leprosy reaction in Thai population: a 20-year retrospective study. *Dermatol Res Pract.* (2015) 2015:253154. doi: 10.1155/2015/253154

29. Noden DM, Trainor PA. Relations and interactions between cranial mesoderm and neural crest populations. *J Anat.* (2005) 207:575–601. doi: 10.1111/j.1469-7580.2005.00473.x

30. Leerunyakul K, Suchonwanit P. Evaluation of hair density and hair diameter in the adult Thai population using quantitative trichoscopic analysis. *Biomed Res Int.* (2020) 2020:2476890. doi: 10.1155/2020/2476890

31. Whiting DA. How real is senescent alopecia? A histopathologic approach. *Clin Dermatol.* (2011) 29:49–53. doi: 10.1016/j.clindermatol.2010.07.007

32. Suchonwanit P, Udompanich S, Thadanipon K, Chanprapaph K. Trichoscopic signs in systemic lupus erythematosus: a comparative study with 109 patients and 305 healthy controls. *J Eur Acad Dermatol Venereol.* (2019) 33:774–80. doi: 10.1111/jdv.15421

33. Sriphojanart T, Khunkhet S, Suchonwanit P. A retrospective comparative study of the efficacy and safety of two regimens of diphenylcyclopropenone in the treatment of recalcitrant alopecia areata. *Dermatol Rep.* (2017) 9:7399. doi: 10.4081/dr.2017.7399

34. Suchonwanit P, Hector CE, Bin Saif GA, McMichael AJ. Factors affecting the severity of central centrifugal cicatricial alopecia. *Int J Dermatol.* (2016) 55:e338–43. doi: 10.1111/ijd.13061

35. Chanprapaph K, Udompanich S, Visessiri Y, Ngamjanyaporn P, Suchonwanit P. Nonscarring alopecia in systemic lupus erythematosus: a cross-sectional study with trichoscopic, histopathologic, and immunopathologic analyses. *J Am Acad Dermatol.* (2019) 81:1319–29. doi: 10.1016/j.jaad.2019.05.053

18

From Macroscopy to Ultrastructure: An Integrative Approach to Pulmonary Pathology

Stijn E. Verleden [1,2,3†], Peter Braubach [4,5†], Christopher Werlein [5], Edith Plucinski [4,5], Mark P. Kuhnel [4,5], Annemiek Snoeckx [6], Haroun El Addouli [6], Tobias Welte [4,7], Axel Haverich [4,8], Florian P. Laenger [4,5], Sabine Dettmer [4,9], Patrick Pauwels [10], Veronique Verplancke [2], Paul E. Van Schil [1,3], Therese Lapperre [2,11], Johanna M. Kwakkel-Van-Erp [2,11], Maximilian Ackermann [12,13], Jeroen M. H. Hendriks [1,3] and Danny Jonigk [4,5*]

[1] Antwerp Surgical Training, Anatomy and Research Centre (ASTARC), Antwerp University, Antwerp, Belgium, [2] Division of Pneumology, University Hospital Antwerp, Edegem, Belgium, [3] Department of Thoracic and Vascular Surgery, University Hospital Antwerp, Edegem, Belgium, [4] Member of the German Center for Lung Research (DZL), Biomedical Research in Endstage and Obstructive Lung Disease Hannover (BREATH), Hannover, Germany, [5] Institute for Pathology, Hannover Medical School, Hannover, Germany, [6] Division of Radiology, University Hospital Antwerp and University of Antwerp, Edegem, Belgium, [7] Division of Pneumology, Hannover Medical School, Hannover, Germany, [8] Division of Thoracic Surgery, Hannover Medical School, Hannover, Germany, [9] Department of Radiology, Hannover Medical School, Hannover, Germany, [10] Division of Pathology, University Hospital Antwerp, Edegem, Belgium, [11] Laboratory of Experimental Medicine and Pediatrics (LEMP), Antwerp University, Antwerp, Belgium, [12] Institute of Pathology and Department of Molecular Pathology, Helios University Clinic Wuppertal, University of Witten-Herdecke, Witten, Germany, [13] Institute of Functional and Clinical Anatomy, University Medical Center of the Johannes Gutenberg University Mainz, Mainz, Germany

*Correspondence:
Danny Jonigk
jonigk.danny@mh-hannover.de

[†]*These authors have contributed equally to this work*

Pathology and radiology are complimentary tools, and their joint application is often crucial in obtaining an accurate diagnosis in non-neoplastic pulmonary diseases. However, both come with significant limitations of their own: Computed Tomography (CT) can only visualize larger structures due to its inherent–relatively–poor resolution, while (histo)pathology is often limited due to small sample size and sampling error and only allows for a 2D investigation. An innovative approach of inflating whole lung specimens and subjecting these subsequently to CT and whole lung microCT allows for an accurate matching of CT-imaging and histopathology data of exactly the same areas. Systematic application of this approach allows for a more targeted assessment of localized disease extent and more specifically can be used to investigate early mechanisms of lung diseases on a morphological and molecular level. Therefore, this technique is suitable to selectively investigate changes in the large and small airways, as well as the pulmonary arteries, veins and capillaries in relation to the disease extent in the same lung specimen. In this perspective we provide an overview of the different strategies that are currently being used, as well as how this growing field could further evolve.

Keywords: microCT, lung, histology, lung disease, imaging

INTRODUCTION

Computed tomography (CT), positron emission tomography (PET) and histopathology are major components in the differential diagnosis and follow-up of patients with acute and chronic non-neoplastic respiratory diseases. Given the diversity in CT and histologic presentation and the inherent morphologic differences in strategies of diagnosis between neoplastic and non-neoplastic disease, we will specifically focus on non-neoplastic diseases. Especially as these tend to result in significant day-to-day challenges in the differential diagnosis.

Particularly in the field of interstitial lung diseases (ILD), there is an important diagnostic and prognostic role for CT and histopathology, with a growing emphasis on the relative weight of chest imaging as a diagnostic tool (1). Thus, the need for an invasive video-assisted or robot- assisted thoracic surgery biopsy to confirm differential diagnosis has drastically reduced. Consequently, lung biopsies are currently only recommended for those challenging cases where major discrepancies are observed between CT and clinical findings and a clear diagnosis cannot be rendered. Given this important role of imaging in the management of ILD, it is primordial to integrate the existing clinical, imaging and histopathologic data as much as possible.

Initially, assessment of remodeling and fibrosis patterns by experienced radiologists was the only way to leverage the available imaging data, but gradually and partly due to the large inter-observer variability, automated image analysis tools for characterization and quantification of CT signs and patterns have been developed of which some are on the verge of making their appearance in routine clinical care. CT can provide 3D insight into the (gross) morphological changes in the lung. However, CT patterns are often nonspecific and may change during the evolution of a disease. Importantly, CT changes may also have more than one (histo-) pathological correlate. For example, a study demonstrated that more than 90% of patients presenting with CT findings that were inconsistent with usual interstitial pneumonia demonstrated histological evidence of usual interstitial pneumonia (2). Additionally, *in vivo* resolution is rather limited with a slice thickness of 1 mm most commonly being used for routine patient CT scans due to radiation concerns. This is sufficient to investigate airways and vessels >1 mm in diameter and gross changes in the secondary pulmonary lobule and the lung parenchyma. However, the small airways, the cellular composition and specific smaller sized structures are impossible to address, although morphologic secondary effects of primary changes such as hyperinflation and air trapping may be observed.

Histopathology on the other hand provides the advantage of a detailed analysis of the morphologic and cellular changes within the lung, whereby structures in the micrometer range can be readily resolved. However, (histo-) pathology is limited due to relatively small tissue samples and only allows for a 2D investigation. This can lead to discordance between initial diagnosis made on transbronchial cryobiopsy or surgical lung biopsy and the final diagnosis made in explant lung specimens at the time of transplantation (15–22 and 12.4% respectively) (3, 4). In addition, the lung is considered quite fragile, making it vulnerable for deformation and distortion during the preparation resulting in histologic artifacts potentially hampering microscopic examination.

As, especially non-neoplastic pulmonary diseases, show a great spatial heterogeneity in disease activity and progression, targeted sampling is essential. It is reasonable to assume that often important patterns/changes in the lung can be overlooked due to sampling bias or sectioning artifacts upon histologic examination.

Proof of concept data of the huge potential of microCT, a tool designed to combine the 3D aspect of CT with almost full histological resolution, to investigate human lung (disease) was provided in 2005. However, at the time, the authors were still struggling to obtain sufficient contrast between air and tissue (5). A subsequent porcine study by Litzlbauer et al. (6) extensively validated the use of microCT with histology, showing great promise in measuring morphological changes such as alveolar surface density and mean linear intercept. Therefore, we and others have further optimized these protocols for *ex-vivo* scanning of human lung tissue to bridge the gap between radiology and histopathology, and thus between macroscopy and near-cellular resolution. In this article, we describe a unique approach of air-inflating whole human lung/lobe explants and subjecting these to a wide spectrum of investigations. We propose to use this macro to micro approach leveraging CT and microCT to bridge the gap between radiologic data and histopathology with illustrative examples. Further, we propose to use this approach to selectively investigate changes in the large and small airways, the interstitial compartment as well as the pulmonary arteries, veins and capillaries in relation to the disease extent in the same lung specimen. In addition, other promising tools are discussed in more detail including their potential applications. We acknowledge that a plethora of techniques has also been investigated in animal studies, which can readily be leveraged to combine imaging data with mechanistical insights (7); however, we deliberately focus on studies in humans that can be implemented more easily into routine clinical practice.

METHODOLOGY OF LUNG PROCESSING

Obtaining sufficient contrast between tissue and air is of major importance in the imaging of lung explants. Therefore, immediately following surgical resection, the lung is collected and cannulated via the main stem bronchus. Applying water-controlled air pressure, inflating the lung with 30 cm of water pressure and subsequently lowering the pressure to 10 cm of water pressure allows for an even and uniform recruitment of the lung specimen. The lungs are then mounted in a styrofoam box and frozen in liquid nitrogen vapors. At this moment, the lungs can be safely stored at −80°C until further use. *Ex vivo* CT scanning can be used to correlate with the last available *in vivo* CT, which already allows a higher spatial resolution due to higher radiation doses that can be used. MicroCT scanning of entire lung specimens is more complicated and a dedicated device is needed, where large samples can be mounted while keeping the lung frozen solid inside a styrofoam box. Depending on the size of the specimen, a resolution of 90–150 micron is feasible, thereby increasing the resolution 6–8 fold compared to conventional *in vivo* CT imaging.

After CT and microCT imaging, which can be used to identify structures of interest, the lung is cut in even slices using a band saw and smaller sized samples with a diameter typically between 12 and 22 mm can be extracted with a core bore or power drill depending on the degree of fibrosis within the samples. These samples can subsequently be re-scanned with high-resolution microCT preferably while keeping the sample frozen (8), where a further increase in resolution can be achieved given the smaller size of the respective specimen, typically up to 5–15 microns.

Subsequently, the lung can be further processed for histopathologic and molecular assessment, e.g., by formalin fixation and dehydration of samples. Our workflow is further illustrated in **Figure 1**. The quality of standard histology is not severely impaired by the prior process of freezing and scanning the lung. Although minor freezing artifacts can be observed, the quality of the histology is much better compared to frozen sections, explained by the fact that the tissue is never in direct contact with ice-cold solutions such as glutaraldehyde. It is very important to emphasize that this process of freezing the lung *in toto* and using microCT also has limited negative impact on further downstream molecular analysis illustrated by e.g., similar gene expression signatures in scanned vs. non-scanned specimens (8). Also bulk RNA-sequencing (9, 10), immunohistochemistry (11), and microbiome sequencing (Einarsson et al. accepted for publication) have already been performed, making ours a valid tool for more molecular-based research.

CT AND MICROCT OF EXPLANT LUNGS

Leveraging CT and whole lung microCT, an easier separation of the lung into morphologically inconspicuous, moderate and severely diseased areas can be made, that can be specifically sampled using the targeted sampling protocol described above. The healthy appearing areas as evident from the imaging can be used as a proxy of early disease. This is valuable given the temporal heterogeneity in non-neoplastic lung diseases, since genuine specimens with early disease features for research purposes are difficult to obtain. There is certainly some ground truth in such a hypothesis as distinct morphological and molecular processes have been demonstrated in minimally affected vs. severely affected regions (9, 10).

Next to pattern and structure analysis, it is also possible to visually identify and segment the entire bronchial tree from the main stem bronchus until the last branch of conducting airways (i.e., terminal bronchioles). This approach can therefore be used to investigate airway abnormalities like airway collapse, airway obstruction or bronchiectasis on a whole lung scale. In addition quantitative data such as the numbers of airways per generation, airway diameters and segment lengths can be generated as has been described already in COPD (12), graft-vs.-host-disease post-allogenic stem cell transplantation (13), lymphangioleiomyomatosis (11) and physiologic aging

(14). The use of a contrast agent, for example osmium staining, also allows for the investigation of (micro-)vascular structures, making the estimation of vascular volumes relative to the total tissue volume possible (15). Specifically in rare pulmonary diseases, whole lung microCT can bridge the gap between research and clinical routine as exemplified in **Figure 2**, where a representative *ex-vivo* CT scan (**Figure 2A**), whole lung microCT scan (**Figure 2B**) and the segmented airway tree based on whole lung microCT (**Figure 2C**) are shown from a patient who underwent pneumonectomy for unilateral congenital emphysema (**Figures 2D,E**). The airway segmentation shows an aberrant airway bifurcation pattern with a marked decrease in the number of visible airways. Remarkably, there are large airway segments without notable airway branching; especially airway segments in severely emphysematous areas show a lack of airway bifurcations (**Figure 2C**).

CORRELATION WITH HISTOPATHOLOGY

Numerous insights can be generated by high-resolution imaging, however the correlation between imaging and histopathology is often difficult, given the inherent differences in spatial resolution. While high-resolution imaging data allows for the investigation of morphological changes, it only provides black and white images and changes at the cellular level or minimal density differences cannot be resolved, making routine pathology still an indispensable tool for both research and routine clinical purposes. Some attempts have, however, been made to correlate imaging with histopathology data, especially with the recent introduction of synchrotron imaging, an extremely powerful source of X-rays, of paraffin embedded samples where sub-stacks of images with (sub)micrometer resolution can be created. Hierarchical phase contrast imaging is another application of synchrotron imaging, where specialized sample preparation and equipment enable the scanning of entire lungs, but also other organs, with a resolution of 25 micron. Furthermore, this technology allows the acquisition of sub-scans with a resolution of 2.5 micron due to the high X-ray photon flux and coherence achieved at modern fourth-generation synchrotron sources (16). This technique has been employed by Ackermann and colleagues to reveal microvascular changes (i.e., broncho-pulmonary shunting) in the bronchial circulation of COVID-19 patients (17). Synchrotron imaging of paraffin embedded samples on the other hand has been used by another group to study morphological changes in the vascularity in pulmonary vascular diseases. Westroo and colleagues leveraged synchrotron imaging to demonstrate a previously unappreciated plexiform lesion heterogeneity, the pathological hallmark of (idiopathic) pulmonary hypertension (18). The same group also used synchrotron-based phase-contrast microCT in combination with vascular dye injection to investigate the vascular morphology in alveolar capillary dysplasia with misaligned pulmonary veins, with vascular dye injection being of significant help in the analysis and further segmentation of the vascular structures (19). A 3D approach for virtual histology and histopathology based on multi-scale phase contrast x-ray tomography has also been

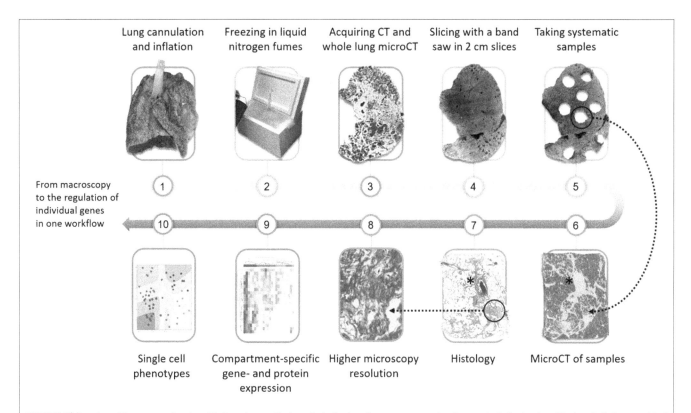

FIGURE 1 | Overview of the proposed protocol that can be used to investigate the lung from macroscopy to microscopical ultrastructure. The lung is firstly cannulated via the main stem bronchus and inflated using a compressed air source and subsequently fixed in liquid nitrogen fumes. Following an *ex-vivo* CT and microCT, the lung is sliced in 2 cm slices and samples are systematically extracted using a core bore or power drill. Pre-selected or randomly selected samples can be scanned with microCT to further improve the spatial resolution. Further validation can be performed with histopathology. More downstream possible molecular analysis includes compartment-specific gene expression analysis or single nuclear analysis which can be used to elucidate specific pathways in pathological areas. *blood vessel.

applied to punches of tissue samples with a maximum cross section of 8 mm derived from COVID-19 victims, which allows the segmentation of individual cells with a minimal resolution of 167 nm (20). Lastly, a 36 M-pixel synchrotron radiation microCT has been successfully used to study the secondary pulmonary lobule from a large human lung specimen (21).

However, this approach is not readily available due to the specific nature of the required equipment for both acquisition and analysis, the need for extensive experience with the interpretation of the images and is therefore not (yet) ready for high-throughput screening.

MICROCT IMAGING AS A SCOUTING TOOL

Histopathologic analysis remains the only reliable option for identifying cellular and morphologic patterns keeping the limitation of small tissue samples and the lack of 3D insight in mind. Serial sectioning of paraffin blocks has been used to extensively demonstrate the correlation between microCT and histology (14), however the process of aligning, matching and cutting the samples is tedious and time-consuming. As an alternative, microCT scanning of paraffin blocks or microCT as a scouting tool have been proposed (22). This can especially

be interesting for retrospective studies, in situations where no whole organ is available or when detailed and fast histopathologic assessment is essential for routine patient care such as surgical lung biopsies in the context of a possible interstitial lung disease or suspicion of neoplasms in a resected lung specimen. Interesting and relevant regions can be selected for further sectioning based on the microCT selection which enables time-efficient preparation of conventional histological sections (22). In that aspect, it is also of interest that a novel X-ray microtomosynthesis of unstained pathology tissue samples has also been proposed. Its unique design maximizes the photon flux density through the sample as no rotation is required and therefore samples can be scanned closer to the source resulting in higher resolution (23).

In addition to its potential as a scouting tool, X-ray imaging can also assist in generating a 3D overview of morphological changes in the lung structure. Jones et al. leveraged microCT of paraffin embedded samples to investigate the 3D morphology of fibroblast foci, a key histologic feature of active fibroproliferation in the context of interstitial lung disease. In contrast to the general belief at that time, the fibroblast foci in the lungs of IPF patients were not interconnected and displayed a wide plasticity (24). Wells et al. also used microCT, histopathology, and immunohistochemistry to investigate necrotic granuloma, a characteristic feature of tuberculosis and showed that necrotic

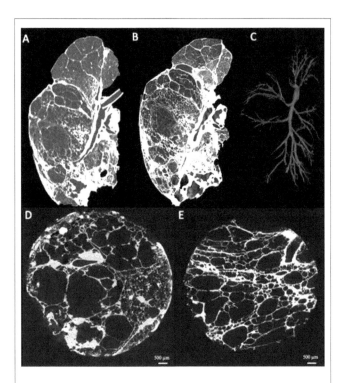

FIGURE 2 | Presentation of a case where clinical routine meets research. Patient with unilateral congenital emphysema that underwent pneumonectomy. The *ex-vivo* clinical CT scan shows severe emphysematous destruction **(A)** with some fibrosis in the lower lung lobe. The whole lung microCT shows greatly improved details providing near alveolar resolution **(B)**. Airway segmentation of the whole lung by microCT demonstrating the simplification of the airway tree characterized by a low number of visible airways and remarkable long airway segments without airway branching **(C)**. MicroCT imaging of extracted lung specimens showing the severe emphysematous destruction in this lung **(D,E)**.

granulomas exhibit more complex shapes than anticipated, including cylindrical, branched morphologies that are connected to the airways and shaped by the bronchi (25).

The 3D overview provided by microCT is not only helpful to investigate morphologic changes but can also be used to investigate structural changes in the airways. Mcdonough et al. were the first to employ microCT to quantify the size and number of terminal bronchioles, the last generation of conducting airways before the respiratory bronchioles and alveoli, in tissue samples removed from explanted lungs from COPD patients. Terminal bronchioles can be visually identified on microCT imaging by the loss of the airway wall and appearance of alveolar buds and are of considerable importance in chronic non-neoplastic lung diseases. A significant decrease in the number and size of terminal bronchioles in end-stage COPD lungs was found compared to controls. Given that repeated sampling of the same lung was possible and given that the tissue volume of the sample could be determined, it not only allowed the assessment of the number of terminal bronchioles in the sample, but by carefully measuring the lung volume, these numbers could be extrapolated to the entire lung. This approach provided quantitative data of the actual small airway involvement in COPD

for the first time, something that was always assumed but never conclusively demonstrated in a quantitative way (26). Later on, this approach has also been successfully leveraged to demonstrate small airway involvement in post lung transplantation rejection, cystic fibrosis and idiopathic pulmonary fibrosis (27–30). Over the last years, this approach has been further refined to allow scanning of the samples in frozen condition, making destructive dehydration which was applied at first, unnecessary. In addition, an improvement in the analysis tools has allowed the researchers to extract additional quantitative parameters such as the number of alveolar attachments, the thickness of the airway wall, the circularity of the lumen, but also size and diameter of the preterminal bronchioles (31).

DISCUSSION

Given the above evidence, it is clear that microCT can serve as a complementary, and in the future perhaps even an indispensable tool for routine pathology (32). Although significant technical advances have been made, there is still some work to be done. Indeed, specific microCT devices have already been optimized for 3D imaging of non-stained soft tissue at a resolution of 5–10 micron. These scans could be implemented in routine care and could assist in histology-guided identification of a range of tissue structures and diagnostically relevant histologic criteria and moreover may allow easy quantification of relevant measures such as for example tissue thickness (33). It is our belief that similar advances could also assist in improving the differential diagnosis, particularly in the field of non-neoplastic diseases. However, these approaches could also be leveraged to better understand neoplastic lung diseases such as micro-metastasis, the role of the tumor micro-environment and the role of the vasculature in neoplastic lung disease. Our approach also allows for structurally targeted molecular investigation with both fresh frozen–or formalin fixed tissue being available after non-destructive imaging, allowing panel-based gene expression analysis or broad next-generation sequencing approaches (34). Additionally, microorganisms such as bacteria from biofilms can be recultivated from native flash frozen tissue and used in *in-vitro* assays.

Applying microCT or synchrotron imaging directly to living patients remains an elusive dream, yet a recent study applied propagation-based phase-contrast CT on a human-scale chest phantom prepped with an inflated fresh porcine lung. The authors demonstrated that a resolution of 100 micron could be obtained in a limited local area of interest with significant less radiation than used in conventional CT scanning (35), indicating the possibilities of *in vivo* high resolution scanning. This indicates that we could dream big and hope to apply similar high-resolution imaging *in vivo*, making it perhaps even possible to avoid invasive biopsies. Caution is however needed as rigorous interpretation of the, often immense, imaging data is needed, which could cause a new wave for artificial intelligence based analysis of microCT scans, similar to the current wave of research in the use of artificial intelligence analysis of conventional CT images (36).

Therefore, the imaging-based approaches to close the gap from macroscopy to ultrastructure seems a safe and trustworthy option, which can be relatively fast implemented in the routine care of patients suffering from acute or chronic lung disease and which can facilitate the differential diagnosis.

REFERENCES

AUTHOR CONTRIBUTIONS

SV, PB, CW, MA, JH, TL, JK-V-E, and DJ: responsible for conception and design of the study. EP, MK, AS, HE, TW, AH, FL, SD, PP, VV, and PV: wrote sections of the manuscript. All authors contribute to sample preparation, processing, contributed to manuscript revision, read, and approved the submitted version.

1. Raghu G, Remy-Jardin M, Myers JL, Richeldi L, Ryerson CJ, Lederer DJ, et al. Diagnosis of idiopathic pulmonary fibrosis. an official ATS/ERS/JRS/ALAT clinical practice guideline. *Am J Respir Crit Care Med.* (2018) 198:e44–68. doi: 10.1164/rccm.201807-1255ST

2. Yagihashi K, Huckleberry J, Colby TV, Tazelaar HD, Zach J, Sundaram B, et al. Radiologic–pathologic discordance in biopsy-proven usual interstitial pneumonia. *Eur Respir J.* (2016) 47:1189–97. doi: 10.1183/13993003.01680-2015

3. Unterman A, Wand O, Fridel L, Edelstein E, Pertzov B, Kramer MR. High diagnostic accuracy of transbronchial cryobiopsy in fibrotic interstitial lung diseases compared to final explant diagnosis. *Respiration.* (2019) 98:421–7. doi: 10.1159/000502893

4. Panchabhai TS, Arrossi AV, Highland KB, Bandyopadhyay D, Culver DA, Budev MM, et al. A single-institution study of concordance of pathological diagnoses for interstitial lung diseases between pre-transplantation surgical lung biopsies and lung explants. *BMC Pulm Med.* (2019) 19:20. doi: 10.1186/s12890-019-0778-x

5. Watz H, Breithecker A, Rau WS, Kriete A. Micro-CT of the human lung: imaging of alveoli and virtual endoscopy of an alveolar duct in a normal lung and in a lung with centrilobular emphysema—initial observations. *Radiology.* (2005) 236:1053–8. doi: 10.1148/radiol.2363041142

6. Litzlbauer HD, Neuhaeuser C, Moell A, Greschus S, Breithecker A, Franke FE, et al. Three-dimensional imaging and morphometric analysis of alveolar tissue from microfocal X-ray-computed tomography. *Am J Physiol Lung Cell Mol Physiol.* (2006) 291:L535–45. doi: 10.1152/ajplung.00088.2005

7. Tielemans B, Dekoster K, Verleden SE, Sawall S, Leszczyński B, Laperre K, et al. From mouse to man and back: closing the correlation gap between imaging and histopathology for lung diseases. *Diagnostics.* (2020) 10:636. doi: 10.3390/diagnostics10090636

8. Vasilescu DM, Phillion AB, Tanabe N, Kinose D, Paige DF, Kantrowitz JJ, et al. Nondestructive cryomicro-CT imaging enables structural and molecular analysis of human lung tissue. *J Appl Physiol (1985).* (2017) 122:161–9. doi: 10.1152/japplphysiol.00838.2016

9. McDonough JE, Ahangari F, Li Q, Jain S, Verleden SE, Herazo-Maya J, et al. Transcriptional regulatory model of fibrosis progression in the human lung. *JCI Insight.* (2019) 4:e131597. doi: 10.1172/jci.insight.131597

10. De Sadeleer LJ, McDonough JE, Schupp JC, Yan X, Vanstapel A, Van Herck A, et al. Lung microenvironments and disease progression in fibrotic hypersensitivity pneumonitis. *Am J Respir Crit Care Med.* (2021) 205:60–74. doi: 10.1164/rccm.202103-0569OC

11. Verleden SE, Vanstapel A, De Sadeleer L, Weynand B, Boone M, Verbeken E, et al. Quantitative analysis of airway obstruction in lymphangioleiomyomatosis. *Eur Respir J.* (2020) 56:1901965. doi: 10.1183/13993003.01965-2019

12. Everaerts S, McDonough JE, Verleden SE, Josipovic I, Boone M, Dubbeldam A, et al. Airway morphometry in COPD with bronchiectasis: a view on all airway generations. *Eur Respir J.* (2019) 54:1802166. doi: 10.1183/13993003.02166-2018

13. Verleden SE, McDonough JE, Schoemans H, Knoop C, Verschakelen J, Dubbeldam A, et al. Phenotypical diversity of airway morphology in chronic lung graft vs. host disease after stem cell transplantation. *Mod Pathol.* (2019) 32:817–29. doi: 10.1038/s41379-019-0203-2

14. Verleden SE, Kirby M, Everaerts S, Vanstapel A, McDonough JE, Verbeken EK, et al. Small airway loss in the physiologically ageing lung: a cross-sectional study in unused donor lungs. *Lancet Respir Med.* (2020) 9:167–74. doi: 10.1016/s2213-2600(20)30324-6

15. Kampschulte M, Schneider C, Litzlbauer H, Tscholl D, Schneider C, Zeiner C, et al. Quantitative 3D micro-CT imaging of human lung tissue. *Fortschr Röntgenstr.* (2013) 185:869–76. doi: 10.1055/s-0033-13 50105

16. Walsh CL, Tafforeau P, Wagner WL, Jafree DJ, Bellier A, Werlein C, et al. Imaging intact human organs with local resolution of cellular structures using hierarchical phase-contrast tomography. *Nat Method.* (2021) 18:1532–41. Available online at: https://www.nature.com/articles/s41592-021-01317-x

17. Ackermann M, Tafforeau P, Wagner WL, Walsh C, Werlein C, Kühnel MP, et al. The bronchial circulation in COVID-19 pneumonia. *Am J Respir Crit Care Med.* (2022) 205:121–5. doi: 10.1164/rccm.202103-0594im

18. Westöö C, Norvik C, Peruzzi N, van der Have O, Lovric G, Jeremiasen I, et al. Distinct types of plexiform lesions identified by synchrotron-based phase-contrast micro-CT. *Am J Physiol Lung Cell Mol Physiol.* (2021) 321:L17–28. doi: 10.1152/ajplung.00432.2020

19. Norvik C, Westöö CK, Peruzzi N, Lovric G, van der Have O, Mokso R, et al. Synchrotron-based phase-contrast micro-CT as a tool for understanding pulmonary vascular pathobiology and the 3-D microanatomy of alveolar capillary dysplasia. *Am J Physiol Lung Cell Mol Physiol.* (2020) 318:L65–75. doi: 10.1152/ajplung.00103.2019

20. Eckermann M, Frohn J, Reichardt M, Osterhoff M, Sprung M, Westermeier F, et al. 3D virtual pathohistology of lung tissue from Covid-19 patients based on phase contrast X-ray tomography. *Elife.* (2020) 9:e60408. doi: 10.7554/eLife.60408

21. Umetani K, Okamoto T, Saito K, Kawata Y, Niki N. 36M-pixel synchrotron radiation micro-CT for whole secondary pulmonary lobule visualization from a large human lung specimen. *Eur J Radiol Open.* (2020) 7:100262. doi: 10.1016/j.ejro.2020.100262

22. Scott AE, Vasilescu DM, Seal KAD, Keyes SD, Mavrogordato MN, Hogg JC, et al. Three dimensional imaging of paraffin embedded human lung tissue samples by micro-computed tomography. Warburton D, editor. *PLoS ONE.* (2015) 10:e0126230. doi: 10.1371/journal.pone.0126230

23. Nguyen DT, Larsen TC, Wang M, Knutsen RH, Yang Z, Bennett EE, et al. X-ray microtomosynthesis of unstained pathology tissue samples. *J Microsc.* (2021) 283:9–20. doi: 10.1111/jmi.13003

24. Jones MG, Fabre A, Schneider P, Cinetto F, Sgalla G, Mavrogordato M, et al. Three-dimensional characterization of fibroblast foci in idiopathic pulmonary fibrosis. *JCI Insight.* (2016) 1:e86375. doi: 10.1172/jci.insight.86375

25. Wells G, Glasgow JN, Nargan K, Lumamba K, Madansein R, Maharaj K, et al. Micro–computed tomography analysis of the human tuberculous lung reveals remarkable heterogeneity in three-dimensional granuloma morphology. *Am J Respir Crit Care Med.* (2021) 204:583–95. doi: 10.1164/rccm.202101-0032OC

26. McDonough JE, Yuan R, Suzuki M, Seyednejad N, Elliott WM, Sanchez PG, et al. Small-airway obstruction and emphysema in chronic obstructive pulmonary disease. *N Engl J Med.* (2011) 365:1567–75. doi: 10.1056/NEJMoa1106955

27. Verleden SE, Vasilescu DM, Willems S, Ruttens D, Vos R, Vandermeulen E, et al. The site and nature of airway obstruction after lung transplantation. *Am J Respir Crit Care Med.* (2014) 189:292–300. doi: 10.1164/rccm.201310-1894OC

28. Verleden SE, Vasilescu DM, McDonough JE, Ruttens D, Vos R, Vandermeulen E, et al. Linking clinical phenotypes of chronic lung allograft dysfunction to changes in lung structure. *Eur Respir J.* (2015) 46:1430–9. doi: 10.1183/09031936.00010615

29. Boon M, Verleden SE, Bosch B, Lammertyn EJ, McDonough JE, Mai C, et al. Morphometric analysis of explant lungs in cystic fibrosis. *Am J Respir Crit Care Med.* (2016) 193:516–26. doi: 10.1164/rccm.201507-1281OC

30. Verleden SE, Tanabe N, McDonough JE, Vasilescu DM, Xu F, Wuyts WA, et al. Small airways pathology in idiopathic pulmonary fibrosis: a retrospective cohort study. *Lancet Respir Med.* (2020) 8:573–84. doi: 10.1016/S2213-2600(19)30356-X

31. Tanabe N, Vasilescu DM, McDonough JE, Kinose D, Suzuki M, Cooper JD, et al. Micro-computed tomography comparison of preterminal bronchioles in centrilobular and panlobular emphysema. *Am J Respir Crit Care Med.* (2017) 195:630–8. doi: 10.1164/rccm.201602-0278OC

32. Bourdin A, Gamez AS, Vachier I, Crestani B. LAM is another small airway disease: lessons from microCT. *Eur Respir J.* (2020) 56:2002162. doi: 10.1183/13993003.02162-2020

33. Katsamenis OL, Olding M, Warner JA, Chatelet DS, Jones MG, Sgalla G, et al. X-ray micro-computed tomography for nondestructive three-dimensional (3D) X-ray histology. *Am J Pathol.* (2019) 189:1608–20. doi: 10.1016/j.ajpath.2019.05.004

34. Ackermann M, Verleden SE, Kuehnel M, Haverich A, Welte T, Laenger F, et al. Pulmonary vascular endothelialitis, thrombosis, and angiogenesis in Covid-19. *N Engl J Med.* (2020) 383:120–8. doi: 10.1056/NEJMoa2015432

35. Wagner WL, Wuennemann F, Pacilé S, Albers J, Arfelli F, Dreossi D, et al. Towards synchrotron phase-contrast lung imaging in patients - a proof-of-concept study on porcine lungs in a human-scale chest phantom. *J Synchrotron Rad.* (2018) 25:1827–32. doi: 10.1107/S1600577518013401

36. Soffer S, Morgenthau AS, Shimon O, Barash Y, Konen E, Glicksberg BS, et al. Artificial intelligence for interstitial lung disease analysis on chest computed tomography: a systematic review. *Acad Radiol.* (2022) 29 Suppl 2:S226–S235. doi: 10.1016/j.acra.2021.05.014

19

SARS-CoV2 Infection and the Importance of Potassium Balance

Helen C. Causton*

Department of Pathology and Cell Biology, Columbia University Irving Medical Center, New York, NY, United States

*Correspondence:
Helen C. Causton
hc2415@cumc.columbia.edu

SARS-CoV2 infection results in a range of symptoms from mild pneumonia to cardiac arrhythmias, hyperactivation of the immune response, systemic organ failure and death. However, the mechanism of action has been hard to establish. Analysis of symptoms associated with COVID-19, the activity of repurposed drugs associated with lower death rates or antiviral activity *in vitro* and a small number of studies describing interventions, point to the importance of electrolyte, and particularly potassium, homeostasis at both the cellular, and systemic level. Elevated urinary loss of potassium is associated with disease severity, and the response to electrolyte replenishment correlates with progression toward recovery. These findings suggest possible diagnostic opportunities and therapeutic interventions. They provide insights into comorbidities and mechanisms associated with infection by SARS-CoV2 and other RNA viruses that target the ACE2 receptor, and/or activate cytokine-mediated immune responses in a potassium-dependent manner.

Keywords: electrolyte, renin-angiotensin system, drug repurposing, SARS-CoV-2 infection, potassium

INTRODUCTION

SARS-CoV2 infects cells *via* interaction with the ACE2 receptor which is found primarily on the surface of the heart, liver, kidney, and lungs (1). ACE2 is a negative regulator of the renin-angiotensin system (RAS) that acts in conjunction with ion transporters and the insulin receptor to protect against hypertension, diabetes, cardiovascular disease, and organ damage (2). It does this by regulating electrolyte balance and blood pressure, cell volume, intercellular signaling, filtering of urine in the kidney, membrane potential, and the firing rate of electrically active cells (3, 4). Binding of ACE2 by the SARS-CoV2 virus and the processes of viral entry and replication, enhance degradation of the receptor, which decreases inhibition of the classical RAS system. The net result is increased reabsorption of sodium and water, and raised blood pressure (5). Hypokalemia/low intracellular potassium can also lead to cellular hyperpolarity, increased resting potential, and depolarization in cardiac and lung cells that can trigger ventricular arrhythmia and respiratory dysfunction (6). In parallel, expression of the viral viroporin, Orf3a protein actively promotes potassium efflux, and stimulates activation of the innate immune response. It does so by triggering the cell-intrinsic Nod-like receptor family, pyrin domain-containing 3 (NLRP3) inflammasome (7–9), which promotes cytokine release. Inflammasome responses play fundamental roles in clearing viruses and promoting tissue repair (10), however, hyperactivation of this immune response, gives rise to the devastating "cytokine storm" that is associated with severe infection, and a major cause of death (11).

This mini-perspective discusses the effects of electrolyte and potassium imbalance in SARS-CoV2 infection, describes how a number of comorbidities of COVID-19 affect ion homeostasis and, identifies some drugs effective against SARS-CoV2 *in vivo* that have also been shown to affect pH or K+ balance. Collectively, these findings highlight the importance of maintaining, and promoting electrolyte homeostasis. They also provide a framework for beginning to understand the broad, and seemingly unrelated, range of symptoms associated with COVID-19 and possibly other RNA viruses, that target the ACE2 receptor and/or those that activate the NRPL3 inflammasome in a potassium-dependent manner.

POTASSIUM IMBALANCE IS COMMON AMONG PATIENTS WITH SEVERE SARS-CoV2 INFECTION

Potassium homeostasis is maintained at a systemic level, in the balance between dietary intake ($\sim$100 mmol/day) and excretion (95% *via* the kidney; 5% *via* the colon) and *via* internal balance of K^+ between intracellular and extracellular fluid compartments (4). Hypokalemia, typically defined as <3.5 mmol/L in plasma, shares many of the features of SARS-CoV2 infection, including muscle weakness, palpitations, cardiac dysrhythmias, and poor diabetic control (4, 12).

In the course of SARS-CoV2 infection, hypokalemia is primarily caused by elevated aldosterone, which promotes excretion of potassium in urine (13). One study involving 1,415 patients, found electrolyte imbalance and hypokalemia were associated with disease severity (Weighted Mean Difference:0.12 mmol/L [95% CI: −0.18 to −0.07 mmol/ L], I21/433%) (14). Another found that hypokalemia around the time of admission was associated with a requirement for invasive mechanical ventilation (15), while a smaller study observed that although only 54% of the patients ($n = 175$) had low potassium levels, of the severely ill patients 85% had hypokalemia (13). A case-controlled study of three emergency rooms in France found that hypokalemia and hyponatremia (sodium <135 mmol/L) were independently associated with COVID-19 infection, but that low sodium, and not potassium levels were associated with ICU admission (16). Disease severity is also related to the degree of response to potassium replacement as mildly ill COVID-19 patients with hypokalemia in the Chen study achieved normokalemia within 5–8 days of potassium replacement (3 g potassium chloride or 40 mEq/day), whereas, it took 10–14 days to achieve homeostasis potassium in severely ill patients (13). Severe hypokalemia may be harder to correct as it is associated with alkalosis (29% had a $\geq$ pH 7.45) (13). This is due to hydrogen-potassium exchange between the intra

and extracellular fluid (4). Patients with COVID-19 are also susceptible to pro-arrhythmic effects (17).

A NUMBER OF COMORBIDITIES FOR COVID-19 AFFECT ION HOMEOSTASIS

Patients with severe symptoms of COVID-19 are more likely to have kidney or cardiovascular disease, hypertension, diabetes mellitus (DM) or other comorbidities than those with milder symptoms (18–22). The association between COVID-19 and a number of these comorbidities is bidirectional (23, 24): patients with diabetes are more likely to develop severe symptoms or die of COVID-19 (12, 22) and acute diabetes or acid-ketosis can develop as a result of SARS-CoV2 infection (25–28). High levels of insulin are found in the olfactory bulb in the brain. Insulin modulates the voltage-dependent potassium channel, Kv1.3, and suppresses the Kv1.3-contributed current in cultured olfactory bulb neurons (OBNs) of rodents (29, 30),while deletion of the Kv1.3 channel results in "super smeller" mice (31). There is little data on the effect of decreased insulin production on the Kv1.3 channel, however it may contribute to the anosmia experienced by some COVID-19 patients (32).

A NUMBER OF REPURPOSED DRUGS EFFECTIVE AGAINST SARS-CoV2 AFFECT POTASSIUM BALANCE

It has been hard to obtain insights into the mechanism by which SARS-CoV2 acts, based on the diversity of symptoms identified in infected individuals. Likewise, FDA approved drugs that act *in vitro* to reduce viral replication and plaque formation, increase cell viability, or are associated with lower death rates in patients target a range of host factors. These drugs are used for a wide range of purposes from treatment of malaria to pancreatitis and diabetes (33–36) (**Table 1**). However, some patterns are emerging: 17 of 66 FDA approved drugs with anti-viral activity were found to target the Sigma-1 receptor (σ1-R) and sigma-2 receptor (σ2-R) (SIGMAR1/SIGMAR2) (34). Sigma receptors are ubiquitously expressed in mammalian tissues and are involved in cellular signaling in a number of conditions including retinal and neurodegenerative disorders (37, 38). A number of σ1-R and σ2-R receptor agonists have been found to inhibit Kv2.1 potassium channel activity in a receptor-independent manner (39), suggesting that they act to modulate potassium currents directly. Another 7 of the 69 drugs inhibit protein synthesis (34). Although the mechanism is not known, protein synthesis, and potassium abundance are inversely correlated in systems as diverse as yeast, algae, and mouse fibroblasts (40–43), such that inhibition of protein synthesis would be expected to result in greater intracellular potassium abundance. A further 17 drugs have been shown to affect osmotic or ion homeostasis. Agonists of potassium channels, angiotensin II, and protein synthesis were also found to be enriched among drugs with anti-SARS-CoV2 activity in an independent study (35).

TABLE 1 | Repurposed drugs with anti-viral activity that also affect potassium balance.

Drug	Human target	Anti-viral activity	Indication	Affects	Reference
Camostat	Cell Entry	(44, 45)	Pancreatitis	Elevates Na+:K+ ratio	(46)
Chloroquine	Cell Entry	(47)	Malaria, immune modulation	Blocks hERG K+ channels	(48)
Hydroxy chloroquine	Cell Entry	(34, 47)	Malaria, immune modulation	Blocks hERG K+ channels	(48)
Loratadine	SLC6A15	(49)	Antihistamine	Kv1.5, outward current	(50, 51)
Nafamostat	Cell Entry	(52)	Pancreatitis	Can induce hyperkalemia, by suppressing the Na-K ATPase dependent pathway	(53)
Pioglitazone	CISD1	(54)	Diabetes	Remodeling of Kv1.5 & Kv4.2	(55)
YH-1238	H+, K+ ATPase Proton Pump	(35)	Phase I	H+,K+-ATPase (ATP4A, ATP4B)	(35)

Some of these repurposed drugs many act to reduce disease severity *via* their effects on the immune system. Sex hormones, such as progesterone, promote immune tolerance, and anti-inflammatory responses and that may account for lower COVID-related disease severity and mortality in women and during pregnancy (56, 57). Clinical studies of drug efficacy also point to the key role of the renin-angiotensin system and electrolyte balance in influencing patient outcomes. A retrospective study of COVID-19 patients taking famotidine, an antiacid, found that hospitalized patients taking the drug were more than twice as likely to survive (33). Famotidine was also identified in a computational screen of drugs likely to have anti-SARS-CoV2 activity (36). Another drug, Nafamostat, acts on potassium balance by reducing urinary excretion of potassium *via* the Na+/K+ ATPase-dependent pathway (58, 59). These data support the idea that restoring potassium balance promotes a better host response against viral infection. Conversely some of these drugs pose a risk as they promote hyperkalemia (48, 60). This is a complication found in a number of patients who die of COVID-19 (37% of those who died (n = 113) compared with 14% (*n* = 161) of those who recovered (61).

Potassium dysregulation is also likely to form part of the mechanism that promotes viral pathogenicity. A study that ectopically expressed the SARS-CoV2 envelope (E) protein in HEK 293 and NIH3T3 cells found that it formed a pH-dependent ion channel permeable to potassium and sodium ions (62 Only a small proportion of the E protein ends up in the viral envelope and most is localized to the endoplasmic reticulum-Golgi complex where it multimerizes to form a virioporin, that promotes an increase in intra-golgi pH (62, 63). The E protein channel is critical for infectivity and for the pathogenicity of SARS-CoV2, as it is for other coronaviruses, and thus presents a good target for therapeutic intervention (63, 64).

DISCUSSION

Taken together, these observations drawn from comorbidities, clinical features of disease and the possible targets of drugs that are effective against viral infection show that symptoms associated with low intracellular potassium are similar to those that result from SARS-CoV2 infection, and that potassium efflux can promote hyperactivation of the innate immune response. Although we do not yet understand how SARS-CoV2 acts in detail, potassium balance is likely to be important for both the propagation and pathogenicity of the virus, *via* effects on both the virus, and on homeostatic mechanisms in the host.

It is likely that this line of enquiry will have relevance for understanding the consequences of viral infection more broadly. Ion disturbance, mediated by virioporins, is central to the mechanism of action of a range of viruses from influenza, and rhinovirus to COVID-19 and HIV (8), and a number of RNA viruses modulate activity of the NLRP3 inflammasome in a potassium-dependent manner (65, 66). In bats, dampening of the inflammasome and proinflammatory responses confers tolerance to a range of RNA viruses, suggesting that modulating the inflammasome may prove a useful therapeutic target for reducing disease severity in humans too (10).

Similarities between SARS-CoV2 and other coronaviruses offer further mechanistic insight and opportunities for drug repurposing. SARS-CoV1 also enters the cell *via* the ACE2 receptor and can cause acute lung failure, cardiac arrhythmia, gastrointestinal disorders, hyperkalemia and diabetes (4, 5, 67, 68). Nafamostat, which induces hyperkalemia, inhibits the activity of SARS-CoV1, 2 and MERS-CoV (52, 53, 60, 69). Approximately 50 FDA-approved drugs are known to have activity against all 3 viruses (70). These results present a strong argument for gaining a fundamental understanding of how electrolyte balance functions in both the healthy host and in response to viral infection. This knowledge is expected to identify strategies for diagnosis and therapeutic intervention in patients suffering from a number of virally induced diseases.

AUTHOR CONTRIBUTIONS

The author confirms being the sole contributor of this work and has approved it for publication.

REFERENCES

1. Hamming I, Timens W, Bulthuis ML, Lely AT, Navis G, van Goor H. Tissue distribution of ACE2 protein, the functional receptor for SARS coronavirus. A first step in understanding SARS pathogenesis. *J Pathol.* (2004) 203:631–7. doi: 10.1002/path.1570

2. Cheng H, Wang Y, Wang GQ. Organ-protective effect of angiotensin-converting enzyme 2 and its effect on the prognosis of COVID-19. *J Med Virol.* (2020) 92:726–730. doi: 10.1002/jmv.25785

3. Santos RA, Ferreira AJ, Simoes AC. Recent advances in the angiotensin-converting enzyme 2-angiotensin(1-7)-Mas axis. *Exp Physiol.* (2008) 93:519–27. doi: 10.1113/expphysiol.2008.042002

4. Unwin RJ, Luft FC, Shirley DG. Pathophysiology and management of hypokalemia: a clinical perspective. *Nat Rev Nephrol.* (2011) 7:75–84. doi: 10.1038/nrneph.2010.175

5. Kuba K, Imai Y, Rao S, Jiang C, Penninger JM. Lessons from SARS: control of acute lung failure by the SARS receptor ACE2. *J Mol Med.* (2006) 84:814–20. doi: 10.1007/s00109-006-0094-9

6. Bielecka-Dabrowa A, Mikhailidis DP, Jones L, Rysz J, Aronow WS, Banach M. The meaning of hypokalemia in heart failure. *Int J Cardiol.* (2012) 158:12–7. doi: 10.1016/j.ijcard.2011.06.121

7. Chen IY, Moriyama M, Chang MF, Ichinohe T. Severe acute respiratory syndrome coronavirus viroporin 3a activates the NLRP3 inflammasome. *Front Microbiol.* (2019) 10:50. doi: 10.3389/fmicb.2019.00050

8. Farag NS, Breitinger U, Breitinger HG, El Azizi, MA. Viroporins and inflammasomes: a key to understand virus-induced inflammation. *Int J Biochemistr Cell Biol.* (2020) 122:105738. doi: 10.1016/j.biocel.2020.105738

9. Xu H, Chitre SA, Akinyemi IA, Loeb JC, Lednicky JA, McIntosh MT, Bhaduri-McIntosh S. SARS-CoV-2 viroporin triggers the NLRP3 inflammatory pathway, *BioRxiv* (2020). doi: 10.1101/2020.10.27.357731

10. Nagaraja S, Jain D, Kesavardhana S. Inflammasome regulation in driving COVID-19 severity in humans and immune tolerance in bats. *J Leukoc Biol.* (2021) 21:93. doi: 10.1002/JLB.4COVHR0221-093RR

11. Hu B, Huang S, Yin L. The cytokine storm and COVID-19. *J Med Virol.* (2021) 93:250–256. doi: 10.1002/jmv.26232

12. Docherty A, Harrison E, Green C, Hardwick H, Pius R, Norman L, et al. Features of 20133 UK patients in hospital with covid-19 using the ISARIC WHO clinical characterisation protocol: prospective observational cohort study. *BMJ.* (2020) 369:m1985.

13. Chen D, Li X, Song Q, Hu C, Su F, Dai J, et al. Assessment of hypokalemia and clinical characteristics in patients with coronavirus disease 2019 in Wenzhou, China. *JAMA Netw Open.* (2020) 3:e2011122. doi: 10.1001/jamanetworkopen.2020.11122

14. Lippi G, South AM, Henry BM. Electrolyte imbalances in patients with severe coronavirus disease 2019 (COVID-19). *Ann Clin Biochem.* (2020) 57:262–265. doi: 10.1177/0004563220922255

15. Moreno-Perez O, Merino E, Leon-Ramirez JM, Andres M, Ramos JMJ, et al. CA.r. group, Post-acute COVID-19 syndrome. Incidence and risk factors: A Mediterranean cohort study. *J Infect.* (2021) 82:378–383. doi: 10.1016/j.jinf.2021.01.004

16. De Carvalho H, Richard MC, Chouihed T, Goffinet NQ, Freund Y, Kratz A, et al. Electrolyte imbalance in COVID-19 patients admitted to the emergency department: a case-control study. *Intern Emerg Med.* (2021) 6:32. doi: 10.1007/s11739-021-02632-z

17. Wu CI, Postema PG, Arbelo E, Behr ER, Bezzina CR, Napolitano C, et al. SARS-CoV-2, COVID-19, and inherited arrhythmia syndromes. *Heart Rhythm.* (2020) 17:1456–62. doi: 10.1016/j.hrthm.2020.03.024

18. Cheng Y, Luo R, Wang K, Zhang M, Wang Z, Dong L, et al. Kidney disease is associated with in-hospital death of patients with COVID-19. *Kidney Int* (2020) 97:829-838. doi: 10.1016/j.kint.2020.03.005

19. Dworakowska D, Grossman AB. Renin-angiotensin system inhibitors in management of hypertension during the COVID-19 pandemic. *J Physiol Pharmacol* (2020) 71:20. doi: 10.26402/jpp.2020.2.01

20. Lim JH, Jung HY, Choi JY, Park SH, Kim CD, Kim YL, et al.. Hypertension and Electrolyte Disorders in Patients with COVID-19. *Electrolyte Blood Press.* (2020) 18:23–30. doi: 10.5049/EBP.2020.18.2.23

21. Zhou F, Yu T, Du R, Fan G, Liu Y, Liu Z, et al. Clinical course and risk factors for mortality of adult inpatients with COVID-19 in Wuhan, China: a retrospective cohort study. *Lancet.* (2020) 395:1054–1062. doi: 10.1016/S0140-6736(20)30566-3

22. Zhu L, She ZG, Cheng X, Qin JJ, Zhang XJ, Cai J, et al. Association of Blood Glucose Control and Outcomes in Patients with COVID-19 and Pre-existing Type 2 Diabetes. *Cell Metabolism.* (2020) 31:1068–1077. doi: 10.1016/j.cmet.2020.04.021

23. Pal R, Bhadada SK. COVID-19 and diabetes mellitus: an unholy interaction of two pandemics. *Diabetes Metab Syndr.* (2020) 14:513-517. doi: 10.1016/j.dsx.2020.04.049

24. Nishiga M, Wang DW, Han Y, Lewis DB, Wu JC. COVID-19 and cardiovascular disease: from basic mechanisms to clinical perspectives. *Nat Rev Cardiol.* (2020) 17:543–558. doi: 10.1038/s41569-020-0413-9

25. Bornstein SR, Rubino F, Khunti K, Mingrone G, Hopkins D, Birkenfeld AL, et al. Practical recommendations for the management of diabetes in patients with COVID-19. *Lancet Diab. Endocrinol.* (2020) 8:546–550. doi: 10.1016/S2213-8587(20)30152-2

26. Chee YJ S.Ng JH, Yeoh E. Diabetic ketoacidosis precipitated by Covid-19 in a patient with newly diagnosed diabetes mellitus. *Diabet Res Clinic Pract.* (2020) 164:108166. doi: 10.1016/j.diabres.2020.108166

27. Li J, Wang X, Chen J, Zuo X, Zhang H, Deng A. COVID−19 infection may cause ketosis and ketoacidosis. *Diabet Obesity Metabol.* (2020) 22:1935–41. doi: 10.1111/dom.14057

28. Rubino F, Amiel SA, Zimmet P, Alberti G, Bornstein S, Eckel RH, et al. New-onset diabetes in Covid-19. *N Engl J Med.* (2020) 383:789–90. doi: 10.1056/NEJMc2018688

29. Fadool DA, Tucker K, Phillips JJ, Simmen JA. Brain insulin receptor causes activity-dependent current suppression in the olfactory bulb through multiple phosphorylation of Kv1.3. *J Neurophysiol.* (2000) 83:2332–48. doi: 10.1152/jn.2000.83.4.2332

30. Das P, Parsons AD, Scarborough J, Hoffman J, Wilson J, Thompson RN, et al. Electrophysiological and behavioral phenotype of insulin receptor defective mice. *Physiol Behav.* (2005) 86:287–96. doi: 10.1016/j.physbeh.2005.08.024

31. Fadool DA, Tucker K, Perkins R, Fasciani G, Thompson RN, et al. Kv1.3 channel gene-targeted deletion produces "Super-Smeller Mice" with altered glomeruli, interacting scaffolding proteins, biophysics. *Neuron.* (2004) 41:389–404. doi: 10.1016/S0896-6273(03)00844-4

32. Lechien JR, Chiesa-Estomba DR, Horoi MSD, Le Bon D, Rodriguez A, Dequanter D, et al. Olfactory and gustatory dysfunctions as a clinical presentation of mild-to-moderate forms of the coronavirus disease (COVID-19): a multicenter European study. *Eur Arch Otorhinolaryngol.* (2020) 277:2251–2261. doi: 10.1007/s00405-020-05965-1

33. Freedberg D, Conigliaro J, Wang T, Tracey K, Callahan M, Abrams J, et al. Famotidine use is associated with improved clinical outcomes in hospitalized covid-19 patients: a propensity score matched retrospective cohort study. *Gastroenterology.* (2020) 159:1129–31. doi: 10.1053/j.gastro.2020.05.053

34. Gordon DE, Jang GM, Bouhaddou M, Xu J, Obernier K, et al. A SARS-CoV-2 protein interaction map reveals targets for drug repurposing. *Nature.* (2020) 583:459–68. doi: 10.1038/s41586-020-2286-9

35. Riva L, Yuan S, Yin X L. Martin-Sancho, Matsunaga N, Pache LS, et al. Discovery of SARS-CoV-2 antiviral drugs through large-scale compound repurposing. *Nature.* (2020) 586:113-119. doi: 10.1038/s41586-020-2577-1

36. Wu C, Liu Y, Yang Y, Zhang P, Zhong W, Wang Y, et al. Analysis of therapeutic targets for SARS-CoV-2 and discovery of potential drugs by computational methods. *Acta Pharm Sin B.* (2020) 10:766–88. doi: 10.1016/j.apsb.2020.02.008

37. Wang J, Saul A, Roon P, Smith SB. Activation of the molecular chaperone, sigma 1 receptor, preserves cone function in a murine model of inherited retinal degeneration. *Proc Natl Acad Sci U S A.* (2016) 113:E3764–72. doi: 10.1073/pnas.1521749113

38. Maurice T, Goguadze N. Sigma-1 (sigma1) receptor in memory and neurodegenerative diseases. *Handbook Experiment Pharmacol.* (2017) 244:81–108. doi: 10.1007/164_2017_15

39. Liu X, Fu Y, Yang H, Mavlyutov T, Li J, McCurdy CR, et al. Potential independent action of sigma receptor ligands through inhibition of the Kv2.1 channel. *Oncotarget.* (2017) 8:59345–59358. doi: 10.18632/oncotarget.19581

40. Mahmoud S, Planes MD, Cabedo M, Trujillo C, Rienzo A, Caballero-Molada M, Sarma SC, Montesinos C, et al. TOR complex 1 regulates the yeast plasma membrane proton pump and pH and potassium homeostasis. *FEBS Lett.* (2017) 591:1993–2002. doi: 10.1002/1873-3468.12673

41. Primo C, Ferri-Blazquez, Leowith R, Yenush L. Reciprocal regulation of target of rapamycin complex 1 and potassium accumulation. *J Biol Chem.* (2017) 292:563–574. doi: 10.1074/jbc.M116.746982

42. O'Neill JS, Hoyle NP, Robertson JB, Edgar R, Frezza C, Day JH, et al. Eukaryotic cell biology is temporally coordinated to support the energetic demands of protein homeostasis. *Nat Commun.* (2020) 14:955521. doi: 10.1101/2020.05.14.095521

43. Stangherlin A, Wong D, Barbiero S, Watson J, Zeng A, Seinkmane E, et al. Compensatory ion transport buffers daily protein rhythms to regulate osmotic balance and cellular physiology. *BioRxiv preprint.* (2020) 28:118398. doi: 10.1101/2020.05.28.118398

44. Sun G, Sui Y, Zhou Y, Ya J, Yuan C, Jiang L, Huang M. Structural Basis of Covalent Inhibitory Mechanism of TMPRSS2-Related Serine Proteases by Camostat. *J Virol.* (2021) 95:e0086121. doi: 10.1128/JVI.00861-21

45. Hoffmann MH, Smith JC, Kruger N, Arora P, Sorensen LK, Sogaard OS, et al. Camostat mesylate inhibits SARS-CoV-2 activation by TMPRSS2-related proteases and its metabolite GBPA exerts antiviral activity. *EBioMedicine.* (2021) 65:103255. doi: 10.1016/j.ebiom.2021.103255

46. Kitamura K, Tomita K. Proteolytic activation of the epithelial sodium channel and therapeutic application of a serine protease inhibitor for the treatment of salt-sensitive hypertension. *Clin Exp Nephrol.* (2012) 16:44–8. doi: 10.1007/s10157-011-0506-1

47. Rakedzon S, Neuberger A, Domb AJ, Petersiel N, Schwartz E. From hydroxychloroquine to ivermectin: what are the anti-viral properties of anti-parasitic drugs to combat SARS-CoV-2? *J Travel Med.* (2021) 28:5. doi: 10.1093/jtm/taab005

48. Szendrey M, Guo J, Li W, Yang T, Zhang S. COVID-19 drugs chloroquine and hydroxychloroquine, but not azithromycin and remdesivir, block hERG potassium channels. *J Pharmacol Experiment Therapeut.* (2021) 377:265–72. doi: 10.1124/jpet.120.000484

49. Hou Y, Ge S, Li X, Wang C, He H, He L. Testing of the inhibitory effects of loratadine and desloratadine on SARS-CoV-2 spike pseudotyped virus viropexis. *Chem Biol Interact.* (2021) 338:109420. doi: 10.1016/j.cbi.2021.109420

50. Lacerda AE, Roy ML, Lewis EW, Rampe D. Interactions of the nonsedating antihistamine loratadine with a Kv1.5-type potassium channel cloned from human heart. *Mol Pharmacol.* (1997) 52:314–22. doi: 10.1124/mol.52.2.314

51. Crumb WJ. Rate-dependent blockade of a potassium current in human atrium by the antihistamine loratadine. *Br J Pharmacol.* (1999) 126:575–80. doi: 10.1038/sj.bjp.0702273

52. Hoffmann M, Schroeder SH, Kleine-Weber H, Muller MA, Drosten C, Pohlmann S. Nafamostat mesylate blocks activation of SARS-CoV-2: new treatment option for COVID-19. *Antimicrob Agents Chemotherap.* (2020) 64:20. doi: 10.1128/AAC.00754-20

53. Ookawara S, Tabei K, Sakurai T, Sakairi Y, Furuya H, Asano Y. Additional mechanisms of nafamostat mesilate-associated hyperkalaemia. *Eur J Clin Pharmacol.* (1996) 51:149–51. doi: 10.1007/s002280050176

54. Imamura K, Sakurai Y, Enami T, Shibukawa R, Nishi Y, Ohta A, Shu T, et al. iPSC screening for drug repurposing identifies anti-RNA virus agents modulating host cell susceptibility. *FEBS Open Bio.* (2021) 11:1452–1464. doi: 10.1002/2211-5463.13153

55. Gu J, Hu W, Liu X. Pioglitazone improves potassium channel remodeling induced by angiotensin II in atrial myocytes. *Med Sci Monit Basic Res.* (2014) 20:153–60. doi: 10.12659/MSMBR.892450

56. Slowik A, Lammerding L, Zendedel A, Habib P, Beyer C. Impact of steroid hormones E2 and P on the NLRP3/ASC/Casp1 axis in primary mouse astroglia and BV-2 cells after in vitro hypoxia. *J Steroid Biochem Mol Biol.* (2018) 183:18–26. doi: 10.1016/j.jsbmb.2018.05.003

57. Pinna G, Sex and COVID-19: a protective role for reproductive steroids. *Trends Endocrinol Metab.* (2021) 32:3–6. doi: 10.1016/j.tem.2020.11.004

58. Muto S, Imai M, Asano Y. Mechanisms of the hyperkalaemia caused by nafamostat mesilate: effects of its two metabolites on Na+ and K+ transport properties in the rabbit cortical collecting duct. *Br J Pharmacol.* (1994) 111:173–8. doi: 10.1111/j.1476-5381.1994.tb14040.x

59. Muto S, Sebata K, Watanabe H, Shoji F, Yamamoto Y, Ohashi M, Yamada T, et al. Effect of oral glucose administration on serum potassium concentration in hemodialysis patients. *Am J Kidney Dis.* (2005) 46:697–

705. doi: 10.1053/j.ajkd.2005.06.013

60. Okajima M, Takahashi Y, Kaji T, Ogawa N, Mouri H. Nafamostat mesylate-induced hyperkalemia in critically ill patients with COVID-19: Four case reports. *World J Clin Cases.* (2020) 8:5320–5325. doi: 10.12998/wjcc.v8.i21.5320

61. Chen T, Wu D, Chen H, Yan W, Yang D, et al. Clinical characteristics of 113 deceased patients with coronavirus disease 2019: retrospective study. *BMJ.* (2020) 368:m1091. doi: 10.1136/bmj.m1091

62. Cabrera-Garcia D, Bekdash R, Abbott GW, Yazawa M, Harrison NL, he envelope protein of SARS-CoV2 increases intra-Golgi pH and forms a cation channel that is regulated by pH. *J Physiol.* (2021) 599:2851–68. doi: 10.1113/JP281037

63. Trobec T. The role of the SARS-CoV-2 envelope protein as a pH-dependent cation channel. *J Physiol.* (2021) 599:3435–3436. doi: 10.1113/JP281785

64. Singh Tomar PP, Arkin IT. SARS-CoV-2 E protein is a potential ion channel that can be inhibited by Gliclazide and Memantine. *Biochem Biophys Res Commun.* (2020) 530:10–14. doi: 10.1016/j.bbrc.2020.05.206

65. da Costa LS, Outlioua A, Anginot A, Akarid K, Arnoult D. RNA viruses promote activation of the NLRP3 inflammasome through cytopathogenic effect-induced potassium efflux. *Cell Death Dis.* (2019) 10:346. doi: 10.1038/s41419-019-1579-0

66. Choudhury S, Ma X, Abdullah SW, Zheng H. Activation and Inhibition of the NLRP3 Inflammasome by RNA Viruses. *J Inflamm Res.* (2021) 14:1145–1163. doi: 10.2147/JIR.S295706

67. Tsang OT, Chau TN, Choi KW, Tso EY, Lim W, Chiu MC, et al. Coronavirus-positive nasopharyngeal aspirate as predictor for severe acute respiratory syndrome mortality. *Emerg Infect Dis.* (2003) 9:1381–7. doi: 10.3201/eid0911.030400

68. Yang JK, Lin SS, Ji XJ, Guo LM. Binding of SARS coronavirus to its receptor damages islets and causes acute diabetes. *Acta Diabetol.* (2010) 47:193–9. doi: 10.1007/s00592-009-0109-4

69. Yamamoto M, Matsuyama S, Li X, Takeda M, Kawaguchi Y, Inoue JI et al. Identification of nafamostat as a potent inhibitor of Middle East Respiratory Syndrome coronavirus S protein-mediated membrane fusion using the split-protein-based cell-cell fusion assay. *Antimicrob Agents Chemotherap.* (2016) 60:6532–39. doi: 10.1128/AAC.01043-16

70. Weston S, Coleman C, Haupt R, Logue J, Matthews K, Frieman M. Broad anti-coronaviral activity of FDA approved drugs against SARS-CoV-2 in vitro and SARS-CoV in vivo. *J.Virol.* (2020) 94:e01218–20. 25:8482. doi: 10.1101/2020.03.25.008482

20

Senescence-Associated Molecules and Tumor-Immune-Interactions as Prognostic Biomarkers in Colorectal Cancer

Franziska Kellers[1], Aurélie Fernandez[1], Björn Konukiewitz[2], Mario Schindeldecker[1], Katrin E. Tagscherer[1], Achim Heintz[3], Moritz Jesinghaus[4], Wilfried Roth[1] and Sebastian Foersch[1]*

[1] Institute of Pathology, University Medical Center Mainz, Mainz, Germany, [2] Institute of Pathology, Christian-Albrecht University of Kiel, Kiel, Germany, [3] Department of General, Visceral and Vascular Surgery, Catholic Hospital Mainz, Mainz, Germany, [4] Department of Pathology, University Hospital Marburg, Marburg, Germany

*Correspondence:
Sebastian Foersch
sebastian.foersch@
unimedizin-mainz.de

Background and Aims: The initiation of cellular senescence in response to protumorigenic stimuli counteracts malignant progression in (pre)malignant cells. Besides arresting proliferation, cells entering this terminal differentiation state adopt a characteristic senescence-associated secretory phenotype (SASP) which initiates alterations to their microenvironment and effects immunosurveillance of tumorous lesions. However, some effects mediated by senescent cells contribute to disease progression. Currently, the exploration of senescent cells' impact on the tumor microenvironment and the evaluation of senescence as possible target in colorectal cancer (CRC) therapy demand reliable detection of cellular senescence *in vivo*. Therefore, specific immunohistochemical biomarkers are required. Our aim is to analyze the clinical implications of senescence detection in colorectal carcinoma and to investigate the interactions of senescent tumor cells and their immune microenvironment *in vitro* and *in vivo*.

Methods: Senescence was induced in CRC cell lines by low-dose-etoposide treatment and confirmed by Senescence-associated β-galactosidase (SA-β-GAL) staining and fluorescence activated cell sorting (FACS) analysis. Co-cultures of senescent cells and immune cells were established. Multiple cell viability assays, electron microscopy and live cell imaging were conducted. Immunohistochemical (IHC) markers of senescence and immune cell subtypes were studied in a cohort of CRC patients by analyzing a tissue micro array (TMA) and performing digital image analysis. Results were compared to disease-specific survival (DSS) and progression-free survival (PFS).

Results: Varying expression of senescence markers in tumor cells was associated with in- or decreased survival of CRC patients. Proximity analysis of p21-positive senescent tumor cells and cytotoxic T cells revealed a significantly better prognosis for patients in which these cell types have the possibility to directly interact. *In vitro*, NK-92 cells (mimicking natural killer T cells) or TALL-104 cells (mimicking both cytotoxic T cells and natural killer T cells) led to dose-dependent specific cytotoxicity in >75 % of the senescent CRC cells but <20 % of the proliferating control CRC cells. This immune cell-mediated senolysis seems to be facilitated via direct cell-cell contact inducing apoptosis and granule exocytosis.

Conclusion: Counteracting tumorigenesis, cellular senescence is of significant relevance in CRC. We show the dual role of senescence bearing both beneficial and malignancy-promoting potential *in vivo*. Absence as well as exceeding expression of senescence markers are associated with bad prognosis in CRC. The antitumorigenic potential of senescence induction is determined by tumor micromilieu and immune cell-mediated elimination of senescent cells.

Keywords: cellular senescence, colorectal cancer, senescence-associated secretory phenotype (SASP), prognostic biomarker, senolysis

INTRODUCTION

Malignant neoplasia of colon and rectum are associated with high morbidity and mortality and account for 10 % of cancer cases and 9.4 % of cancer deaths (1). Molecular mechanisms of colorectal carcinogenesis are increasingly understood, yet the role of cellular senescence and its contribution to survival and treatment outcome of cancer patients remain unclear.

One mechanism in tumor biology that only recently started to gain more attention due to its role in carcinogenesis is cellular senescence. Cellular senescence describes a permanent cell cycle arrest following potentially protumorigenic DNA-damaging incidents in premalignant cells, thereby counteracting malignant progression (2). There is a multitude of trigger mechanisms leading to the initiation of cellular senescence. Eroded telomeres which occur after repetitive cell divisions (3) or cumulative DNA erosions due to sublethal stressful conditions such as oxidative stress (4), proliferative stress due to oncogene-induced mitogenic hyperstimulation (5–7), loss of tumor suppressors (8, 9) or the presence of DNA damaging agents can induce a DNA damage response, arresting the cell cycle of impaired cells (10). Anticancer treatment such as chemotherapeutic agents, ionizing radiation (11–15) as well as targeted therapies are capable of evoking cellular senescence (16–21). Therapy-induced senescence (TIS) has been observed in tumor cells both *in vitro* and *in vivo* (15). Apart from ceasing proliferation, senescent transformation involves characteristic morphological and metabolic changes (22). *In vitro*, senescent cells adopt a characteristic flat, enlarged "fried egg" morphology as well as nuclear alterations (23–26). Increased lysosomal activity, detected by visualization of the lysosomal enzyme Senescence-associated β-galactosidase (SA-β-GAL) at pH 6, is a widely established biomarker of senescent cells (27). While detection of SA-β-GAL may be used for identification of cellular senescence in fresh or frozen cells (28, 29), the enzyme activity-dependent assay cannot be carried out on formalin-fixed, paraffin-embedded (FFPE) tissues (29) and therefore this distinctive feature may not be used to study cellular senescence

in vivo to a large extent. Due to the irreversible proliferation arrest, the senescent state is strongly associated with an absence of proliferation markers such as Ki-67 and the expression of anti-proliferative proteins (30). The onset of the senescence program involves cell cycle suppressors such as p53, p21, and p16 (22). The extent to which these features are displayed may vary (23) and none of these characteristics are exclusively linked to cellular senescence. Consequently only a combination of markers allows for distinctive identification of senescent cells (31). Recently, there have been approaches to identify novel markers of senescence (32, 33).

Although no longer proliferating, senescent cells remain highly metabolically active and display an altered secretory and signaling activity. Apart from autocrine enforcement of the senescent state, senescent cells induce non-cell-autonomous effects via direct cell-cell contact with nearby cells, paracrine signaling, and secretion of a multitude of factors affecting angiogenesis and immune surveillance of the tissue environment. The SASP, adopted by arrested cells in the presence of DNA impairment, consists of a distinct composition of secreted molecules involving signaling factors like inflammatory cytokines, enzymes and extracellular matrix components (34). The SASP highly depends on the cell type (34) and enables senescent cells to attract immune cells such as macrophages, NK cells and T cells to the site of a tumorous lesion, activating them to specifically eliminate senescent cells and thus promoting the immunosurveillance of the tumor (35, 36). While some senescent cells remain in the tissue for years (29, 37, 38) and eventually contribute to age-related diseases (39, 40), there are settings where the SASP signaling activates an immediate immune response, resulting in the installation of a proinflammatory micromilieu and eventually the removal of the senescent cells (41, 42), termed "senolysis." This immune cell driven clearance of senescent cells involves the innate (41, 42) as well as the adaptive immune cells (43, 44). There is evidence that senescent cells under senescence surveillance are eliminated by macrophages (45) or NK cell-mediated induction of granule exocytosis (46, 47).

Cellular senescence has been linked to colorectal carcinogenesis (40). The silencing of the senescence-regulating cell cycle suppressors p16 and p53 typically involved in cellular senescence induction (22) is a crucial step to overcome cellular senescence in colorectal carcinogenesis (48, 49). There is first evidence that measurement of cellular senescence might be a predictive parameter in CRC patients (50) but the clinical implications of the contribution of cellular senescence to colorectal carcinogenesis have not yet been studied in a large patient cohort. Since TIS occurs during various CRC therapies, the influence of this biomechanism on disease progression in CRC needs to be investigated in a clinical setting. Furthermore, it might be a promising approach in colorectal cancer therapy to use the potential of the senescence-induced immunosurveillance to counteract malignant progression (51). Evaluating the impact of cellular senescence and the potential of therapy-induced senescence in CRC demands reliable detection methods and biomarkers applicable to FFPE tissue to explore this key mechanism in colorectal carcinogenesis *in vivo*. We further explored the potential of senescence-associated molecules as prognostic and predictive biomarkers in CRC and conducted both *in vitro* and *in vivo* studies to gain a better understanding of the functional role of the interaction between senescent colorectal tumor cells and the immune system.

MATERIALS AND METHODS

Material

A list of antibodies and inhibitors used in this study can be found in **Supplementary Table 1**.

CRC Cell Culture

After preliminary experiments with various CRC cell lines, Caco-2 cells were cultivated in MEM (+15 % fetal bovine serum + 1 % pyruvate, 1 % NEAA, 1 % glutamine, 1 % penicillin, 1% streptomycin) at 37°C and 5% CO_2 on 12-well-plates. Senescence was induced by low dose (5 μM) Etoposide treatment. 24 h after seeding, the growth medium was replaced by medium containing 5 μM Etoposide. Cells treated with equal volumes of Dimethyl Sulfoxide (DMSO) were used as negative control. After 48 h the medium was replaced by growth medium, and cells were allowed to recover. Analyses were performed after 72 h.

Cytoblocks of Etoposide-treated and control cells were generated after harvesting using Accutase (Sigma Aldrich) treatment, formalin (Sigma Aldrich) fixation and embedding in 1 % Agarose. For following analyses, samples were transferred to paraffin and standard sectioning (2 μm) and subsequent staining was performed according to standard protocols used for routine pathology or as published previously (52). Furthermore, transmission electron microscopy (TEM) was performed according to protocols established for routine diagnostics at our institute (53).

Immune and CRC Cell Culture

NK-92 cells were cultivated in α-MEM + 12.5% fetal bovine serum + 12.5% horse serum + 1% penicillin + 1% streptomycin + 100–200 U/ml IL-2 (48 h)/ 5 ng/ml IL-2 (every 48 h) at 37°C

and 5% CO_2. TALL-104 cells were cultivated in Iscove's Modified Dulbecco's Medium (ATCC) + 20% fetal bovine serum, 2.5 μg /ml human albumin, 0.5 μg/ml D-manitol + 50–100 U/ml recombinant human IL-2 (48 h) at 37°C and 5% CO_2. For co-culture experiments, Caco-2 cells were cultivated on 6-well-plates and senescence was induced as according to 3.1. After 72 h of recovery, the growth medium was replaced by immune cell growth medium containing immune cells in different target-to-effector ratios. Cells were co-cultivated for up to 180 min. Following 120 min of co-incubation, cells were washed, and non-adherent cells (immune cells and non-vital Caco-2 cells) were removed. The quantity of remaining adherent Caco-2 cells after Co-culture was measured using cell viability assays such as crystal violet (CRV) staining of the remaining adherent cells.

Senescence and Cell Viability Assays

Cellular senescence was detected by SA-β-Gal staining using the Senescence β-Galactosidase Staining kit according to the manufacturer's instructions (Cell Signaling). In addition, cells were subjected to FACS analysis using the cellular senescence live cell analysis assay (Enzo) and a Becton Dickinson FACScalibur cytometer and Cell Quest Software (BD Bioscience). For viability analysis, Caco-2 cells were treated as described. At the indicated times, cells were washed with PBS, fixed with methanol:ethanol (2:1) and stained with 0.1 % crystal violet for 30 min. The plates were washed in running tap water and air dried for 24 h. Crystal violet was solubilized using 33 % acetic acid for 30 min. The absorbance was measured at 600 nm using a microplate reader (Tecan).

Live Cell Imaging

Immune cells were added to Etoposide-treated Caco-2 cells as described above. Cells were incubated at 32°C for 180 min. Cell-cell interactions were observed using a Jenoptik GRYPHAX SUBRA camera system in 100 x magnification. Pictures of representative areas were taken with a 30 s interval.

Patient Cohort

The patient cohort consisted of up to 598 patients diagnosed with primary colorectal carcinoma at the Institute of Pathology of the University Medical Center, Mainz. These patients had not received neoadjuvant treatment prior to their surgery and were treated according to national and WHO guidelines in place at the time. Patients with a hereditary cancer syndrome or history of inflammatory bowel disease were not included in this study. Retrospective use of these and other patients' data as well as material for research purposes was approved by the ethical committee of the medical association of the State of Rhineland-Palatinate [ref. no. 837.075.16 (10394)]. All experiments were in accordance with the Declaration of Helsinki. Characteristics of the patients can be found in **Supplementary Table 2**.

Human Tissue Analyses

From each patient, FFPE tissue samples containing tissue of the primary tumor and non-cancerous tissue were obtained from routine procession of the surgery specimens. Clinical data such as age, DSS, PFS, localization and stage of the tumor were obtained. Representative areas of tumor center, invasive margin and non-cancerous epithelium were identified by review of hematoxylin and eosin (H&E)-stained sections from each sample and cores of 1 mm in diameter were obtained using the TMArrayer (Pathology Devices, San Diego, USA) and included in the TMA. From each patient, 3 samples containing representative areas of the primary tumor were included. TMA sections were stained for various senescence-associated molecules and other cell types. Staining of the slides was carried out using an automated staining system (Agilent Technologies) and its respective reagents. IHC-stained TMA sections were digitalised using a Hamamatsu Nanozoomer Series scanner (Hamamatsu Photonics, Hamamatsu, Japan) at 20 x magnification. Slides were thoroughly annotated by a pathology expert, thereby cancerous epithelium and stroma were marked. Digital image analysis was performed using HALO (Indica Labs, Albuquerque, USA). A random forest classifier was trained to discern (cancerous) epithelium and stroma. The percentage of positive cells within the classified tumor cells was obtained. Consecutive sequential TMA sections were co-registered for additional comprehensive morphometric analyses such as distance-measurements.

Statistical Analyses

Statistical analyses were carried out using GraphPad Prism version 9. Cell viability data was compared with the control group using t-test or ordinary one-way ANOVA. Dunnett T3 test (statistical hypothesis testing) was used to correct for multiple testing. For each marker, the values' distribution was analyzed, and cutoff values were chosen to represent meaningful biological groups, while at the same time finding optimal cutoff values. This was done similar to the method proposed by Budczies et al. where "[t]he optimal cutoff is defined as the point with the most significant (log-rank test) split." These authors have implemented their approach as open source software named the Charité Cutoff Finder (54). Additionally, we also applied the surv_cutpoint capability of the R survminer package which functions in a similar fashion (54). Cutoff values can be found in **Supplementary Table 3**. Survival analyses were performed using Kaplan-Meier-plots, differences in survival were calculated by performing log-rank Mantel-Cox test.

RESULTS

Low dose Etoposide treatment induces senescence-related morphological changes and SA-ß-Gal activity. Morphological changes commonly found in senescent cells such as enlarged size and vacuolation could be detected in cells treated with Etoposide using white light microscopy and electron microscopy (**Figure 1A**). Increased SA-β-GAL activity was observed in 71.9 % of Etoposide-treated Caco-2 cells but only 1.1 % of control cells ($p < 0.0001$) (**Figure 1B**). Senescence induced by Etoposide treatment was also confirmed by FACS analysis (**Figure 1C**).

To assess the prognostic potential of senescence-associated molecules suggested by previous studies (32, 33) in a clinical setting, we evaluated various markers in our cohort of CRC patients immunohistochemically (**Figure 2A**) and observed mixed effects. For NTAL, ARMCX3, p21, and EBP50 the

percentage of positive tumor cells showed a statistically significant prognostic effect. High expression of NTAL was linked to a better DSS and PFS (**Supplementary Figure 1**). A high expression of p21 was linked to a higher PFS (**Supplementary Figure 1**), underlining the important role of p21-mediated senescence in tumor defense. Evaluating expression of ARMCX3 and EBP50 (**Supplementary Figure 1**), we found that a high expression was associated with a decreased DSS compared to the group of patients with lower expression levels. This surprising finding led us to try a three-tier cutoff system into excessive, moderate, and low expression (**Figures 2B–F**, cutoffs on the right and in **Supplementary Table 3**). Interestingly, for all markers (including gH2AX), using this approach showed that moderate expression was associated with the best prognosis, while both low and excessive expression showed a worse prognosis. This was statistically significant for NTAL, ARMCX3, and EBP50 (**Figures 2B–E, Supplementary Figure 1**). Taken together, this highlights the dual role of cellular senescence, with both low and excessive expression of senescence-associated markers showing worse DSS and PFS.

In search of an explanation for this plurivalent effect we hypothesized that the negative prognosis in patients with large numbers of senescent cells might result from a defective interaction between senescent cells and the tumor micromilieu. The excessive numbers of senescent cells in patients with a negative prognosis might reflect accumulation of these cells within the tumor tissue due to an ineffective tumor immunosurveillance and a failure of the immune system to clear of senescent cells. To investigate the immunosurveillance of senescent cells in our clinical cohort and analyse immune cells targeting senescent cells, we visualized the spatial relationship of senescent cells and cytotoxic T cell as stained by CD8 (**Figure 3A**). Using digital image analysis, consecutive sections with cores of one patient stained for different molecules were co-registered and corresponding tissue areas on the different sections were identified. The average distance between these two cell populations as well as the percentage of CD8-positive cells within 100 μm of p21-positive cells were determined (**Figure 3C**). To identify a possible impact on survival, proximity data was correlated with DSS and PFS. Interestingly, both a lower average distance between these two cell populations as well as a higher percentage of CD8-postive cells within 100 μm of p21-positive cells were linked to a significantly increased DSS and PFS (**Figures 3B,D**). This suggests that a closer immunosurveillance of the lesion improves the prognosis of CRC patients.

To explore the senescence-induced immunosurveillance of colonic cancer cells in depth, we conducted a series of co-culture experiments. After 2 h of co-incubation, the number of adherent senescent Caco-2 cells decreased depending on the ratio of immune cells that was added. Addition of NK-92 (displaying properties of natural killer cells) or TALL-104 cells (displaying properties of both cytotoxic T cells and NKT cells) to Caco-2 cells lead to dose-dependent detaching of adherent Caco-2 cells and cell death in >75 % of senescent cells but <20 % of proliferating control cells which was confirmed by CRV staining. This dose-dependent cytotoxicity was not

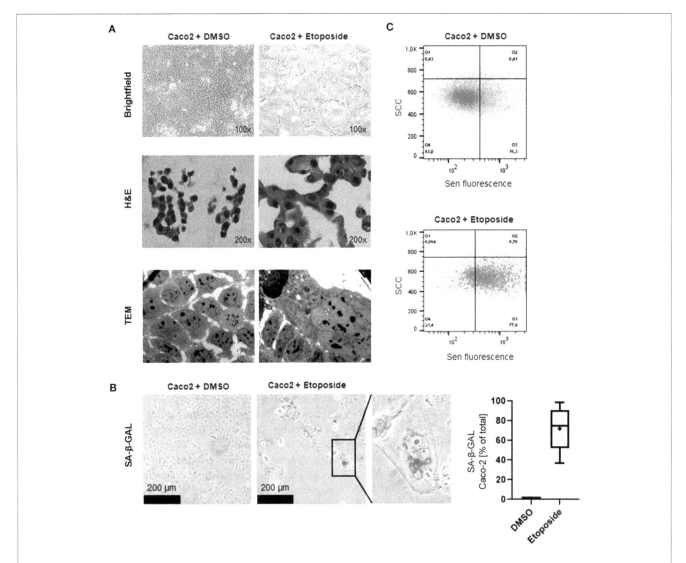

FIGURE 1 | Induction of cellular senescence *in vitro* by Etoposide treatment. **(A)** Morphological appearance of Etoposide (Eto)-treated and control (DMSO) Caco2 cells using brightfield microscopy (upper panel), normal H&E-stained sections of cytoblocks (middle panel) and TEM (lower panel). Senescent cells adopt a characteristic "fried egg" morphology, including an enlarged shape and nucleus. Cytoplasmatic vacuolation is apparent. **(B)** Increased senescence SA-β-GAL staining indicates senescence induction. SA-β-GAL-positive cells were counted after DMSO and Etoposide-treatment. **(C)** FACS analysis confirms senescence induction in Etoposide-treated cells.

observed in the control group of proliferating cells that had not been exposed to Etoposide (**Figures 4A,B**). To discern whether this specific elimination of senescent cells was facilitated via factors secreted into the growth medium by the immune cells, we incubated senescent Caco-2 cells with immune cell supernatant. Importantly, addition of conditioned supernatant of TALL-104 or NK-92 cells to Etoposide-pre-treated Caco-2 cells did not decrease cell viability measured by CRV absorption (**Figures 4C,D**). To confirm the hypothesis that direct cell-cell contact with immune cells accounts for the cell death of senescent Caco-2 cells and to visualize this interaction, we conducted electron microscopy and live cell imaging during co-incubation. Live cell imaging proves directed movement of immune cells toward senescent cells followed by detaching of senescent cells.

Non-senescent cells in the environment of senescent cells were not eliminated by the immune cells to the same extent. Electron microscopy of the co-culture experiments shows direct cell-cell contact between TALL-104 cells and senescent Caco-2 cells (**Figures 4E,F, Supplementary Video 1**).

To determine how immune cells execute the elimination of senescent cells, a set of co-culture experiments was conducted under inhibition of different pathways of cell death. By adding inhibitors of apoptosis, granule exocytosis and necroptosis, the relevance of those pathways for immune cell-mediated elimination was determined. ZVAD has been demonstrated to decrease death receptor mediated cell death in senescent cells (46). Previous studies had not found an impact of caspase-dependent apoptosis on NK cell-mediated senolysis (46).

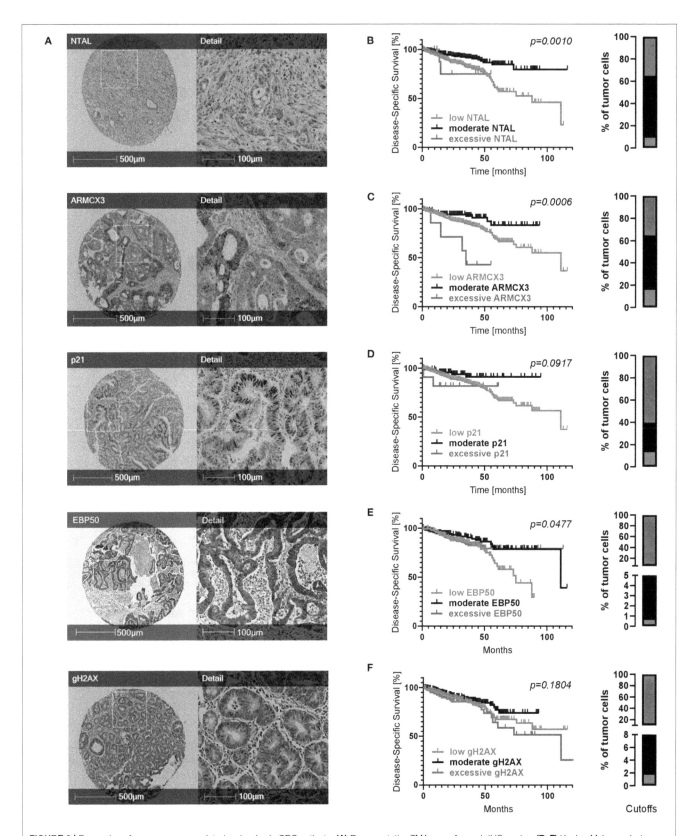

FIGURE 2 | Expression of senescence-associated molecules in CRC patients. **(A)** Representative TMA cores for each IHC marker. **(B–F)** Kaplan-Meier survival analyses regarding expression of senescence markers when divided into three subcohorts: low expression (petrol), moderate expression (black) and excessive expression (red). Cutoffs are displayed as bar graphs on the right of each curve and were calculated using a modification of the Charité Cutoff Finder from (54). Disease-specific survival is shown. Two tier subdivision, progression-free survival and detailed individual cutoff values can be found in the **Supplementary Material**.

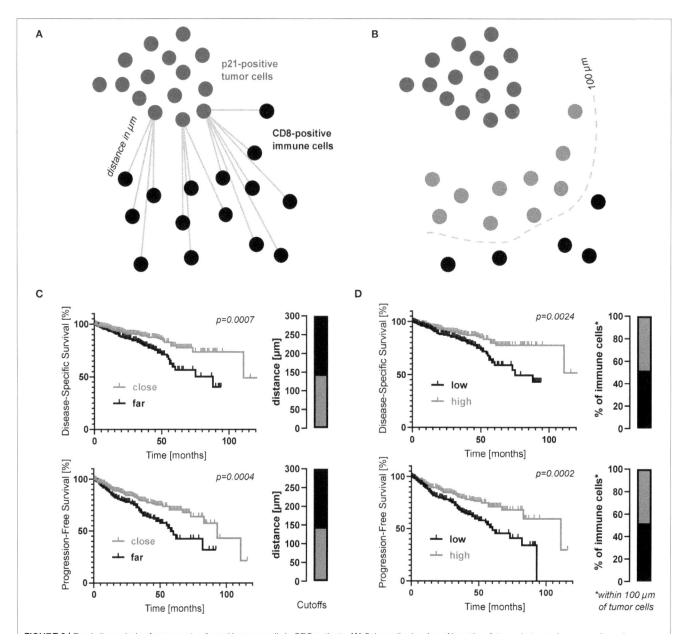

FIGURE 3 | Proximity analysis of senescent cells and immune cells in CRC patients. **(A)** Schematic drawing of how the distance between immune cells and senescent tumor cells was measured. **(B)** Kaplan-Meier survival analyses regarding the average distance between CD8- and p21-positive cells. **(C)** Schematic drawing of how the proportion of immune cells within close proximity (within 100 μm) of senescent tumor cells was measured. **(D)** Kaplan-Meier survival analyses regarding the percentage of CD8-positive cells within 100 μm of p21-positive cells. Again, cutoff values are displayed as bar graphs.

However, we found that using pan-caspase inhibitor ZVAD to block death-receptor-mediated apoptosis resulted in significantly higher quantity of remaining adherent senescent cells after co-incubation resulting from abrogated senolysis of both NK-92 and TALL-104 cells ($p < 0.0001$). Addition of the SMAC-mimetic and apoptosis-sensitizer BV6 however did not have a measurable effect. Inhibiting the necroptosis pathway using Necrostatin-1, an allosteric inhibitor of RIP1, did not reverse the cytotoxicity of TALL-104 or NK-92 cells, suggesting a necroptosis-independent mechanism responsible for the targeted elimination of senescent

cells. To assess the role of granule exocytosis for the immune-mediated depletion of senescent cells, we conducted a set of experiments in the presence of Concanamycin A (Conc A) which inhibits perforin-based cytolytic activity by inhibition of vacuolar type H^+-ATPase. Conc A decreased the cytotoxic effect of TALL-104 cells ($p < 0.0001$) but did not significantly prevent killing of senescent cells by NK-92 cells. HMGB1-Inhibititor glycyrrhizinic acid (Gly. Acid) was used to address HMGB1-dependent metabolic cell death. Spautin-1 ($p < 0.0230$) was used to address autophagy-associated cell death mechanisms.

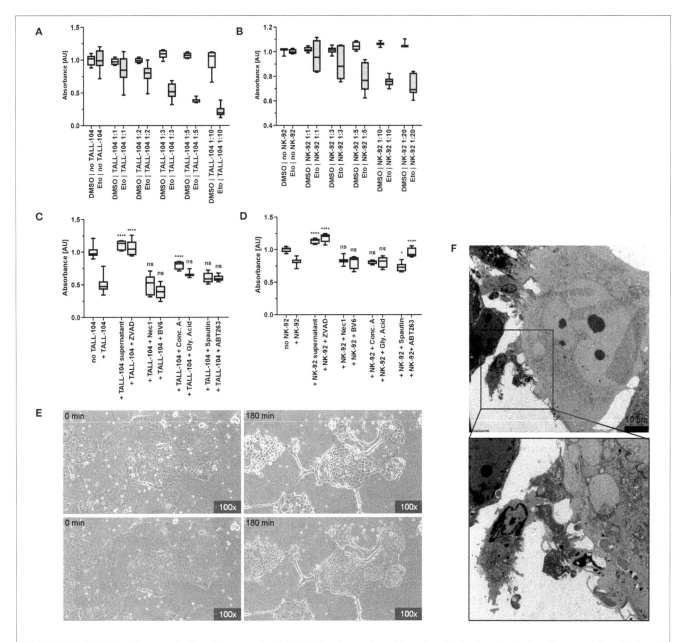

FIGURE 4 | Co-incubation of senescent cells and immune cells. **(A,B)** CRV absorbance of remaining adherent cells after co-incubation of senescent Caco-2 cells and immune cells. Co-incubation with TALL-104 **(A)** or NK-92 **(B)** immune cells lead to dose-dependent elimination of senescent cells. **(C,D)** Elimination of senescent cells under the influence of immune cell conditioned supernatant and various inhibitors of cellular clearance mechanisms as measured by CRV absorbance. TALL-104 **(C)** and NK-92 **(D)** experiments are shown. $^*p \leq 0.05$, $^{**}p \leq 0.01$, $^{***}p \leq 0.001$, $^{****}p \leq 0.0001$, ns = not significant. **(E)** Life cell imaging of co-incubation of senescent cells and immune cells. Specific elimination of senescent cells (blue) by NK-92 cells while proliferating cells (orange) are spared. **(F)** Electron microscopy. Cell-cell contact of TALL-104 cells (red) and a senescent cell (blue).

ABT263 partly abrogated the cytotoxic effect of NK-92 cells ($p < 0.0001$) but did not significantly prevent killing of senescent cells by TALL-104 cells. Altogether, our co-incubation, electron microscopy and live cell imaging results indicate that direct cell-cell contact between immune cells and targeted senescent cells is a key mechanism for immune-cell-mediated senolysis. In the presence of inhibitors of apoptosis or (to some extent) granule exocytosis, immune cell-mediated elimination of senescent cells is decreased, suggesting that killing of senescent cells is mainly facilitated via apoptosis induction and via induction of granule exocytosis (**Figures 4C,D**).

DISCUSSION

Arresting the cell cycle of premalignant cells as a response to oncogenic signaling and DNA impairment strongly supports the idea of senescence as a beneficial anti-cancer-mechanism (55–57). A premalignant cell's ability to senesce involves major tumor-suppressor pathways and has been proven crucial to fight neoplastic transformation *in vivo* (6, 9, 58–60) and affects treatment outcome of cancer patients (61, 62). Recent studies point to a crucial role of cellular senescence in gastrointestinal diseases including colorectal carcinogenesis (40). Studies report that oncogene-induced senescence (OIS) prevents progression of benign KRAS-mutated sessile serrated adenomas to invasive carcinomas and provides an important barrier opposing malignancy in these early lesions. Malignant transformation to serrated adenocarcinoma requires overcoming this OIS-facilitated cell cycle arrest by downregulation of p16Ink4a (49). There is evidence to suggest that senescence detection might be of predictive value for CRC patients (50), however an extensive clinical study to evaluate the prognostic potential of senescence markers had been missing.

Our study reflects the important and complex role of cellular senescence in colorectal carcinogenesis. In many previous studies, cellular senescence has been described as a "double-edged sword" (34), referring to both the pro- and antitumorigenic effects senescent cells do have on disease progression. We demonstrate that absence of intratumoral senescence and therefore the lack of a basic antitumor defense mechanism is linked with a negative prognosis. Regarding the expression of p21, NTAL, EBP50 and ARMCX3, our results show the important role of senescence induction in tumor defense and underline the relevance of cell cycle regulator p21 and p21-mediated senescence. Moreover, we show that the occurrence of extremely high percentages of senescent cells in CRC is linked to a negative prognosis when compared to patients with moderate expression of senescence markers. These findings point to a complex role of cellular senescence in CRC, suggesting that both non-existent and extensive detection of senescent cells correlate with a negative prognosis. However, further analyses in the context of various molecular and disease subtypes are also necessary to validate our findings.

Senescent cells within the tumor do not automatically imply an effective tumor defense. An effect contributing to the negative outcome of those patients with large numbers of senescent cells might be the inflammatory micromilieu developing in close distance to senescent cells as a driver of further cell damage and therefore accelerating disease progression. While some of the factors secreted after SASP initiation contribute to maintaining the cell cycle arrest and reinforce the senescence program in premalignant cells (63–66) the SASP-driven proinflammatory alterations to the micromilieu–despite enhancing immune surveillance –do as well have malignancy-promoting effects (67).

Secreted factors may provide protumorigenic conditions and stimulate growth, dedifferentiation, and invasiveness of premalignant epithelial cells (68–70). Senescent fibroblasts signaling might contribute to growth-enabling changes to the microenvironment of dormant metastases (71). Increased VEGF expression by senescent cells increases angiogenesis in lesions at risk of malignant transformation and facilitates tumor vascularization, hereby contributing to malignant transformation (72). In CRC, VEGFR2 signaling silences the tumor-antagonizing effect of cellular senescence by actively bypassing p21 (73). There is evidence that the SASP-mediated inflammatory response

enhances immune control of senescent tumorous lesions in colorectal carcinoma and prevents malignant transformation in the presence of functional p53 but is protumorigenic in p21/p53-deficient lesions (74).

The perception of senescence as a beneficial anticancer mechanism (55–57) depends on the ability of the immune system to clear senescent cells and prevent negative effects mediated by senescent cells that remain in the tissue (39). Disruption of the tumor immunosurveillance results in accumulation of senescent cells (39), which might be the cause for the negative prognosis we observed in patients with extensive expression of senescence markers. Our study demonstrates that a dichotomous classification does not apply when describing the impact of cellular senescence detection on CRC prognosis. Senescence-associated molecules do have significant prognostic value concerning the outcome of patients with CRC. Moreover, we demonstrate that immune cells *in vitro* specifically eliminate senescent colon cancer cells while somewhat sparing proliferating cells. As Sagiv et al. showed for liver fibrosis in mice (46), we could demonstrate that NK cell-mediated clearance of senescent colorectal carcinoma cells is dependent on granule exocytosis. However, in contrast to Sagiv et al. (46) we found that suppression of the death receptor pathway by ZVAD abrogated the immune cell-mediated elimination of senescent cells in both the NK cell and the cytotoxic T cell model. Thus, our findings lead to the conclusion that induction of both apoptosis and granule exocytosis contribute to the targeted elimination of senescent cells by the immune system.

To reflect this interaction in the clinical setting, proximity analyses of the spatial relation of senescent tumor cells and immune cells are of prognostic relevance and could constitute a prognostic tool in colorectal cancer. Interestingly, we found that the spatial relation of p21-positive tumor cells and cytotoxic T cells is indicative of prognosis regarding DSS and PFS of CRC patients. There is evidence for an immune-infiltration-preventing effect of SASP signaling under certain circumstances (75). High percentage of senescent cells within the tumor–indicative of a negative prognosis as demonstrated in our study–might be the result of impeded tumor immune infiltration due to SASP signaling by senescent cells inhibiting immune cells (75). Furthermore, we showed that patients with close distance of senescent tumor cells and cytotoxic T cells do have a significant better survival which might indicate an antitumorigenic, preferable SASP signaling in these patients. How to impact SASP and induce the preferable, immunosurveillance-promoting secretory activity in senescent cells needs further evaluation and bares great potential in future therapy development. There is *in vitro* (18, 76, 77) and *in vivo* (78–80) evidence for a therapeutic approach inducing cellular senescence in cancerous lesions, evoking immune-cell mediated elimination of cancer cells and enhancing tumor surveillance (41, 44, 81). There are first therapeutic approaches of altering the senescence-induced immune response to induce an antitumorigenic microenvironment (51). Furthermore, therapeutic agents specifically eliminating senescent cells, called senolytics, have demonstrated great potential in various age-associated diseases, including cancer (82).

Taken together, cellular senescence is a key mechanism in opposing malignant transformation of impaired cells. The antitumorigenic effect of cellular senescence is dependent on an intact immune surveillance of the lesion. Therefore, the interaction of immune cells and senescent cells within the tumor microenvironment is of crucial prognostic relevance and provides targets for CRC therapy.

AUTHOR CONTRIBUTIONS

FK and SF: conception and design. FK, SF, AF, and AH: acquisition and data. FK, SF, BK, KT, and MJ: analysis, interpretation of data, and critical revision of the manuscript. FK, SF, and KT: drafting of the manuscript. FK, SF, and MS: statistical analysis. SF: obtaining funding, administrative, and technical, or material support. SF and WR: supervision.

ACKNOWLEDGMENTS

Aspects of this work are part of the MD thesis of FK.

SUPPLEMENTARY MATERIAL

Supplementary Figure 1 | Additional Kaplan-Meier curves showing **(A)** disease-specific survival with a two-tier cutoff and **(B)** complementary progression-free survival. Cutoffs are displayed as bar graphs and were calculated using a modification of the Charité Cutoff Finder from (54).

Supplementary Table 1 | Antibodies and inhibitors used in this study.

Supplementary Table 2 | Clinicopathological characteristics of the patient cohort.

Supplementary Table 3 | Cutoff values for survival analysis as calculated using a modification of the Cutoff Finder from (54).

Supplementary Video 1 | Elimination of senescent Caco-2 cells by TALL-104 immune cells.

REFERENCES

1. Sung H, Ferlay J, Siegel RL, Laversanne M, Soerjomataram I, Jemal A, et al. Global cancer statistics 2020: GLOBOCAN estimates of incidence and mortality worldwide for 36 cancers in 185 countries. *CA Cancer J Clin.* (2021) 71:209–49. doi: 10.3322/caac.21660

2. Hayflick L. The limited *in vitro* lifetime of human diploid cell strains. *Exp Cell Res.* (1965) 37:614–36. doi: 10.1016/0014-4827(65)90211-9

3. Harley CB, Futcher AB, Greider CW. Telomeres shorten during ageing of human fibroblasts. *Nature.* (1990) 345:458–60. doi: 10.1038/345458a0

4. von Zglinicki T. Oxidative stress shortens telomeres. *Trends Biochem Sci.* (2002) 27:339–44. doi: 10.1016/S0968-0004(02)02110-2

5. Serrano M, Lin AW, McCurrach ME, Beach D, Lowe SW. Oncogenic ras provokes premature cell senescence associated with accumulation of p53 and p16INK4a. *Cell.* (1997) 88:593–602. doi: 10.1016/S0092-8674(00)81902-9

6. Bartkova J, Rezaei N, Liontos M, Karakaidos P, Kletsas D, Issaeva N, et al. Oncogene-induced senescence is part of the tumorigenesis barrier imposed by DNA damage checkpoints. *Nature.* (2006) 444:633–7. doi: 10.1038/nature05268

7. Di Micco R, Fumagalli M, Cicalese A, Piccinin S, Gasparini P, Luise C, et al. Oncogene-induced senescence is a DNA damage response triggered by DNA hyper-replication. *Nature.* (2006) 444:638–42. doi: 10.1038/nature05327

8. Shamma A, Takegami Y, Miki T, Kitajima S, Noda M, Obara T, et al. Rb Regulates DNA damage response and cellular senescence through E2F dependent suppression of N-ras isoprenylation. *Cancer Cell.* (2009) 15:255–69. doi: 10.1016/j.ccr.2009.03.001

9. Chen Z, Trotman LC, Shaffer D, Lin HK, Dotan ZA, Niki M, et al. Crucial role of p53-dependent cellular senescence in suppression of Pten-deficient tumorigenesis. *Nature.* (2005) 436:725–30. doi: 10.1038/nature03918

10. d'Adda di Fagagna F, Reaper PM, Clay-Farrace L, Fiegler H, Carr P, Von Zglinicki T, et al. A DNA damage checkpoint response in telomere-initiated senescence. *Nature.* (2003) 426:194–8. doi: 10.1038/nature02118

11. Chang BD, Broude EV, Dokmanovic M, Zhu H, Ruth A, Xuan Y, et al. A senescence-like phenotype distinguishes tumor cells that undergo terminal proliferation arrest after exposure to anticancer agents. *Cancer Res.* (1999) 59:3761–7.

12. te Poele RH, Okorokov AL, Jardine L, Cummings J, Joel SP. DNA damage is able to induce senescence in tumor cells *in vitro* and *in vivo*. *Cancer Res.* (2002) 62:1876–83.

13. Chang BD, Swift ME, Shen M, Fang J, Broude EV, Roninson IB. Molecular determinants of terminal growth arrest induced in tumor cells by a chemotherapeutic agent. *Proc Natl Acad Sci U S A.* (2002) 99:389–94. doi: 10.1073/pnas.012602599

14. Roninson IB. Tumor cell senescence in cancer treatment. *Cancer Res.* (2003) 63:2705–15.

15. Ewald JA, Desotelle JA, Wilding G, Jarrard DF. Therapy-induced senescence in cancer. *J Natl Cancer Inst.* (2010) 102:1536–46. doi: 10.1093/jnci/djq364

16. Cadoo KA, Gucalp A, Traina TA. Palbociclib: an evidence-based review of its potential in the treatment of breast cancer. *Breast Cancer.* (2014) 6:123–33. doi: 10.2147/BCTT.S46725

17. Yoshida A, Lee EK, Diehl JA. Induction of therapeutic senescence in vemurafenib-resistant melanoma by extended inhibition of CDK4/6. *Cancer Res.* (2016) 76:2990–3002. doi: 10.1158/0008-5472.CAN-15-2931

18. Rader J, Russell MR, Hart LS, Nakazawa MS, Belcastro LT, Martinez D, et al. Dual CDK4/CDK6 inhibition induces cell-cycle arrest and senescence in neuroblastoma. *Clin Cancer Res.* (2013) 19:6173–82. doi: 10.1158/1078-0432.CCR-13-1675

19. Sherr CJ. A new cell-cycle target in cancer - inhibiting cyclin D-dependent kinases 4 and 6. *N Engl J Med.* (2016) 375:1920–3. doi: 10.1056/NEJMp1612343

20. Acosta JC, Gil J. Senescence: a new weapon for cancer therapy. *Trends Cell Biol.* (2012) 22:211–9. doi: 10.1016/j.tcb.2011.11.006

21. Dabritz JH, Yu Y, Milanovic M, Schonlein M, Rosenfeldt MT, Dorr JR, et al. CD20-targeting immunotherapy promotes cellular senescence in B-cell lymphoma. *Mol Cancer Ther.* (2016) 15:1074–81. doi: 10.1158/1535-7163.MCT-15-0627

22. von Zglinicki T, Saretzki G, Ladhoff J, d'Adda di Fagagna F, Jackson SP. Human cell senescence as a DNA damage response. *Mech Ageing Dev.* (2005) 126:111–7. doi: 10.1016/j.mad.2004.09.034

23. Matsumura T, Zerrudo Z, Hayflick L. Senescent human diploid cells in culture: survival, DNA synthesis and morphology. *J Gerontol.* (1979) 34:328–34. doi: 10.1093/geronj/34.3.328

24. Narita M, Nunez S, Heard E, Narita M, Lin AW, Hearn SA, et al. Rb-mediated heterochromatin formation and silencing of E2F target genes during cellular senescence. *Cell.* (2003) 113:703–16. doi: 10.1016/S0092-8674(03)00401-X

25. Mehta IS, Figgitt M, Clements CS, Kill IR, Bridger JM. Alterations to nuclear architecture and genome behavior in senescent cells. *Ann N Y Acad Sci.* (2007) 1100:250–63. doi: 10.1196/annals.1395.027

26. Zhang R, Chen W, Adams PD. Molecular dissection of formation of senescence-associated heterochromatin foci. *Mol Cell Biol.* (2007) 27:2343–58. doi: 10.1128/MCB.02019-06

27. Kurz DJ, Decary S, Hong Y, Erusalimsky JD. Senescence-associated (beta)-galactosidase reflects an increase in lysosomal mass during

replicative ageing of human endothelial cells. *J Cell Sci.* (2000) 113:3613–22. doi: 10.1242/jcs.113.20.3613

28. Itahana K, Campisi J, Dimri GP. Methods to detect biomarkers of cellular senescence: the senescence-associated beta-galactosidase assay. *Methods Mol Biol.* (2007) 371:21–31. doi: 10.1007/978-1-59745-361-5_3

29. Dimri GP, Lee X, Basile G, Acosta M, Scott G, Roskelley C, et al. A biomarker that identifies senescent human cells in culture and in aging skin in vivo. *Proc Natl Acad Sci U S A.* (1995) 92:9363–7. doi: 10.1073/pnas.92.20.9363

30. Sharpless NE, Sherr CJ. Forging a signature of in vivo senescence. *Nat Rev Cancer.* (2015) 15:397–408. doi: 10.1038/nrc3960

31. Campisi J. Aging, cellular senescence, and cancer. *Annu Rev Physiol.* (2013) 75:685–705. doi: 10.1146/annurev-physiol-030212-183653

32. Althubiti M, Lezina L, Carrera S, Jukes-Jones R, Giblett SM, Antonov A, et al. Characterization of novel markers of senescence and their prognostic potential in cancer. *Cell Death Dis.* (2014) 5:e1528. doi: 10.1038/cddis.2014.489

33. Wagner J, Damaschke N, Yang B, Truong M, Guenther C, McCormick J, et al. Overexpression of the novel senescence marker beta-galactosidase (GLB1) in prostate cancer predicts reduced PSA recurrence. *PLoS ONE.* (2015) 10:e0124366. doi: 10.1371/journal.pone.0124366

34. Coppe JP, Desprez PY, Krtolica A, Campisi J. The senescence-associated secretory phenotype: the dark side of tumor suppression. *Annu Rev Pathol.* (2010) 5:99–118. doi: 10.1146/annurev-pathol-121808-102144

35. Burton DGA, Stolzing A. Cellular senescence: immunosurveillance and future immunotherapy. *Ageing Res Rev.* (2018) 43:17–25. doi: 10.1016/j.arr.2018.02.001

36. Kuilman T, Peeper DS. Senescence-messaging secretome: SMS-ing cellular stress. *Nat Rev Cancer.* (2009) 9:81–94. doi: 10.1038/nrc2560

37. Michaloglou C, Vredeveld LC, Soengas MS, Denoyelle C, Kuilman T, van der Horst CM, et al. BRAFE600-associated senescence-like cell cycle arrest of human naevi. *Nature.* (2005) 436:720–4. doi: 10.1038/nature03890

38. Bayreuther K, Francz PI, Gogol J, Hapke C, Maier M, Meinrath HG. Differentiation of primary and secondary fibroblasts in cell culture systems. *Mutat Res.* (1991) 256:233–42. doi: 10.1016/0921-8734(91)90014-3

39. Ovadya Y, Landsberger T, Leins H, Vadai E, Gal H, Biran A, et al. Impaired immune surveillance accelerates accumulation of senescent cells and aging. *Nat Commun.* (2018) 9:5435. doi: 10.1038/s41467-018-0 7825-3

40. Frey N, Venturelli S, Zender L, Bitzer M. Cellular senescence in gastrointestinal diseases: from pathogenesis to therapeutics. *Nat Rev Gastroenterol Hepatol.* (2018) 15:81–95. doi: 10.1038/nrgastro. 2017.146

41. Xue W, Zender L, Miething C, Dickins RA, Hernando E, Krizhanovsky V, et al. Senescence and tumour clearance is triggered by p53 restoration in murine liver carcinomas. *Nature.* (2007) 445:656–60. doi: 10.1038/nature05529

42. Iannello A, Thompson TW, Ardolino M, Lowe SW, Raulet DH. p53-dependent chemokine production by senescent tumor cells supports NKG2D-dependent tumor elimination by natural killer cells. *J Exp Med.* (2013) 210:2057–69. doi: 10.1084/jem.20130783

43. Hoenicke L, Zender L. Immune surveillance of senescent cells–biological significance in cancer- and non-cancer pathologies. *Carcinogenesis.* (2012) 33:1123–6. doi: 10.1093/carcin/bgs124

44. Kang TW, Yevsa T, Woller N, Hoenicke L, Wuestefeld T, Dauch D, et al. Senescence surveillance of pre-malignant hepatocytes limits liver cancer development. *Nature.* (2011) 479:547–51. doi: 10.1038/nature10599

45. Lujambio A, Akkari L, Simon J, Grace D, Tschaharganeh DF, Bolden JE, et al. Non-cell-autonomous tumor suppression by p53. *Cell.* (2013) 153:449–60. doi: 10.1016/j.cell.2013.03.020

46. Sagiv A, Biran A, Yon M, Simon J, Lowe SW, Krizhanovsky V. Granule exocytosis mediates immune surveillance of senescent cells. *Oncogene.* (2013) 32:1971–7. doi: 10.1038/onc.2012.206

47. Krizhanovsky V, Yon M, Dickins RA, Hearn S, Simon J, Miething C, et al. Senescence of activated stellate cells limits liver fibrosis. *Cell.* (2008) 134:657–67. doi: 10.1016/j.cell.2008.06.049

48. Leggett B, Whitehall V. Role of the serrated pathway in colorectal cancer pathogenesis. *Gastroenterology.* (2010) 138:2088–100. doi: 10.1053/j.gastro.2009.12.066

49. Carragher LA, Snell KR, Giblett SM, Aldridge VS, Patel B, Cook SJ, et al. V600EBraf induces gastrointestinal crypt senescence and promotes tumour

50. Haugstetter AM, Loddenkemper C, Lenze D, Grone J, Standfuss C, Petersen I, et al. Cellular senescence predicts treatment outcome in metastasised colorectal cancer. *Br J Cancer.* (2010) 103:505–9. doi: 10.1038/sj.bjc.6605784

51. Toso A, Revandkar A, Di Mitri D, Guccini I, Proietti M, Sarti M, et al. Enhancing chemotherapy efficacy in Pten-deficient prostate tumors by activating the senescence-associated antitumor immunity. *Cell Rep.* (2014) 9:75–89. doi: 10.1016/j.celrep.2014.08.044

52. Radspieler MM, Schindeldecker M, Stenzel P, Forsch S, Tagscherer KE, Herpel E, et al. Lamin-B1 is a senescence-associated biomarker in clear-cell renal cell carcinoma. *Oncol Lett.* (2019) 18:2654–60. doi: 10.3892/ol.2019.10593

53. Musayeva A, Manicam C, Steege A, Brochhausen C, Straub BK, Bell K, et al. Role of alpha1-adrenoceptor subtypes on corneal epithelial thickness and cell proliferation in mice. *Am J Physiol Cell Physiol.* (2018) 315:C757–65. doi: 10.1152/ajpcell.00314.2018

54. Budczies J, Klauschen F, Sinn BV, Gyorffy B, Schmitt WD, Darb-Esfahani S, et al. Cutoff Finder: a comprehensive and straightforward Web application enabling rapid biomarker cutoff optimization. *PLoS ONE.* (2012) 7:e51862. doi: 10.1371/journal.pone.0051862

55. Collado M, Serrano M. The senescent side of tumor suppression. *Cell Cycle.* (2005) 4:1722–4. doi: 10.4161/cc.4.12.2260

56. Braig M, Schmitt CA. Oncogene-induced senescence: putting the brakes on tumor development. *Cancer Res.* (2006) 66:2881–4. doi: 10.1158/0008-5472.CAN-05-4006

57. Campisi J, d'Adda di Fagagna F. Cellular senescence: when bad things happen to good cells. *Nat Rev Mol Cell Biol.* (2007) 8:729–40. doi: 10.1038/nrm2233

58. Lazzerini Denchi E, Attwooll C, Pasini D, Helin K. Deregulated E2F activity induces hyperplasia and senescence-like features in the mouse pituitary gland. *Mol Cell Biol.* (2005) 25:2660–72. doi: 10.1128/MCB.25.7.2660-2672.2005

59. Braig M, Lee S, Loddenkemper C, Rudolph C, Peters AH, Schlegelberger B, et al. Oncogene-induced senescence as an initial barrier in lymphoma development. *Nature.* (2005) 436:660–5. doi: 10.1038/nature03841

60. Collado M, Gil J, Efeyan A, Guerra C, Schuhmacher AJ, Barradas M, et al. Tumour biology: senescence in premalignant tumours. *Nature.* (2005) 436:642. doi: 10.1038/436642a

61. Childs BG, Durik M, Baker DJ, van Deursen JM. Cellular senescence in aging and age-related disease: from mechanisms to therapy. *Nat Med.* (2015) 21:1424–35. doi: 10.1038/nm.4000

62. Nardella C, Clohessy JG, Alimonti A, Pandolfi PP. Pro-senescence therapy for cancer treatment. *Nat Rev Cancer.* (2011) 11:503–11. doi: 10.1038/nrc3057

63. Acosta JC, O'Loghlen A, Banito A, Guijarro MV, Augert A, Raguz S, et al. Chemokine signaling via the CXCR2 receptor reinforces senescence. *Cell.* (2008) 133:1006–18. doi: 10.1016/j.cell.2008.03.038

64. Kuilman T, Michaloglou C, Vredeveld LC, Douma S, van Doorn R, Desmet CJ, et al. Oncogene-induced senescence relayed by an interleukin-dependent inflammatory network. *Cell.* (2008) 133:1019–31. doi: 10.1016/j.cell.2008.03.039

65. Wajapeyee N, Serra RW, Zhu X, Mahalingam M, Green MR. Oncogenic BRAF induces senescence and apoptosis through pathways mediated by the secreted protein IGFBP7. *Cell.* (2008) 132:363–74. doi: 10.1016/j.cell.2007.12.032

66. Bartek J, Hodny Z, Lukas J. Cytokine loops driving senescence. *Nat Cell Biol.* (2008) 10:887–9. doi: 10.1038/ncb0808-887

67. Campisi J. Senescent cells, tumor suppression, and organismal aging: good citizens, bad neighbors. *Cell.* (2005) 120:513–22. doi: 10.1016/j.cell.2005.02.003

68. Krtolica A, Parrinello S, Lockett S, Desprez PY, Campisi J. Senescent fibroblasts promote epithelial cell growth and tumorigenesis: a link between cancer and aging. *Proc Natl Acad Sci U S A.* (2001) 98:12072–7. doi: 10.1073/pnas.211053698

69. Parrinello S, Coppe JP, Krtolica A, Campisi J. Stromal-epithelial interactions in aging and cancer: senescent fibroblasts alter epithelial cell differentiation. *J Cell Sci.* (2005) 118:485–96. doi: 10.1242/jcs.01635

70. Coppe JP, Patil CK, Rodier F, Sun Y, Munoz DP, Goldstein J, et al. Senescence-associated secretory phenotypes reveal cell-nonautonomous functions of oncogenic RAS and the p53 tumor suppressor. *PLoS Biol.* (2008) 6:2853–68. doi: 10.1371/journal.pbio.0060301

71. Joyce JA, Pollard JW. Microenvironmental regulation of metastasis. *Nat Rev*

Cancer. (2009) 9:239–52. doi: 10.1038/nrc2618

72. Coppe JP, Kauser K, Campisi J, Beausejour CM. Secretion of vascular endothelial growth factor by primary human fibroblasts at senescence. *J Biol Chem.* (2006) 281:29568–74. doi: 10.1074/jbc.M603307200

73. Foersch S, Sperka T, Lindner C, Taut A, Rudolph KL, Breier G, et al. VEGFR2 signaling prevents colorectal cancer cell senescence to promote tumorigenesis in mice with colitis. *Gastroenterology.* (2015) 149:177–89 e10. doi: 10.1053/j.gastro.2015.03.016

74. Pribluda A, Elyada E, Wiener Z, Hamza H, Goldstein RE, Biton M, et al. A senescence-inflammatory switch from cancer-inhibitory to cancer-promoting mechanism. *Cancer Cell.* (2013) 24:242–56. doi: 10.1016/j.ccr.2013.06.005

75. Choi YW, Kim YH, Oh SY, Suh KW, Kim YS, Lee GY, et al. senescent tumor cells build a cytokine shield in colorectal cancer. *Adv Sci.* (2021) 8:2002497. doi: 10.1002/advs.202002497

76. Michaud K, Solomon DA, Oermann E, Kim JS, Zhong WZ, Prados MD, et al. Pharmacologic inhibition of cyclin-dependent kinases 4 and 6 arrests the growth of glioblastoma multiforme intracranial xenografts. *Cancer Res.* (2010) 70:3228–38. doi: 10.1158/0008-5472.CAN-09-4559

77. Thangavel C, Dean JL, Ertel A, Knudsen KE, Aldaz CM, Witkiewicz AK, et al. Therapeutically activating RB: reestablishing cell cycle control in endocrine therapy-resistant breast cancer. *Endocr Relat Cancer.* (2011) 18:333–45. doi: 10.1530/ERC-10-0262

78. Leonard JP, LaCasce AS, Smith MR, Noy A, Chirieac LR, Rodig SJ, et al. Selective CDK4/6 inhibition with tumor responses by PD0332991 in patients with mantle cell lymphoma. *Blood.* (2012) 119:4597–607. doi: 10.1182/blood-2011-10-388298

79. Guha M. Blockbuster dreams for Pfizer's CDK inhibitor. *Nat Biotechnol.* (2013) 31:187. doi: 10.1038/nbt0313-187a

80. Dickson MA, Tap WD, Keohan ML, D'Angelo SP, Gounder MM, Antonescu CR, et al. Phase II trial of the CDK4 inhibitor PD0332991 in patients with advanced CDK4-amplified well-differentiated or dedifferentiated liposarcoma. *J Clin Oncol.* (2013) 31:2024–8. doi: 10.1200/JCO.2012. 46.5476

81. Ventura A, Kirsch DG, McLaughlin ME, Tuveson DA, Grimm J, Lintault L, et al. Restoration of p53 function leads to tumour regression in vivo. *Nature.* (2007) 445:661–5. doi: 10.1038/nature05541

82. Wang L, Leite de. Oliveira R, Wang C, Fernandes Neto JM, Mainardi S, Evers B, et al. High-throughput functional genetic and compound screens identify targets for senescence induction in cancer. *Cell Rep.* (2017) 21:773–83. doi: 10.1016/j.celrep.2017.09.085

21

Gastrointestinal Manifestations of COVID-19 Infection: Clinicopathologic Findings in Intestinal Resections Performed at Single Institution

Alison E. Burkett[1†], Sophia B. Sher[1†], Chirag R. Patel[1], Isam Ildin-Eltoum[1], Deepti Dhall[1], Camilla Margaroli[2], Shajan Peter[3], Goo Lee[1], Prachi Bajpai[1], Paul V. Benson[1], Upender Manne[1,4] and Sameer Al Diffalha[1,4*]

[1] Department of Pathology, University of Alabama at Birmingham, Birmingham, AL, United States, [2] Division of Pulmonary, Allergy and Critical Care Medicine, Department of Medicine, University of Alabama at Birmingham, Birmingham, AL, United States, [3] Division of Gastroenterology, Department of Medicine, University of Alabama at Birmingham, Birmingham, AL, United States, [4] O'Neal Compressive Cancer Center, Birmingham, AL, United States

*Correspondence:
Sameer Al Diffalha
saldiffalha@uabmc.edu

† These authors have contributed equally to this work and share first authorship

It is now known that COVID-19 not only involves the lungs, but other organs as well including the gastrointestinal tract. Although clinic-pathological features are well-described in lungs, the histopathologic features of gastrointestinal involvement in resection specimens are not well characterized. Herein, we describe in detail the clinicopathologic features of intestinal resection specimens in four patients with COVID-19 infection. COVID-19 viral particles by *in situ* hybridization and immunofluorescence studies are also demonstrated. All four patients were males, aged 28–46 years, with comorbidities. They initially presented with a severe form of pulmonary COVID-19 and showed gastrointestinal symptoms, requiring surgical intervention. Histopathologic examination of resected GI specimens, mostly right colectomies, revealed a spectrum of disease, from superficial mucosal ischemic colitis to frank transmural ischemic colitis and associated changes consistent with pneumatosis cystoides intestinalis. Three patients were African American (75%), and one was Caucasian (25%); three patients died due to complications of their COVID-19 infection (75%), while one ultimately recovered from their GI complications (25%), but experienced prolonged sequela of COVID-19 infection including erectile dysfunction. In conclusion, COVID-19 infection, directly or indirectly, can cause ischemic gastrointestinal complications, with predilection for the right colon.

Keywords: COVID-19, gastrointestinal manifestations, pneumatosis cystoides intestinalis, ischemic colitis, ISH

INTRODUCTION

In December 2019, a new human coronavirus (SARS-CoV-2) type emerged in Wuhan, China. COVID-19, the infectious disease caused by SARS-CoV-2, is now a pandemic affecting countries throughout the world. Since spring 2020, the United States has seen a dramatic rise in number of cases, and currently the number of deaths attributable to COVID-19 infection is more than 500,000 (1).

Although the most common presentation of the infection is the development of respiratory symptoms 2–14 days following exposure, gastrointestinal (GI) presentation is becoming increasingly recognized. The receptor of SARS-CoV-2, angiotensin converting enzyme 2 (ACE2) is highly expressed both in GI epithelial cells and in liver (2). Almost the entire GI tract, including the stomach, small intestine, and rectal epithelial cells express the SARS-CoV-2 nucleocapsid protein and the ACE2 protein (3). The SARS-CoV-2 nucleocapsid protein, which encapsulates the viral genome, is essential for SARS-CoV-2 replication (4). High levels of these two proteins in cells of the GI tracts of SARS-CoV-2 infected patients can explain the concomitant digestive symptoms, including diarrhea, nausea, vomiting, and abdominal pain (3).

TABLE 1 | Patients' demographic, laboratory values and pathologic findings.

	Demographics				Laboratory values						Pathologic findings	
Case #	Age	Sex	Race	Comorbidities	CRP (mg/L)	D-dimer (ng/ml)	LDH (Units/L)	Lactic acid (mMol/L)	Troponin I (ng/L)	Hgb/Hct	Gross findings	Histology
Case 1	47	M	AA	HTN, Obesity (BMI 33.08 kg/m^2)	176.3	4,064	NA	4.0	39	9.9/26	Large patches of erythematous colonic mucosa with focal loss of mucosal folds.	Ischemic colitis showing transmural acute and chronic inflammation and serositis. Features suggestive of pneumatosis.
Case 2	37	M	AA	HTN, Obesity, Insulin Dependent DM	282.6	978	556	NA	44	11/33	Cecum showed several areas of ulceration ranging in size from 0.6 to 1.0 cm	Focal mucosal ulceration, with associated acute and chronic inflammation. Features suggestive of pneumatosis. Focal serositis.
Case 3	40	M	C	Obesity (BMI 33.2 kg/m^2)	NA	>20,000	NA	7.1	1,838	15.6/46	Cecum: Necrotic with dark-brown discoloration. Ascending colon is hemorrhagic and dusky with obvious air bubbles	Mucosal hemorrhagic ischemia, fibrin microthrombi, and pneumatosis cystoides intestinalis
Case 4	28	M	AA	DM	24.87	1,380	681	10.6	98	7.3/22	Small intestine: Granular/gritty brown mucosa with diffuse gray-brown exudate	Transmural ischemia with pseudomembrane formation and acute serositis. Features suggestive of pneumatosis.

Here, we present a series of four SARS-CoV-2 patients who were admitted to the University of Alabama at Birmingham (UAB) Medical Center during June to August 2020 and who underwent GI resections. The course of their SARS-CoV-2 infections was remarkable for the development of GI complications, which necessitated surgical management by right hemicolectomy or segmental small bowel resection; three of the four patients ultimately died as a result of the complications of their COVID-19 infection. The clinical, macroscopic and histopathologic findings are described, which adds to the pathophysiology of SARS-CoV-2 infection and contributes to the ongoing management of the COVID-19 disease.

MATERIALS AND METHODS

The Institutional Review Board of UAB approved the study. A retrospective review of surgical pathology archives for COVID-19 related intestinal resections was performed during the period of June to August 2020. There were four patients with bowel resections, three of whom underwent right hemicolectomies and one a segmental small bowel resection. The hematoxylin and eosin (H&E)-stained slides were reviewed by GI pathologists (SA, IE, DD, and CRP).

In this study, for detection of SARS-CoV2 virus, both immunofluorescence and *in situ* hybridization (ISH) assays were performed as follows: 5-μm formalin-fixed paraffin-embedded (FFPE) tissues sections on Plus Slides (VWR, Radnor, PA) were cut at 5μm and baked for 2h at 60°C. Tissues were then deparaffinized and rehydrated with sequential 5-min incubations in xylene (three times), twice in 100% ethanol, and twice in 95% ethanol. Slides were washed three times, for 5min each, with distilled water. Antigen retrieval was then performed in Tris-EDTA pH-9 buffer at 70°C for 20min in a steamer, followed by three 5-min washes in distilled water. Tissues were balanced with PBS for 10min and blocked with 3% w/v bovine serum albumen (BSA) in PBS for 40min at room temperature. Slides were then blotted dry, and antibody against SARS-CoV-2 nucleocapsid protein (clone GTX135361, GeneTex, Irvine, CA) was applied at a 1:500 dilution in PBS+3% w/v BSA for 1h at room temperature. Tissues were then rinsed with PBS three times for 5min under gentle agitation. 4′,6-Diamidino-2-phenylindole (100 ng/mL in PBS) staining was performed for 5min in the dark at room temperature, followed by three 5-min washes in PBS under gentle agitation. Slides were then mounted with ProLong Gold antifade mounting media (Thermofisher) and stored in the dark until image acquisition. Confocal immunofluorescence images were acquired with a Nikon A1R confocal microscope.

ISH assay was performed using RNAscope® kit and ISH probes according to the manufacturer's instructions (Advanced Cell Diagnostics, ACD, Newark, CA). RNA probe, in C2 channel

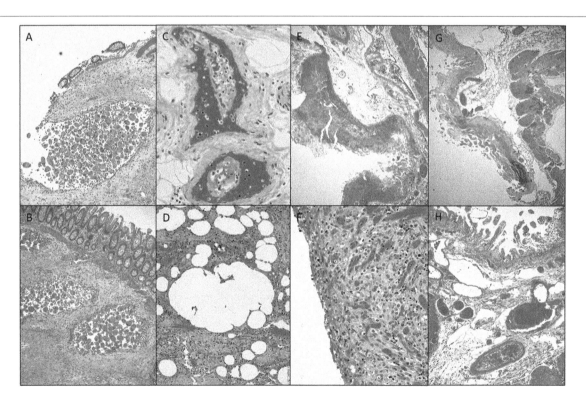

FIGURE 1 | Photomicrographs of a hemicolectomy specimen. Aggregates of multinucleated giant cells lining the cysts. H&E stain 20x **(A,B)**. Fibrin thrombi, H&E staining 40x **(C)**. Micro-cyst lined with multinucleated giant cells, H&E staining 10x **(D)**. Pseudomembrane, H&E 10x **(E)**. Acute serositis, H&E staining 40x **(F)**. Ischemic enteritis, H&E 10x **(G)**. Submucosal thrombi, H&E 10x **(H)**.

targeting SARS-CoV-2 replicative RNA intermediate, was used to detect the replicating virus as red signal (nCoV2019-orf1ab-sense-C2, cat. no. 859151-C2). RNAscope® 2.5 Duplex Reagent Kit (cat. no 322430) along with Human (Hs) Positive Control Probes for housekeeping genes PPIB-C1/ POLR2A-C2, (cat. no 321641) were used to assess the integrity of the RNA. Simultaneously, consecutive sections were probed with probes targeting dihydrodipicolinate reductase B mRNA of a *Bacillus subtilis* strain (DapB) as a negative control, (cat. no. 320751) to assess the specificity of the assay.

RESULTS

Clinical Data

Our cohort included four patients aged 28–46 years with a mean age of 38 years. Three of four patients were African-American (AA); one was non-Hispanic Caucasian. All patients had comorbidities that included essential hypertension (HTN), diabetes mellitus (DM, insulin-dependent or insulin-resistant), and obesity (BMI 33.08–34.8 kg/m^2). All patients initially presented with respiratory symptoms, including fever, dyspnea, and/or flu-like symptoms which developed into acute respiratory distress syndrome (ARDS) requiring intubation, ventilation,

and critical care management. The length of time between a positive COVID-19 test and significant GI symptomatology and resection varied widely from 1 to 53 days, with an average of 21.5 days. GI symptoms occurred on a spectrum, beginning as constipation, abdominal pain, or a lower GI bleed before progressing to ischemia and necrosis requiring surgical intervention. COVID-19 infections were confirmed by the presence of SARS-CoV-2 RNA, determined by PCR. The patients were enrolled in a clinical trial of remdesivir. Despite the treatment, they subsequently developed complications, such as lower extremity deep vein thrombosis, pulmonary thromboembolism, septicemia with septic shock (due to *Cutibacterium/Propionibacterium avidum*), multi-organ failure, hypotension, pulseless electrical activity and encephalopathy. For all four patients, acute renal failure was a complication, and all underwent continuous renal replacement therapy. Furthermore, the course of their disease was complicated by the development of GI symptoms, such as GI bleeding in the form of hematochezia, as well as an ileus. All patients underwent CT scans of the abdomen and pelvis, which showed changes compatible with GI bleeding with various degrees of intestinal pneumatosis and bowel ischemia. These findings were corroborated by the frank ischemia, ulceration, cecal dilation, and necrosis

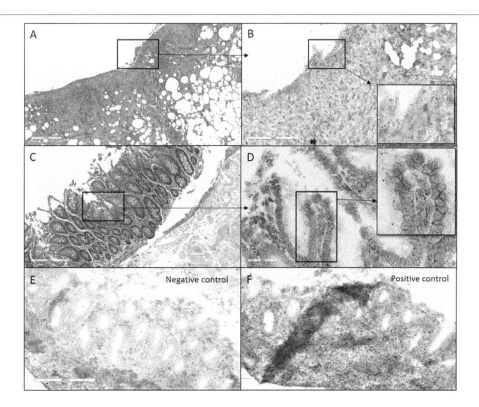

FIGURE 2 | H&E and ISH images of patient #1 in focal mucosal ulcer with granulation tissue formation along with adjacent uninvolved mucosa. **(A)** H&E images of ulcerated colon tissue at 4X magnification **(B)** Images at 20X magnification after *in situ* hybridization using V-nCOV2019—orf1ab–sense probe (cat # 859151-C2), ACD, Bio-techne, detecting replicating SARS-COV-2 RNA (red chromogen) in ulcerated colon tissue sections. **(C)** H&E images at 10x magnification of adjacent uninvolved mucosa **(D)**. Higher magnification images at 40X after *in situ* hybridization using V-nCOV2019—orf1ab-detected as red signal in adjacent uninvolved mucosa. **(E)** Negative control images at 10X after *in situ* hybridization using probe (cat # 320751), ACD, Bio-techne, targeting DapB (Bacillus subtilis stain) which did not detect any staining **(F)**. Positive control images at 10X after *in situ* hybridization using probe (cat # 321641), ACD, Bio-techne, demonstrated strong positive staining (red chromogen) in sections probed for the housekeeping gene POLR2A.

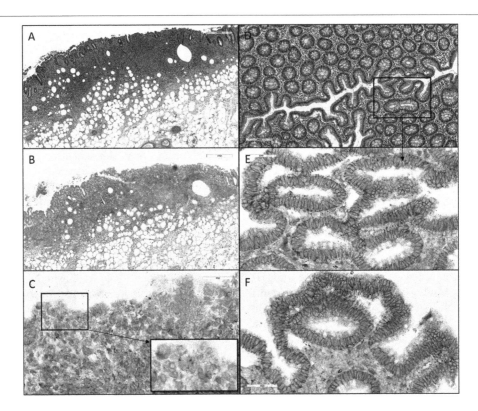

FIGURE 3 | H&E and ISH images of patient #2 in focal mucosal ulcer with granulation tissue formation along with adjacent uninvolved mucosa. **(A)** H&E images of ulcerated colon tissue at 4X magnification **(B,C)** Images after *in situ* hybridization using V-nCOV2019—orf1ab–sense probe (red chromogen) at lower 4X and higher magnification 40x, respectively. **(D)** H&E images at 10X magnification of adjacent uninvolved mucosa **(E,F)** *in situ* hybridization using V-nCOV2019—orf1ab- sense probe detected as red signal in adjacent intact epithelium of uninvolved mucosa at higher magnification images at 40x. Images show pronounced viral load in the surface epithelial lining and the crypts (Basal cytoplasmic localization).

encountered intraoperatively. Additionally, laboratory findings were remarkable for elevated C-reactive protein (ranging from 24.87 to 282.6 mg/L), d-dimer (ranging from 978 to > 20,000 ng/mL), lactate dehydrogenase (556–681 U/L), lactic acid (4.0–10.6 mMol/L), and troponin I (39–1838 ng/L). Most patients were also anemic (Hgb between 7.3 and 11 g/dL; Hct 22–33%). The three patients who expired due to the infection demonstrated the most dramatic clinical courses, with pronounced laboratory, gross, and microscopic abnormalities (**Table 1**). For all four patients with SARS-CoV-2 infection confirmed by nasal swap PCR testing, there was colonic pneumatosis with or without ischemic changes for whom CT scans of the abdomen showed evidence of gas in the mesentery, or features suggestive of lower GI bleeding.

Gross and Microscopic Characteristics

Three patients had right hemicolectomies and one had a segmental small bowel resection. All four specimens showed variable degrees of ischemic changes. Gross examination of one of sample showed transmural ischemic necrosis with hemorrhage, resulting in perforation. The mucosa showed, microscopically, deep ulceration and focal pseudomembrane formation. In an additional patient, there was diffuse transmural

acute and chronic inflammation with necrosis and hemorrhage, and associated acute serositis. The lamina propria demonstrated congestion and edema (in all patients); rare vascular fibrin thrombi were identified (in 2 patients). Pneumatosis cystoides intestinalis (cyst formation with associated multinucleated giant cells lining) were also recognized in two patients (**Figures 1–5** and **Table 1**).

ISH with a V-nCOV2019-sense probe detected replicating SARS-COV-2 RNA. Furthermore, all four samples were positive on immunofluorescence for antibody against SARS-CoV-2 nucleocapsid protein with a distinctive pattern and a variable viral load (**Figures 2–4**). All patients underwent exploratory laparotomies for GI complications of COVID-19 disease, and three of the four patients underwent a right hemicolectomy procedure. The morphologic findings in all specimens included ischemic changes, acute and chronic inflammation, and fibrin microthrombi in small blood vessels in underlying areas of mucosal ulceration. Moreover, all cases, regardless of extent of the disease, showed changes consistent with pneumatosis cystoides intestinalis, including prominent submucosal edema with occasional cyst formation and aggregates of multinucleated giant cells.

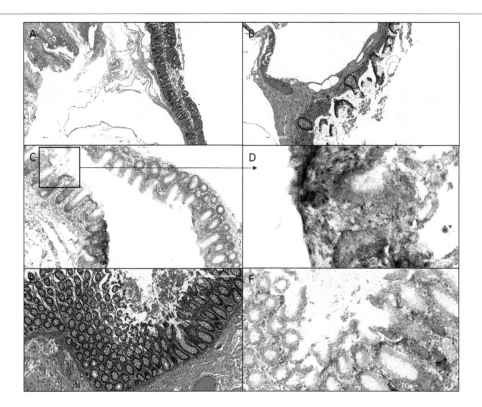

FIGURE 4 | H&E and ISH images of patient #3 in focal mucosal ulcer with granulation tissue formation along with adjacent uninvolved mucosa. **(A,B)** H&E images of ischemic colon tissue sections at 4X and 10X magnification, respectively. **(C,D)** Images at lower (10X) and higher magnification (40X), respectively, after *in situ* hybridization using V-nCOV2019—orf1ab–sense probe (red chromogen) More viral load of replicating SARS-COV-2 RNA was detected in this ischemic section as compared to its uninvolved mucosa represented in **(F)**. **(E)** H&E images at 10X of adjacent uninvolved mucosa **(F)** *in situ* hybridization using V-nCOV2019—orf1ab-sense probe detected as red signal in adjacent intact epithelium of uninvolved mucosa at 20X magnification.

DISCUSSION

GI symptoms associated with COVID-19 are present in up to 30% of patients, with diarrhea, abdominal pain, and hematochezia occasionally evident as the initial presentation (5). Although patients with significant pulmonary disease have detectable SARS-CoV-2 RNA in fecal samples, a substantial number of patients with GI manifestations also have SARS-CoV-2 RNA in fecal samples (6). Others have now individualistically established that the virus can be cultured from the feces during an active infection (7). In the present study, we demonstrated by immunofluorescence (**Figure 6**) and ISH studies (**Figures 2–5**) evidence of the virus in affected area of the intestine.

Notably, neither of the patients had a medical history of established GI disease, nor etiology for colitis. Extensive infectious work up including *Clostridium difficile* serology was conducted on two of the four patients, which was negative. Reactivity for CMV IgG was noted in the serum of one patient indicating a previous infection; however, no evidence of viral cytopathic effects were noted on histology. One patient had clinical and microbiological evidence of septicemia due to *Cutibacterium (Propionibacterium) avidum*, the commensal skin microorganism, which is unlikely to be implicated as a primary agent in the etiology of hemorrhagic colitis. One

patient developed HIT following anticoagulation, resulting in septic shock. While this further exacerbated the bowel ischemia and thrombosis, it was a contributing factor rather than a primary cause. Moreover, extensive chart review failed to reveal definitive evidence of mesenteric thrombosis, radiologically or intraoperatively, to explain the segmental ischemic findings.

The target viral receptor for SARS-CoV-2 is ACE2, which is highly expressed on type II alveolar epithelial cells, as well as in glandular cells of gastric, duodenal, and rectal epithelia (8). This suggests that the SARS-CoV-2 gains entry into, and potentially damages, host GI tissue, explaining the digestive symptoms. Microthrombi also contribute to GI insults (9).

Although several studies have attempted to identify histologic findings indicative of SARS-CoV-2 infection, the presentation and expression of SARS-CoV-2 RNA remains variable (10). In our cohort, not all GI specimens demonstrated findings of coagulopathy and ischemia, but all samples revealed changes consistent with pneumatosis cystoides intestinalis. While pneumatosis cystoides is commonly associated with bacterial infection, its pathogenesis is poorly understood and multifocal, and can also be attributed to mechanical and pulmonary causes (11). In our cohort, those patients that underwent infectious work-up for gas producing bacteria were negative. Moreover, these patients were acutely ill, requiring repeated surgical

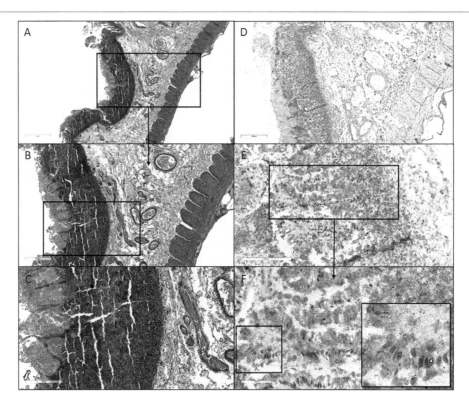

FIGURE 5 | H&E and ISH images of patient #4 in focal mucosal ulcer with granulation tissue formation. **(A–C)** H&E images of ischemic colon tissue sections at 2X, 4X, and 10X magnification, respectively. **(D–F)** Images at lower (4X) and higher magnification (20X and 40X), respectively, after *in situ* hybridization using V-nCOV2019—orf1ab–sense probe (red chromogen) illustrating replicating SARS-COV-2 RNA was detected.

intervention, intubation and ventilation. This suggested that the etiology of pneumatosis could be the result of iatrogenic trauma or manipulation increasing intraluminal pressure (11), or the result of free air entering the perivascular spaces of the intestinal wall following alveolar rupture in the setting of pulmonary obstruction (12); the clinical significance failed to be elucidated. The pathogenic pathway of COVID-19 remains largely undetermined, and its relationship with the gastrointestinal findings remains a challenge. It is widely accepted that the viral infection results in microthrombi which can lead to ischemic injury; however, in the setting of critical illness, HIT, and intragenic interventions (ECMO) it is difficult to quantify the exact role SARS-CoV-2 virus plays. The clinicopathologic findings in our cohort caused us to consider the relationship between the ischemic enterocolitis and hypercoaguable state of our patients with COVID-19 infection; however, comparison with non-COVID associated acute ischemic bowels should be performed to further characterize and ultimately define the histopathological features of the virus.

Moreover, each GI specimen demonstrated SARS-CoV-2 positivity via ISH, regardless of the extent of disease. Coronaviruses are also found by electron microscopy in intestinal cells of animals (13). Comparable to our study, SARS-CoV-2 RNA ISH is reported to be positive in a few mucosal epithelial cells and lymphocytes of the GI tract in humans (7). Also what supports our findings is that SARS-Cov-2

RNA in stool, determined by amplification is now widely accepted (7).

In a recent study that included a large number of SARS-CoV-2 patients (n=95), 58 patients experienced GI symptoms including diarrhea, anorexia and nausea (14). Fecal samples of 65 hospitalized patients were tested for SARS-CoV-2, including 42 patients with and 23 without GI symptoms, of which 22 (52.4%) and 9(39.1%) were positive, respectively. Six of the patients who had GI symptoms underwent endoscopic examination; one showed erosion/ulcer. In two, SARS-CoV-2 RNA was detected in the esophagus, stomach, duodenum, and rectum (14).

In the present study, there were pathologic findings for the four patients with confirmed SARS-CoV-2, for whom CT scans of the abdomen showed either evidence of colonic pneumatosis with or without ischemic changes and evidence of gas in the mesentery, or features suggestive of lower GI bleeding. All four patients underwent exploratory laparotomies and three of the four were subjected to a right hemicolectomy procedure for COVID-19 GI related complications. The presence of microthrombi in the watershed area suggested that SARS-CoV-2 demonstrates partiality toward the right colon. Moreover, all cases, regardless of extent of the disease, showed pathologic changes consistent with pneumatosis cystoides intestinalis.

For some patients, GI symptoms may be associated with pulmonary SARS-CoV-2 infection, and surgical management of

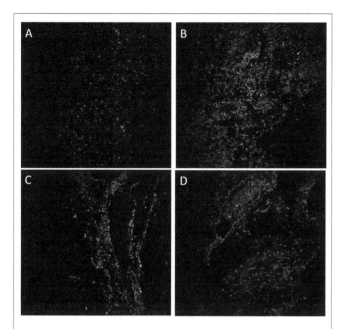

FIGURE 6 | Immunofluorescence for antibody against SARS-CoV-2 nucleocapsid protein. A negative control using a probe targeting DapB (Bacillus subtilis strain) did not detect any staining **(A)**; a positive control demonstrated strong positive staining in sections probed with the housekeeping gene **(B)**. These findings suggest that the GI tract is infected with SARS-CoV-2 **(C)**. A unique observation in our case study is the presence of the virus within the blood vessels **(D)**.

with fibrin microthrombi. Changes consistent with pneumatos cystoides intestinalis were also evident. In conclusion, COVID-19 disease, directly or indirectly, can cause ischemic GI complications, with a predilection for the right colon. Awareness of these morphologic changes may prompt pathologists to include potential SARS-CoV-2 infection to the differential diagnosis when the etiology for ischemic colitis is unclear.

AUTHOR CONTRIBUTIONS

SA principal investigator and corresponding author, conceptualized the study with SS and AB, finalized the manuscript with the assistance of AB. CM, PB, and UM performed the *in-situ* Hybridization and reviewed the results and critically reviewed the manuscript. SP reviewed and revised the manuscript. CP, II, DD, GL, and PVB, contributed in data collection. All authors approved the final manuscript as submitted and agree to be accountable for all aspects of the work.

ACKNOWLEDGMENTS

We thank the UAB Tissue Biorepository (UAB-TBR), UAB Pathology Core Research Laboratory and OCCC Tissue Procurement Shared Resource (TPRO) for their assistance with the processing of the histological specimens, as well Dr. Robert Grabski at the UAB High Resolution Imaging Facility.

GI complications, including bleeding, is sometimes necessary. The morphologic findings observed in the resection specimens varied from superficial acute colitis with or without hemorrhage and ischemic changes, to a frank transmural necrotic colitis

REFERENCES

1. Symptoms of COVID-19: The Center for Disease Control and Prevention (2020). Available online at: https://www.cdc.gov/coronavirus/2019-ncov/symptoms-testing/symptoms.html (accessed February 22, 2021).

2. Hoffmann M, Kleine-Weber H, Schroeder S, Kruger N, Herrler T, Erichsen S, et al. SARS-CoV-2 cell entry depends on ACE2 and TMPRSS2 and Is blocked by a clinically proven protease inhibitor. *Cell.* (2020) 181:271–80 e8. doi: 10.1016/j.cell.2020.02.052

3. Carvalho A, Alqusairi R, Adams A, Paul M, Kothari N, Peters S, et al. SARS-CoV-2 gastrointestinal infection causing hemorrhagic colitis: implications for detection and transmission of COVID-19 disease. *Am J Gastroenterol.* (2020) 115:942–6. doi: 10.14309/ajg.0000000000000667

4. Savastano A, Ibanez de Opakua A, Rankovic M, Zweckstetter M Nucleocapsid protein of SARS-CoV-2 phase separates into RNA-rich polymerase-containing condensates. *Nat Commun.* (2020) 11:6041. doi: 10.1038/s41467-020-19843-1

5. Buscarini E, Manfredi G, Brambilla G, Menozzi F, Londoni C, Alicante S, et al. GI symptoms as early signs of COVID-19 in hospitalised Italian patients. *Gut.* (2020) 69:1547–8. doi: 10.1136/gutjnl-2020-321434

6. Su S, Shen J, Zhu L, Qiu Y, He JS, Tan JY, et al. Involvement of digestive system in COVID-19: manifestations, pathology, management and challenges. *Therap Adv Gastroenterol.* (2020) 13:1756284820934626. doi: 10.1177/1756284820934626

7. Shi X, Gong E, Gao D, Zhang B, Zheng J, Gao Z, et al. Severe acute respiratory syndrome associated coronavirus is detected in intestinal tissues of fatal cases. *Am J Gastroenterol.* (2005) 100:169–76. doi: 10.1111/j.1572-0241.2005.40377.x

8. Xiao F, Tang M, Zheng X, Liu Y, Li X, Shan H. Evidence for gastrointestinal infection of SARS-CoV-2. *Gastroenterology.* (2020) 158:1831–3 e3. doi: 10.1053/j.gastro.2020.02.055

9. Bhayana R, Som A, Li MD, Carey DE, Anderson MA, Blake MA, et al. Abdominal imaging findings in COVID-19: preliminary observations. *Radiology.* (2020) 297:E207–E15. doi: 10.1148/radiol.2020201908

10. Westerhoff M, Jones D, Hrycaj SM, Chan MP, Pantanowitz L, Tu H, et al. Gastrointestinal pathology in samples from coronavirus disease 2019 (COVID-19)-positive patients. *Arch Pathol Lab Med.* (2021) 145:1062–8. doi: 10.5858/arpa.2021-0137-SA

11. Azzaroli F, Turco L, Ceroni L, Galloni SS, Buonfiglioli F, Calvanese C, et al. Pneumatosis cystoides intestinalis. *World J Gastroenterol.* (2011) 17:4932–6. doi: 10.3748/wjg.v17.i44.4932

12. St Peter SD, Abbas MA, Kelly KA. The spectrum of pneumatosis intestinalis. *Arch Surg.* (2003) 138:68–75. doi: 10.1001/archsurg.138.1.68

13. Cimolai N. Features of enteric disease from human coronaviruses: implications for COVID-19. *J Med Virol.* (2020) 92:1834–44. doi: 10.1002/jmv.26066

14. Lin L, Jiang X, Zhang Z, Huang S, Zhang Z, Fang Z, et al. Gastrointestinal symptoms of 95 cases with SARS-CoV-2 infection. *Gut.* 69:997–1001. doi: 10.1136/gutjnl-2020-321013

22

The Mechanism of Lung and Intestinal Injury in Acute Pancreatitis

Dongling Liu[1†], Linlin Wen[2,3†], Zhandong Wang[2], Yang Hai[4], Dan Yang[2], Yanying Zhang[4,5], Min Bai[5], Bing Song[4,5] and Yongfeng Wang[5*]

[1] *School of Pharmacy, Gansu University of Chinese Medicine, Lanzhou, China,* [2] *School of Traditional Chinese and Western Medicine, Gansu University of Chinese Medicine, Lanzhou, China,* [3] *County People's Hospital, Pingliang, China,* [4] *Gansu University of Chinese Medicine/Scientific Research and Experimental Center, Lanzhou, China,* [5] *Gansu Provincial Engineering Laboratory for Research and Promotion of Quality Standardization of Authentic Medicinal Materials in Gansu Province/Provincial Key Laboratory of Pharmaceutical Chemistry and Quality Research in Colleges and Universities in Gansu Province/Gansu Provincial Laboratory Animal Industry Technology Center, Lanzhou, China*

*Correspondence:
Yongfeng Wang
wyf@gszy.edu.cn

[†] *These authors have contributed equally to this work*

Acute pancreatitis (AP), as a common cause of clinical acute abdomen, often leads to multi-organ damage. In the process of severe AP, the lungs and intestines are the most easily affected organs aside the pancreas. These organ damages occur in succession. Notably, lung and intestinal injuries are closely linked. Damage to ML, which transports immune cells, intestinal fluid, chyle, and toxic components (including toxins, trypsin, and activated cytokines to the systemic circulation in AP) may be connected to AP. This process can lead to the pathological changes of hyperosmotic edema of the lung, an increase in alveolar fluid level, destruction of the intestinal mucosal structure, and impairment of intestinal mucosal permeability. The underlying mechanisms of the correlation between lung and intestinal injuries are inflammatory response, oxidative stress, and endocrine hormone secretion disorders. The main signaling pathways of lung and intestinal injuries are TNF-α, HMGB1-mediated inflammation amplification effect of NF-κB signal pathway, Nrf2/ARE oxidative stress response signaling pathway, and IL-6-mediated JAK2/STAT3 signaling pathway. These pathways exert anti-inflammatory response and anti-oxidative stress, inhibit cell proliferation, and promote apoptosis. The interaction is consistent with the traditional Chinese medicine theory of *the lung being connected with the large intestine* (fei yu da chang xiang biao li in Chinese). This review sought to explore intersecting mechanisms of lung and intestinal injuries in AP to develop new treatment strategies.

Keywords: acute pancreatitis, lung injury, intestinal injury, inflammation response, oxidative stress, endocrine disorders

Abbreviations: AP, acute pancreatitis; ALI, acute lung injury; DAMPs, damage-associated molecular patterns; HMGB1, high-mobility group box protein 1; ML, mesenteric lymph; MMPs, matrix metalloproteinases; TNF-α, tumor necrosis factor-α; IL-17, interleukin-17; IL-6, interleukin-6; IL-1β, interleukin-1β; TNF-R1, tumor necrosis factor-R1; TRADD, tumor necrosis factor receptor 1 related death domain protein; TRAF2, tumor necrosis factor receptor related factor 2; TLR4, Toll-like receptors 4; NLRP3, NOD-like receptor protein 3; STAT3, signal transducer and activator of transcription 3; AP-1, activator protein-1; MAPK, mitogen-activated protein kinases; NF-κB, nuclear factor kappa B; SIRS, systemic inflammatory response syndrome; MODS, multiple organ dysfunction syndrome; Nrf2, Related factor 2; ARE, antioxidant response element; AQPs, Water channel proteins; Ang, angiopoietin; IEC, intestinal epithelial cells; AMPs, antimicrobial peptides; JAM-C, junctional adhesion molecule-C; GSH, glutathione; SOD, superoxide dismutase; ROS, reactive oxygen species; VIP, blood vessel active intestinal peptide.

INTRODUCTION

Acute pancreatitis (AP) is one of the common causes of acute abdomen in clinical practice (1, 2). It is closely caused by two predisposing factors – gallstones and alcohol misuse (3). These two factors stimulate the pancreas to secrete a large amount of digestive enzymes, leading to autodigestion, inflammation, edema, and bleeding, and even necrosis of the pancreas or surrounding fatty tissue. Some studies have demonstrated that AP is associated with fat necrosis around the peripancreatic and intra-pancreatic areas. The necrosis develops because adipocytes in the peritoneum are destroyed and digested by inappropriately activated pancreatic enzymes (4). Stored triglycerides in the adipocytes are released and split by pancreatic lipases into fatty acids and glycerol molecules, and the unsaturated free fatty acids increase damage to the surrounding tissues, and systemic inflammation develops (5). Necrosis of adipocytes serves as an important inflammatory source by the release of a huge number of inflammatory mediators (6). In AP, various inflammatory factors trigger the waterfall cascade of inflammatory mediators through the "trigger-like action." Subsequently, which causes the systemic inflammatory response syndrome (SIRS), and eventually leads to multiple organ dysfunction syndrome (MODS), both of which contribute to the high mortality rate of AP (7).

The lungs and intestine are generally considered to be the most directly targeted organs of AP, and resulting in lung injury and intestinal injury are the main causes of early death in AP patients, with a mortality rate of 60% (8, 9). In AP, intestinal injury is an early event involving damage of intestinal mucosa barrier and altered intestinal mucosal permeability that occurs in AP (10). This injury increase intestinal permeability and cause massive cell death in the intestinal epithelium and basement membrane, leading to the activation of the local response and inducing bacterial translocation out of the gastrointestinal tract. These phenomena contribute substantially to MODS and systemic inflammatory response, being able to damage distant organs (11–13). Of these multiple organs, the lung appears to be the earliest remote organ affected by AP (14). Acute lung injury (ALI) is the dominant death-associated factor in patients who have diffuse alveolar damage on chest X-ray with early-stage AP (8). The generation of inflammatory mediators, including cytokines and chemokines, as well as reactive oxygen species (ROS), is a fundamental cause of AP-induced lung injury. These mediators contribute to the accumulation of macrophages and neutrophils and, later, trigger a cascade of pathological changes in pulmonary microcirculation of the lungs, leading to the occurrence and aggravation of AP-induced lung injury (15, 16). Noteworthy, lung injury is one of the most important components of the MODS triggered by intestinal injury (14). Both lung and intestinal injury can together worsen the severity of AP, eventually resulting in death. Interestingly, it is consistent with the traditional Chinese medicine theory of *the lung being connected with the large intestine* (17).

There are some close connections between the physiology of lungs and intestine and also between the pathological changes and molecular mechanism of intestinal and lung injury caused by

AP. Thus, it is necessary to investigate a common intervention strategy for pulmonary and intestinal injuries. This review summarized the AP-related lung and intestinal injury and their mechanisms, and subsequently discussed the intersections of these mechanisms. This review also aimed to explore the underlying co-mechanisms of multiorgan AP injury and find the novel clinical treatment methods as well as provide the valuable insights into clinical practice.

THE MECHANISM OF ACUTE PANCREATITIS

Acute pancreatitis is a relatively common pancreatic inflammatory disorder, leading to local and systemic inflammation. The main pathological mechanism of AP is activated trypsin-induced self-digestive acute inflammatory response in the pancreas (18, 19). Once pancreatic acinar cells are damaged, acinar cells would release many pro-inflammatory mediators, such as cytokines and chemokines, and stimulate the recruitment and activation of immune cells, including innate immune cells (neutrophils, macrophages, dendritic cells, mast cells, and NK cells), and adaptive immune cells (T cells and B cells), which will consequently exacerbate the pancreatic injury, resulting in necrosis of the pancreas (18, 20, 21). The necrotized pancreatic acinar cells release various kinds of damage-associated molecular patterns (DAMPs), such as high-mobility group box protein 1 (HMGB1), and activate infiltrating immune-associated cells to generate more inflammatory mediators, which in turn accelerate more immune cell infiltration and aggravate inflammation, even contributing to systemic inflammation (20, 21).

Numerous studies have shown that acinar cell necrosis and inflammation are induced by oxidative stress, Ca^{2+} overload, a disorder of organelles, early activation of trypsin, activation of Toll-like receptors 4 (TLR4), nuclear factor kappa B (NF-κB), NOD-like receptor protein 3 (NLRP3), signal transducer and activator of transcription 3 (STAT3), activator protein-1 (AP-1), and mitogen-activated protein kinases (MAPK) signaling pathways, and accumulation of inflammatory cells (16, 22). Extensive studies have suggested that Ca^{2+} overload and oxidative stress are early events in AP. Toxic by-products of AP (such as bile acids or alcohol metabolites) promote the production of ROS and the release of Ca^{2+}, affecting pancreatic cell structure and function (23). ROS can also increase the activation of inflammatory signals, such as AP-1, STAT3, and MAPKs (24).

Acute pancreatitis-related multiorgan injury by activating STAT3 pathway. HMGB1, released in stress, promotes pancreatic injury and pro-inflammatory cytokine release and induces the Janus kinase 2 (JAK2)/STAT3 signal pathway, further intensifying the inflammatory reaction (25). TLRs, especially TLR4, are the first factors to become activated. Activated TLR4 and the NF-κB pathway promote cell synthesis, secreting pro-inflammatory cytokines, such as tumor necrosis factor-alpha (TNF-α), interleukin-1β (IL-1β), and IL-6, which can also stimulate NF-κB, leading to its further activation, thus,

TABLE 1 | Targeted pathways in AP.

Targeted pathways	Influence	Function	References
Nrf2 pathway	up-regulation	antioxidant	(31)
NF-κB, P38MAPK pathways	up-regulation	Inflammation	(26)
ATF6/p53/AIFM2 pathway	up-regulation	Apoptosis and injury	(29)
TLR signaling pathway	up-regulation	Inflammation; apoptosis	(26, 27)
NLRP3 inflammasome pathway	up-regulation	Inflammation; Pyroptosis	(20, 27, 28)
VCAM-1 and the E-selectin regulation pathway	up-regulation	oxidative stress	(30)
STAT pathway	up-regulation	inflammation	(32, 33)

resulting in persistent and intensified inflammation (26). TLR9 is expressed in resident immune cells of the pancreas, which are predominantly represented by macrophages, and it is an important DAMP receptors upstream of inflammasome activation, and caspase-1, and NLRP3 inflammasome are required for the development of inflammation in AP (20, 27). A recent study demonstrated that NLRP3 inflammasome and gasdermin D (GSDMD) activation-mediated pyroptosis in acinar cells is closely linked to pancreatic necrosis and systemic inflammation in AP (28). Another study recently indicated a new mechanism in which the p53-apoptosis-inducing factor (AIFM2) pathway regulates AP with multiorgan injury via activating transcription factor 6 (ATF6)-mediated apoptosis, suggesting that endoplasmic reticulum (ER)-mitochondrial-nuclear crosstalk plays an important role in AP development (29). Additionally, the inflammatory process is amplified following further secretion and overexpression of adhesion molecules including intercellular adhesion molecule 1 (ICAM-1) and vascular adhesion molecule 1 (VCAM-1), which represent ligands for lymphocyte function-associated antigen 1 on leukocytes and lymphocytes, αLβ2 and CD11a-CD18 on monocytes and integrin macrophage 1 antigen (Mac-1) on neutrophils, while their secretion is promoted by ROS generation and TNF-α itself (30). The potential targeted pathways in AP are shown in **Table 1**.

MECHANISMS OF LUNG INJURY IN ACUTE PANCREATITIS

Lung injury is the most common feature and the main cause of early death in AP (8). The pathological changes are closely related to an increase in vascular endothelial cell space and permeability, aggregation of marginal concentration of leukocytes, and profuse expression of ICAM-1 (15, 16). During AP, the accumulation of inflammatory cells and inflammatory mediators in the lung destroys the blood-air barrier. Several studies have demonstrated that that the accumulation of a lot of neutrophils in the lungs enhanced generation of ROS and increased the production of pro-inflammatory cytokines, including HMGB1, endotoxin,

TNF-α, IL-1β, and IL-6, which activate various intracellular signaling pathways (e.g., NF-κB, NLRP3, STAT3, MAPK, and AP-1) and adhesion molecules, thus, releasing inflammatory mediators, which exacerbate the damage and result in lung injury (16, 34). According to the relevant literature, the pathological reactions and their molecular mechanisms of AP-related lung injury can be summarized by mainly including inflammatory response outbreak, oxidative stress damage, and endocrine disorders (**Figure 1**).

Inflammatory Response of Lung Injury in Acute Pancreatitis

Inflammatory response plays a key role and has a major effect on the outcome of lung injury in AP (35). Pro-inflammatory factors play a key role in lung injury (36). Pro-inflammatory cytokines are considered to initiate and maintain lung injury (37), and they mainly influence human lung microvascular endothelial cells (HPMECs). Their effect leads to increased alveolar permeability, alveolar tissue fluid extravasation, pulmonary edema, and declined blood oxygen saturation (38). TNF-α, IL-17A, IL-6, IL-1β, and HMGB1 are some of the most important pro-inflammatory cytokines in AP-ALI (**Figures 1, 2**). The possible cytokines of lung injury in AP are shown in **Table 2**.

TNF-α, which is released by macrophages and activated fixed circulating monocytes in activated fixed tissues, appears early and plays an important role in the occurrence and development of lung injury in AP (50). It first binds to TNF receptor 1 (TNF-R1) and interacts with adaptor proteins, such as TNF-R1-related death domain (TRADD) protein, TNF-R-related factor 2 (TRAF2), and receptor-interacting protein (RIP). Then, it docks and binds to the mentioned proteins, triggers the intracellular cascade reaction; and finally activates NF-κB (51, 52). NF-κB activation can enhance the transcription of TNF-α genes, thus, creating a vicious feedback loop that amplifies early inflammatory signals and exacerbates the initial inflammatory effects (53) (**Figure 1**).

IL-17A is closely associated with the pathogenesis of lung injury in AP, and it is mainly expressed by adaptive immune cells populations (39, 54). Study have shown that the expression level of IL-17A is elevated in serum and bronchoalveolar lavage fluid (BALF) in AP-related lung injury (55). Although IL-17A causes lung damage through neutrophil aggregation, which directly leads to pulmonary and pancreatic edema (40), it also acts through synergy with other inflammatory factors, including ligands for TNF-α, IL-1β, and TLRs, and can induce the production of other pro-inflammatory cytokines and chemokines (56). Studies have demonstrated that IL-17A stimulates IL-8 production through synergy with TNF-α and induces an accelerated secretion of IL-6 from human peripancreatic myofibroblasts, which can increase the production of CXCL family of chemokines (neutrophil recruitment) in alveolar type II epithelial cells, and exacerbate airway inflammation and lung ischemia-reperfusion injury (42, 57).

IL-6 is mostly produced by monocytes, macrophages, and dendritic cells (58). It is a multifunctional cytokine with clear pro-inflammatory and anti-inflammatory properties that inhibit

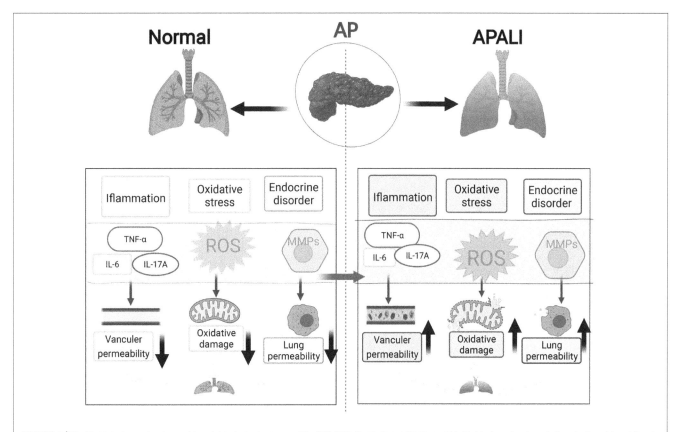

FIGURE 1 | The three main mechanisms of lung injury in acute pancreatitis (AP). This figure shows three most highlighted mechanisms in the studies of lung injury in AP, which include inflammatory response outbreak, oxidative stress damage, and endocrine disorders represented by matrix metalloproteinases (MMPs).

proliferation and promote apoptosis and lung injury by activating the JAK2/STAT3 signaling pathway (59, 60). In the early stages of pancreatic lung injury, IL-6 is rapidly synthesized and plays a protective role in host defense. As the injury persists and leukocyte IL-6 production by leukocytes continues to increase, extravasation of alveolar tissue fluid and pulmonary edema occur, leading to impaired lung function, progression of AP, and increased mortality (61).

IL-1β is a member of the IL1 cytokine family. It is produced by activated macrophage preproteins and is hydrolyzed by cystathionine 1 (CASP1/ICE) protein. This cytokine is an important mediator of inflammatory response, and it is involved in various cellular activities, including cell proliferation, differentiation, and apoptosis (62). In lung injury, it is mainly produced upon activation of the NF-κB and JAK2/STAT3 signaling pathways, which intensifies the acute injury process by activating the aggregation of monocytes and macrophages (63, 64). It is expressed only on the surface of activated vascular endothelial cells and initiates the adhesion of leukocytes to vascular endothelial cells, playing an important role in the early development of lung injury in AP (65, 66).

High-mobility group box protein 1 has been proposed as a potent inflammatory mediator in ALI, and the blockade of HMGB1 has led to a significant reduction in lung inflammatory reaction. Luan et al. (34) and Ding et al. (67) demonstrated that the downregulation of HMGB1 can inhibit the activity of NF-κB,

inhibit the expression of TNF-α, IL-1β, ICAM-1, and matrix metalloproteinase (MMP) 9 in the lung tissue, and tissue, and therefore decrease the severity of AP-associated ALI. Qu et al. (68) indicated that HMGB1 binds to certain receptors, such as receptor for advanced glycation end products (RAGE) and TLR4, activates the ROS and phosphatidylinositol-3 kinase (PI3K) pathways and myeloid differentiating factor 88 (MyD88), and results in the release of TNF-α, IL-1β, IL-6, and other cytokines contributing to ALI, suggesting that blocking HMGB1 may provide an effective treatment strategy for AP-associated ALI.

Oxidative Stress in Lung Injury in Acute Pancreatitis

Oxidative stress plays a crucial role in the development of lung injury in AP. An excessive amount of ROS can be generated by activating neutrophils, leading to severe oxidative stress damage (44, 69). Oxidative stress damage not only plays a role in the local damage of the pancreas but also plays a dominant role in damage to other organs, accelerating the occurrence and development of the SIRS and MODS (70, 71). Nuclear factor erythroid 2-related factor 2 (Nrf2) is a redox-sensitive transcription factor of the alkaline locking chain and a major regulator of resistance to oxidative stress, and thus the Nrf2/antioxidant response element (ARE) pathway is the most important endogenous antioxidant signaling pathway in the body

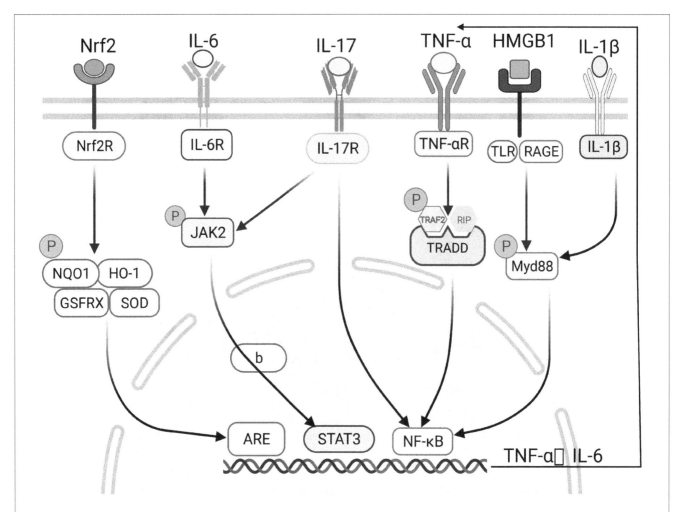

FIGURE 2 | The signaling pathways of lung and intestinal injuries in acute pancreatitis (AP) in different environments and under certain physiological conditions. Several inflammatory activators, such as TNF-α, HMGB1, and proinflammatory factors, activate various intracellular signaling pathways – particularly NF-κB, STAT3, and ARE – by binding specific receptors, thereby releasing a range of inflammatory mediators and promoting each other, forming a vicious cycle.

TABLE 2 | The cytokines of lung and intestinal injuries in AP.

Cytokines	Model	Influence	Function	References
TNF-a	*In vivo*	Upregulation	Promotes the production of inflammatory factors by T cells	(39, 40)
IL-17A	*In vivo*	Upregulation	Enables the body's immune response	(41, 42)
IL-8	*In vivo/In vitro*	Upregulation	Chemotaxis and activation of neutrophils	(43)
IL-1β	*In vivo*	Upregulation	Increase inflammatory cytokines	(16, 34, 44)
HMGB1	*In vivo*	Upregulation	Promotes the release of inflammatory mediators	(45–47)
TXA2, PAF, ET-1, PLA2	*In vivo*	Upregulation	Causes vasospasm, leukocyte and platelet aggregation, thrombosis and vascular endothelial cell damage	(48, 49)

(72). Nrf2 can upregulate antioxidant genes and exert antioxidant effects by binding to the promoter sequence, ARE, and activation of Nrf2 can reduce neutrophilic airway inflammation by the upregulation of antioxidants and downregulation of inflammatory cytokines in the airways (73, 74). In AP, Nrf2 dysfunction and function abnormalities of key enzymes in the Nrf2/ARE pathway, such as heme oxygenase-1 (HO-1), quinone oxidoreductase-1 (NQO1), glutathione peroxidase (GSH-Px) and superoxide dismutase (SOD) occur, resulting

in loss of antioxidant function and consequent lung tissue damage (75).

Endocrine Disorders Involving Matrix Metalloproteinases in Lung Injury in Acute Pancreatitis

HPMEs are damaged by inflammatory factors and inflammatory mediators of lung injury in AP (76). HPMECs can secrete MMPs, which are a type of zinc-dependent endopeptidases (77). MMP-2 and MMP-9 are the most extensively studied MPPs. They degrade extracellular basement membrane collagen and alter lung permeability, exacerbating lung injury (78, 79). MMP-2 and MMP-9 have been found to play an important role in ALI, acute respiratory distress syndrome (ARDS), and pulmonary fibrosis (80–82). MMP-9 is mainly involved in the ALI phase, whereas MMP-2 is mainly involved in the subsequent repair and fibrosis phase (83). MMP-9 levels in BALF have been reported to increase in patients with ARDS secondary to septic shock compared to normal controls, suggesting that MMP-9 plays an important role in the development of lung injury in AP (84).

Other Mechanisms of Lung Injury in Acute Pancreatitis

Abnormalities in the lysosomal degradation pathway, which underlie the emergence of differentiation disorders, can cause impairments in cell development, homeostasis, and survival (85). Studies have shown that abnormalities in the lysosomal degradation pathway, represented by impaired autophagy, play an important role in the evolution of lung injury in AP (86–88). Pulmonary intravascular macrophages (PIMs) damage lung endothelial cells, and they may play a role in another pathogenetic pathway of lung injury in AP (89). Water channel proteins (aquaporins) are a family of membrane proteins involved in the selective transport of water across cell membranes and play a key role in the development of acute pulmonary edema (47). Additional mechanisms, such as activation of ICAM-1 and alteration of circulating protease and phospholipase concentration, have been associated with AP-induced remote lung injury (90). Studies have indicated that ICAM-1 and E-selectin as important inflammatory cytokines are involved in the pathogenesis of AP-associated lung injury, which lead to increased leukocytic infiltration, permeability, proliferation, migration, pulmonary microcirculatory dysfunction and acute respiratory distress syndrome (91, 92).

The Experimental Animal Models of Acute Pancreatitis-Associated Acute Lung Injury

The experimental animal models of AP and AP-associated ALI have been relatively well-established. Sodium taurocholate, caerulein, or L-arginine are primarily used to create the models (**Table 3**).

Where rats are were starved overnight and anesthetized with ketamine 40 mg/kg intraperitoneally. The hepatic portal of the bile duct is clamped, and 3.5% sodium taurocholate in a volume of 1 mL/kg is retrogradely injected into the biliopancreatic conduit at a steady pace (0.1 mL/min) (93). The animal models caused by caerulein and LPS have been made. Mice are treated intraperitoneally (i.p.) with 50 μg/kg body weight caerulein (10 mL/kg of body weight) twice every hour (seven injections in total) and 10 mg/kg of lipopolysaccharide (LPS) (10 mL/kg of body weight, i.p.) following the last dosage of caerulein immediately (74). The AP-associated ALI rat model has been

established by administering two intraperitoneal injections (1 h apart) of L-arginine at a dose of 4 g/kg body weight (96).

MECHANISMS OF INTESTINAL INJURY IN ACUTE PANCREATITIS

In intestinal injury caused by AP, the intestinal barrier becomes damaged the earliest. The pathological changes are closely related to the destruction of the intestinal mucosal structure and an increase in intestinal mucosal permeability (97, 98). The effects of intestinal barrier failure in AP manifest as intestinal immune deficiency, intestinal microflora disturbance, increased intestinal permeability, and excessive release of inflammatory mediators (like endotoxin, cytokines, chemokines, DAMPs, and mRNAs) (16, 97). Based on the relevant literature, this review summarizes the mechanisms of intestinal injury, including inflammatory response burst, oxidative stress injury, and endocrine disruption represented by angiopoietin (Ang) and mitochondrial injury (**Figure 3**).

Inflammatory Response to Intestinal Injury in Acute Pancreatitis

The inflammatory response plays a major role in the development and prognosis of intestinal injury in AP (16). Inflammatory cells and factors accumulate and infiltrate during the development of AP, leading to the disruption of the intestinal barrier and intestinal mucosal structure and an increase in intestinal mucosal permeability. The disruption of the intestinal barrier function is mainly manifested in two aspects: intestinal mucosal epithelial barrier dysfunction (mechanical, chemical, immunological, and biological barrier dysfunction) and intestinal capillary endothelial barrier dysfunction (99). In contrast, most of the inflammatory responses are caused by mechanical and chemical barrier dysfunction.

The intestinal mechanical barrier comprises intestinal epithelial cells (IECs) and tight intercellular junctions. IECs separate the intestinal lumen from the lamina propria. The tight junctions are the main determinants of paracellular permeability (100). IECs ensure proper digestion and barrier function with a high turnover rate of 4–5 days (101). Uncontrolled inflammatory response of the intestinal epithelium is a characteristic feature of intestinal barrier failure in severe AP. The caspase-3 pathway can be stimulated by an inflammatory factor, TNF-α, leading to severe apoptosis of intestinal mucosal cells and destruction of intestinal mucosal structures (102). Another inflammatory factor, HMGB1, activates RAGE and TLRs, which, in turn, activate the NF-κB signaling, release inflammatory mediators, and enhance the binding of ARE elements to downstream target mRNAs (such as those for TNF-α, IL-6, and IL-8), and maintain the stability of target mRNAs. As a result, they increase the translation of related proteins and induce a strong pro-inflammatory effect (16).

The intestinal chemical barrier consists of mucin (MUC), antimicrobial peptides (AMPs), and other digestive enzymes. AMPs have sterilizing and anti-inflammatory functions. Additionally, they promote tissue repair. In the intestine, AMPs, especially β-defensins, in the intestine are reduced due to

TABLE 3 | The experimental animal models of pancreatitis-associated ALI.

Models induced	Model	Function	References
Sodium taurocholate	Rat	Emodin protects against acute pancreatitis associated lung injury by Inhibiting NLPR3 inflammasome activation via Nrf2/HO-1 signaling	(93)
Deoxycholic acid sodium salt	Rat	The ICAM-1-mediated JAK2/STAT3 signaling cascade was able to enhance inflammatory responses	(94)
Caerulein	Rat	Inhibition of MMP-9 activity with doxycycline reduced pancreatitis-associated lung injury	(95)
Caerulein and LPS	Mouse	Activation of Nrf2/ARE may be a promising therapeutic target	(74)
L-arginine	Mouse	Reduces acute lung injury by reducing the infiltration of inflammatory cells and inhibiting inflammatory cytokine secretion and cell apoptosis by inhibiting the activation of JAK2-STAT3 signaling	(96)

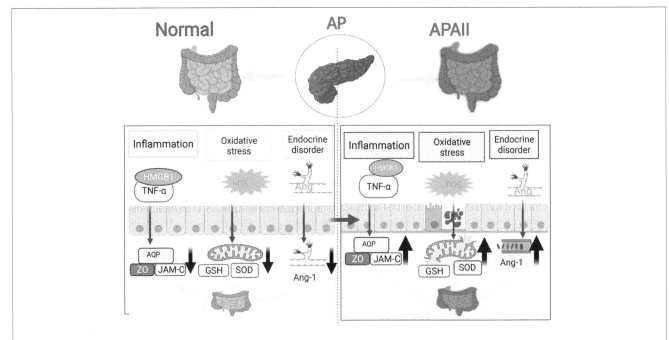

FIGURE 3 | The three main mechanisms of intestinal injury in acute pancreatitis (AP). The three most highlighted mechanisms of intestinal injury in AP are inflammatory response outbreak, oxidative stress damage, and endocrine disorders.

the aggregation and infiltration of inflammatory cells in AP, increasing the rate of intestinal bacterial translocation and the possibility of retrograde infection (103). MUC2, one of the most common forms present of MUC, is the main component of the intestinal chemical barrier covering IECs and forms the intestinal mucus layer. It is the first line of defense of the intestinal mucosal barrier; therefore, it is the most vulnerable to inflammatory reactions and loss of barrier function (104) (**Table 2**).

The intestinal capillary endothelial barrier is a semi-selective barrier composed of a single layer of endothelial cells surrounding the vascular lumen and basement membrane. The occurrence of intestinal capillary endothelial barrier impairs capillary permeability, which affects intestinal mucosal permeability and causes intestinal edema. Capillary permeability is determined by three factors: endothelial cells, inter-endothelial connections, and basement membrane (49). Studies have shown that aquaporin 1 (AQP-1), MMP-9, and junctional adhesion molecule-C (JAM-C) play key roles in the regulation of capillary permeability in AP (105). Under the stimulation of inflammatory factors, intestinal permeability can increase when AQP-1 is

downregulated, leading to an imbalance in water transfer and homeostasis between the cells and blood vessels. Microvascular permeability can increase when MMP-9 is decreased, leading to damage to the basement membrane. JAM-C is localized at cell junctions, increasing intercellular permeability when affected, which, in turn, increases intestinal mucosal permeability and causes intestinal edema (95).

Oxidative Stress of Intestinal Injury in Acute Pancreatitis

During oxidative stress, an imbalance between oxidative and antioxidant action occurs in the body. Inflammatory infiltration of neutrophils, increased secretion of proteases, and production of oxidative intermediates, such as oxygen radicals and lipid peroxides, lead to IEC damage in the early stages of AP (106). Oxygen radicals and lipid peroxides can be produced in damaged intestinal tissues by activated immune cells and alveolar cells, which can activate the Nrf2/ARE antioxidant signaling pathway (79), resulting in a decrease in total GSH and SOD levels

(107, 108). As a result, intestinal barrier function, intestinal mucosal structure, and intestinal mucosal permeability become disrupted (109).

Endocrine Disorders of Intestinal Injury in Acute Pancreatitis

Ang has an important role in the pathology of intestinal capillary leakage syndrome in SAP. Normally, Ang-1 not only promotes endothelial cell chemotaxis and aggregation but also inhibits apoptosis, inflammation, exudation, and leukocyte adhesion (110). Additionally, it regulates the proliferation of endothelial cells and vascular smooth muscle cells, and promotes vascular maturation, which is important for maintaining vascular stability and integrity (111). In AP, a significant decrease in serum Ang-1 levels, a significant increase in the number of inflammatory factors in the serum, an increase in capillary permeability of the tissues, an increase in alveolar fluid, and the appearance of pulmonary edema are all observed. Related studies have shown that Ang1 not only effectively alleviated intestinal capillary leakage in a rat model of AP but also played a positive role in the protection of intestinal microcirculation. Additionally, it significantly upregulated the expression of AQP-1 and downregulated the expression of MMP-9 and JAM-C protein to provide intestinal protection (49).

Other Mechanisms of Intestinal Injury in Acute Pancreatitis

Mitochondria are central to cellular viability and function, controlling control many physiological metabolic processes (112, 113). Disorders of ROS and cytochrome C metabolism, which occur in mitochondria, can lead to abnormalities in intestinal metabolism (114). Significant mitochondrial dysfunction occurs in the jejunum in the early stages of severe AP in rat models (115). Additionally, swelling of mitochondria in the colonic mucosal epithelium occurs. In edematous pancreatitis, degeneration and rupture of colonic mitochondria are present in necrotizing pancreatitis, suggesting that the damage to the mitochondria is closely related to intestinal injury in AP (116).

COMMON MECHANISMS OF LUNG AND INTESTINAL INJURIES IN ACUTE PANCREATITIS

The lungs and intestine are organs that are directly damaged organs in AP. Mesenteric lymph (ML) is the direct axial connection between the intestine and lungs (117). Physiologically, the lungs and large intestine can interact with each other to promote homeostasis, whereas pathologically, the balance and interaction between the two axes are disturbed. Lung-gut syndrome is a condition in which the lungs and large intestine become affected concurrently; respiratory and digestive tract disorders occur together (118). This interaction is consistent with the theory of *the lung being connected with the large intestine* in Chinese medicine. Inflammatory mediators reaching the lung and intestinal tissues cause an inflammatory response, oxidative stress, and endocrine hormone secretion disorders, impairing the balance axis between the lung and intestine.

Inflammatory Response in the Imbalance of the Lung-Gut Axis

Acute pancreatitis is an acute necrotic and inflammatory process that suddenly occurring around and inside the pancreas (119). Overactivation of the inflammatory response is important in the course of pancreatitis, including the production and activation of inflammatory factors and the accumulation of pro-inflammatory mediators. The main inflammatory factors, including TNF-α, IL-17, IL-1, and IL-8, are released into the bloodstream. They accumulate in the lungs and intestine, activating the NF-κB signaling pathway, amplifying the inflammatory effect, and inducing a systemic inflammatory response. These processes lead to inflammatory injury in the lungs and intestine (120). Thromboxane A2 (TXA2), platelet-activating factor (PAF), endothelin 1 (ET-1), phospholipase A2 (PLA2), and IL-1β can cause vasospasm, white blood cell and platelet aggregation, thrombosis, and vascular endothelial cell damage, leading to the loss of the intestinal barrier, which in turn causes lung injury (121). The main pro-inflammatory mediators include HMGB1 and TLR-4. HMGB1 is released by necrotic acinar cells and acts on its receptors, ARGE and TLR (122). Chen et al. (123) found that the expression of HMGB1 is positively related to intestinal barrier failure and inhibition of HMGB1 can significantly improve intestinal injury. Furthermore, HMGB1 activates the NF-κB signaling pathway and releases several downstream inflammatory factors by myd88 and appears during an early inflammatory response (124). Relevant studies have shown that the levels of HMGB1 and TLR-4 can be used as important indicators of AP progress (125) (**Figure 2** and **Table 2**).

Oxidative Stress in the Imbalance of the Lung-Gut Axis

During AP, Ca^{2+} overload, inflammatory mediators, and zymogen activation can damage the arterial muscles and vascular endothelial cells in the pancreatic lobules, resulting in pancreatic vasoconstriction, shunting, and insufficient perfusion. Intestinal mucosal tissue is the most susceptible to insufficient perfusion (126). When the intestinal mucosa is signaled by ischemia and hypoxia, xanthine oxidase and hypoxanthine accumulate in the intestinal tissue, leading to adenosine triphosphate (ATP) depletion due to insufficient oxidative phosphorylation. In the subsequent reperfusion, the body converts hypoxanthine to xanthine, and then releases superoxide ions to generate more free oxygen radicals. The Nrf2/ARE antioxidant signal pathway is activated, causing lipid peroxidation and cell membrane damage, which accelerate intestinal barrier loss and lung function impairment (127). Liu et al. (43) have found that SAP can change the hemodynamics of rats, leading to severe microcirculation disturbances in the pancreas and other organs (especially the lungs) and causing redox imbalance. These changes result in hyperosmotic edema of the lungs and increased alveolar fluid level (10, 15), as well as other pathological changes, including the destruction of intestinal mucosal structure and changes in intestinal mucosal permeability (35) (**Figure 2**).

Endocrine Disorders in the Imbalance of the Lung-Gut Axis

The intestine is not simply a digestive organ: it has certain endocrine functions. The endocrine hormones secreted by the intestine play important roles in gastric content transport and digestion. Hormones, such as secreted cholecystokinin octapeptide (CCK-8) and blood vessel active intestinal peptide (VIP), can cause lung and intestinal damage in AP under pathological conditions (48). Blood CCK is mainly derived from intestinal secretory endothelial cells. Related studies have shown that it not only promotes gall bladder contraction but also relaxes the sphincter of Oddi and protects the gastric mucosa. Additionally, it can relax tracheal muscles, activate pulmonary interstitial macrophages (PIM), and reduce the occurrence of endotoxemia-related pneumonia. Although CCK is derived from enteroendocrine endothelial cells, it can cause lung and intestinal damage concurrently. VIP is a linear peptide widely distributed in the gastrointestinal tract and lungs. Its function is mainly to promote glandular secretion. It is negatively correlated with gastrointestinal motility. It can dilate systemic and pulmonary blood vessels, and inhibit the proliferation of pulmonary artery smooth muscle cells (128). Animal experiments have proven that VIP can reduce pulmonary hypertension by reducing pulmonary vascular resistance (45).

Other Mechanisms in the Imbalance of the Lung-Gut Axis

Water channel proteins play a vital role in maintaining the water homeostasis of the lungs and intestine. AQPs are a type of membrane water channels, consisting of six transmembrane spiral segments and two shorter spiral segments that do not span the entire membrane. Their main function is to promote water transport in passive transport, and AQPs are widely distributed in mammalian organs (46). Currently, 13 AQPs have been discovered, and at least eight AQPs have been shown to transport water in humans and rodents (47). It was previously shown that the expression levels of AQP-1 and AQP-5 were decreased in patients with pulmonary edema after a viral infection were decreased (129). Sakai et al. (130) that the genes of *AQP4* and *AQP8* are mainly expressed in the mouse colon. The regulation of transepithelial fluid transport in the gastrointestinal tract is based on ion and water transport by AQPs (131). Additionally, the appearance of pulmonary and bowel dysfunction is closely related to intra-abdominal hypertension (IAH) and/or abdominal cavity syndrome (ACS). Reduced IAH maintains the integrity of the intestinal barrier, promotes the recovery of intestinal function, inhibits inflammation, and increases blood oxygen saturation (SpO_2) (132). To reduce tissue damage of the intestines and lungs (133), thus, other mechanisms of lung and bowel damage in AP can be targeted to reduce damage to the intestine and lungs (133).

POTENTIAL TARGETS FOR THE PROTECTION OF LUNG AND INTESTINAL INJURIES IN ACUTE PANCREATITIS

Studies have shown that lipoxin A4 inhibits the activation of TNF-α/TNF-R1 and downstream signals, such as TRADD, TRAF2, and RIP. The inhibition influences the activity of the NF-κB pathway, and consequently inhibits the production of inflammatory mediators and the impairment of pulmonary intestinal injury (94, 134). According to another study, TLR4, which is a key receptor for the recognition of pathogen-associated molecular patterns (PAMPs), may provide valuable guidance for the treatment of pulmonary intestinal injury in SAP (135).

BML-111, which is a commercially synthesized lipoxin receptor agonist, protects against emotion-induced LAI in mice by modulating the Nrf2/ARE signaling pathway (74). Isoglycyrrhizinate alleviates AP in mice by inhibiting oxidative stress and modulating the Nrf2/HO1 pathway (31). The protective effect of tanshinone IIA in AP in mice occurs by inhibiting oxidative stress through the Nrf2/ROS pathway (136). Protective effects of rhodopsin against AP-induced lung injury occur by the inhibition of NLRP3 inflammasome activation specifically activated by the Nrf2/HO-1 pathway (93). HMGB1 inhibitors reduce the severity of SAP by reducing intestinal permeability through the reduction in claudin-2 and occludin expression (25). Moreover, hydrostatin-SN10 significantly reduces IL-6 levels, reduces inflammatory response, and improves lung tissue injury by inhibiting JAK2/STAT3 phosphorylation (137).

CONCLUSION AND FUTURE PERSPECTIVES

This review described the three common mechanisms of lung and intestinal injury in AP. The common mechanisms of lung and intestinal injury in AP are inflammatory response, oxidative stress, and endocrine hormone secretion disorder. However, few studies have reported concurrent treatment options for lung and intestinal injury in AP. Therefore, future studies are required to investigate common treatment options for lung and intestinal injury in AP. The mechanism of inflammatory response is the most important element in lung and intestinal injury, because it is generally considered to be effective in the common prevention and treatment of lung and intestinal injury in AP. However, details regarding the involved pro-inflammatory mediators and cells are still lacking.

Mesenteric lymph can concurrently cause lung and intestinal injury in AP. Therefore, surgical diversion of ML represents a treatment option. An inflammatory response is an unclear mechanism of lung and intestinal injury in AP. Therefore, currently, the greatest challenge of studies on lung and intestinal injury in AP is the elucidation of the specific mechanisms and their precise targets. Accurate detection of these mechanisms and targets and demonstration of the remarkable effects of multitarget integration will be useful for lung and intestinal injury in AP in clinical practice. Additionally, immunotherapy is also a promising approach, and it could be an effective strategy targeting and altering the activities of immune cells in AP, which might have long-term therapeutic effects.

AUTHOR CONTRIBUTIONS

YW and DL organized thoughts for the manuscript and revised the manuscript. LW drafted the manuscript and gathered information for the manuscript. DY revised the first manuscript. ZW, YH, and MB translated and revised the manuscript. YZ, DY, and BS offered opinions for the drawing of diagrams and charts in the manuscript. All authors read and approved the final version of the manuscript.

ACKNOWLEDGMENTS

We acknowledge Gansu Provincial Engineering Laboratory for Research and Promotion of Quality Standardization of Authentic Medicinal Materials in Gansu Province, Provincial Key Laboratory of Pharmaceutical Chemistry and Quality Research in Colleges and Universities in Gansu Province, and Gansu Experimental Animal Industry Technology Center for providing support and assistance for this review article.

REFERENCES

1. Gao E, Jiang Y, Li Z, Xue D, Zhang W. Association between high mobility group box-1 protein expression and cell death in acute pancreatitis. *Mol Med Rep.* (2017) 15:4021–6. doi: 10.3892/mmr.2017.6496

2. Yan TY, Li YX, Sun Y, Wang H, Wang J, Wang W, et al. Hospital acquired lower respiratory tract infections among high risk hospitalized patients in a tertiary care teaching hospital in China: an economic burden analysis. *J Infect Public Health.* (2018) 11:507–13. doi: 10.1016/j.jiph.2017.10.003

3. Lankisch PG, Apte M, Banks PA. Acute pancreatitis. *Lancet.* (2015) 386:85–96. doi: 10.1016/S0140-6736(14)60649-8

4. Franco-Pons N, Gea-Sorlí S, Closa D, Chen T, Tian JY, Si HR. Release of inflammatory mediators by adipose tissue during acute pancreatitis. *J Pathol.* (2010) 221:175–82. doi: 10.1002/path.2691

5. Hussain N, Wu F, Zhu L, Thrall RS, Kresch MJ. Neutrophil apoptosis during the development and resolution of oleic acid-induced acute lung injury in the rat. *Am J Respir Cell Mol Biol.* (1998) 19:867–74. doi: 10.1165/ajrcmb.19.6.3118

6. Dal M, Ulutas K. Assessment of visceral and subcutaneous obesity to understand the efficiency of adipose tissue in acute pancreatitis. *Niger J Clin Pract.* (2021) 24:993–993. doi: 10.4103/njcp.njcp_370_19

7. Qiao SF, Sun JB, Li F. Analysis of related factors and prevention measures of pancreatic infection in patients with severe acute pancreatitis. *Clin Med Ch.* (2006) 22:252–3.

8. Samanta J, Singh S, Arora S, Muktesh G, Aggarwal A, Dhaka N, et al. Cytokine profile in prediction of acute lung injury in patients with acute pancreatitis. *Pancreatology.* (2018) 18:878–84. doi: 10.1016/j.pan.2018.10.006

9. Chen H, Su H, Yuan l. Mechanism of lung and intestinal injury in rats with acute pancreatitis. *Needle Res.* (2018) 43:353–9. doi: 10.1186/s12906-017-1789-X

10. Ijaz M, Adrish M. Outcomes in patients with acute lung injury/ARDS vs cardiogenic pulmonary edema. *Chest.* (2015) 148:e194. doi: 10.1378/chest.14-3052

11. Tamura H, Reich J, Nagaoka I. Bacterial endotoxin assays relevant to host defense peptides. *Juntendo Med J.* (2016) 62:132–40. doi: 10.14789/jmj.62.132

12. Garg PK, Singh VP. Organ failure due to systemic injury in acute pancreatitis. *Gastroenterology.* (2019) 156:2008–23. doi: 10.1053/j.gastro.2018.12.041

13. Pasari LP, Khurana A, Anchi P, Saifi MA, Annaldas S, Godugu C. Visnagin attenuates acute pancreatitis via Nrf2/NFκB pathway and abrogates associated multiple organ dysfunction. *Biomed Pharmacother.* (2019) 112:108629. doi: 10.1016/j.biopha.2019.108629

14. Rubenfeld GD, Caldwell E, Peabody E, Weaver J, Martin DP, Neff M, et al. Incidence and outcomes of acute lung injury. *N Engl J Med.* (2005) 353:1685–93. doi: 10.1056/NEJMoa050333

15. Sarr MG, Banks PA, Bollen TL, Dervenis C, Gooszen HG, Johnson CD, et al. The new revised classification of acute pancreatitis. *Surg Clin North Am.* (2012) 93:549–62.

16. Ge P, Luo Y, Okoye CS, Chen H, Liu J, Zhang G, et al. Intestinal barrier damage, systemic inflammatory response syndrome, and acute lung injury: a troublesome trio for acute pancreatitis. *Biomed Pharmacother.* (2020) 132:110770. doi: 10.1016/j.biopha.2020.110770

17. Shao N. The theory and practice of "lung and large intestine being exterior-interior relationship". *Henan Prov Tradit Chin Med.* (2020) 40:1768–72. doi: 10.16367/j.issn.1003-5028.2020.11.0446

18. Al Mofleh IA. Severe acute pancreatitis: pathogenetic aspects and prognostic factors. *World J Gastroenterol.* (2008) 14:675–84. doi: 10.3748/wjg.14.675

19. Chen C, Hu H, Li X, Zheng Z, Wang Z, Wang X, et al. Rapid detection of anti-SARS-CoV-2 antibody using a selenium nanoparticle-based lateral flow immunoassay. *IEEE Trans Nanobioscience.* (2022) 21:37–43. doi: 10.1109/TNB.2021.3105662

20. Lu G, Pan Y, Kayoumu A, Zhang L, Yin T, Tong Z, et al. Indomethacin inhibits the NLRP3 inflammasome pathway and protects severe acute pancreatitis in mice. *Biochem Biophy Res Commun.* (2017) 493:827–32. doi: 10.1016/j.bbrc.2017.08.060

21. Peng C, Li Z, Yu X. The role of pancreatic infiltrating innate immune cells in acute pancreatitis. *Int J Med Sci.* (2021) 18:534–45. doi: 10.7150/ijms.51618

22. Choudhury S, Ghosh S, Gupta P, Mukherjee S, Chattopadhyay S. Inflammation-induced ROS generation causes pancreatic cell death through modulation of Nrf2/NF-κB and SAPK/JNK pathway. *Free Radic Res.* (2015) 49:1371–83. doi: 10.3109/10715762.2015.1075016

23. Maléth J, Hegyi P. Ca2+ toxicity and mitochondrial damage in acute pancreatitis: translational overview. *Philos T R Soc B.* (2016) 371:20150425. doi: 10.1098/rstb.2015.0425

24. Yu JH, Kim H. Oxidative stress and inflammatory signaling in cerulein pancreatitis. *World J Gastroenterol.* (2014) 20:17324–9. doi: 10.3748/wjg.v20.i46.17324

25. Huang L, Zhang D, Han W, Guo C. High-mobility group box-1 inhibition stabilizes intestinal permeability through tight junctions in experimental acute necrotizing pancreatitis. *Inflamm Res.* (2019) 68:677–89. doi: 10.1007/s00011-019-01251-x

26. Chen ZP, Huang HP, He XY, Wu BZ, Liu Y. Early continuous blood purification affects TNF–α, IL-1β, and IL-6 in patients with severe acute pancreatitis via inhibiting TLR4 signaling pathway. *Kaohsiung J Med Sci.* (2022) 2022:1–7. doi: 10.1002/kjm2.12497

27. Hoque R, Sohail M, Malik A, Sarwar S, Luo Y, Shah A, et al. TLR9 and the NLRP3 inflammasome link acinar cell death with inflammation in acute pancreatitis. *Gastroenterology.* (2011) 141:358–69. doi: 10.1053/j.gastro.2011.03.041

28. Gao L, Dong X, Gong W, Huang W, Xue J, Zhu Q, et al. Acinar cell NLRP3 inflammasome and gasdermin D (GSDMD) activation mediates pyroptosis and systemic inflammation in acute pancreatitis. *Br J Pharmacol.* (2021) 178:3533–52. doi: 10.1111/bph.15499

29. Tan JH, Cao RC, Zhou L, Zhou ZT, Chen HJ, Xu J, et al. ATF6 aggravates acinar cell apoptosis and injury by regulating p53/AIFM2 transcription in

severe acute pancreatitis. *Theranostics.* (2020) 10:8298–314. doi: 10.7150/thno.46934

30. Gulla A, Gulbinas A, Dambrauskas Z, Strupas K. Heme oxygenase-1 polymorphism is associated with the development of necrotic acute pancreatitis via vascular cell adhesion molecule-1 and the E-selectin expression regulation pathway. *Pancreas.* (2019) 48:787–91. doi: 10.1097/MPA.0000000000001328

31. Liu XN, Zhu QT, Zhang M, Yin T, Xu R, Xiao W, et al. Isoliquiritigenin ameliorates acute pancreatitis in mice via inhibition of oiative stress and modulation of the Nrf2/HO-1 pathway. *Oxid Med Cell Longev.* (2018) 2018:7161592. doi: 10.1155/2018/7161592

32. Liu Z, Qi M, Tian S, Yang Q, Liu J, Wang S, et al. Ubiquitin-Specific Protease 25 Aggravates Acute Pancreatitis and Acute Pancreatitis-Related Multiple Organ Injury by Destroying Tight Junctions Through Activation of The STAT3 Pathway. *Front Cell Dev Biol.* (2021) 9:806850. doi: 10.3389/fcell.2021.806850

33. Qiu Z, Xu F, Wang Z, Yang P, Bu Z, Cheng F, et al. Blockade of JAK2 signaling produces immunomodulatory effect to preserve pancreatic homeostasis in severe acute pancreatitis. *Biochem Biophys Rep.* (2021) 28:101133. doi: 10.1016/j.bbrep.2021.101133

34. Luan ZG, Zhang XJ, Yin XH, Ma XC, Zhang H, Zhang C, et al. Downregulation of HMGB1 protects against the development of acute lung injury after severe acute pancreatitis. *Immunobiology.* (2013) 218:1261–70. doi: 10.1016/j.imbio.2013.04.013

35. Guo H, Suo DW, Zhu HP, Sun XM, Chen J. Early blood purification therapy of severe acute pancreatitis complicated by acute lung injury. *Eur Rev Med Pharmacol Sci.* (2016) 20:873–8.

36. Zhang Y, Yan L, Han W. Elevated level of miR-551b-5p is associated with inflammation and disease progression in patients with severe acute pancreatitis. *Ther Apher Dial.* (2018) 22:649–55. doi: 10.1111/1744-9987.12720

37. Pastor CM, Matthay MA, Frossard JL. Pancreatitis associated acute lung injury: new insights. *Chest.* (2003) 124:2341–51. doi: 10.1378/chest.124.6.2341

38. Yi L, Huang X, Guo F, Zhou Z, Chang M, Jingning H. GSK-3 beta-dependent activation of GEF-H1/ROCK signaling promotes LPS-induced lung vascular endothelial barrier dysfunction and acute lung injury. *Front Cell Infect Microbiol.* (2017) 7:357. doi: 10.3389/fcimb.2017.00357

39. McGeachy MJ, Cua DJ, Gaffen SL. The IL-17 family of cytokines in health and disease. *Immunity.* (2019) 50:892–906. doi: 10.1016/j.immuni.2019.03.021

40. Tang RM, Qiu L, Sun R, Sun R, Cheng L, Ma X, et al. Increased interleukin-23/17axis and C-reactive protein are associated with severity of acute pancreatitis in patients. *Pancreas.* (2015) 44:321–5.

41. Ahmed N, Naif OA, Sheikh FA, Mohammed MA, Abdullah SA, Ali SA, et al. Blockade of interleukin-2-inducible T-cell kinase signaling attenuates acute lung injury in mice through adjustment of pulmonary Th17/Treg immune responses and reduction of oxidative stress. *Int Immunopharmacol.* (2020) 83:106369. doi: 10.1016/j.intimp.2020.106369

42. Liu Y, Mei J, Gonzales L, Yang G, Dai N, Wang P, et al. IL-17A and TNF-α exert synergistic effects on expression of CXCL5 by alveolar type II cells in vivo and in vitro. *J Immunol.* (2011) 186:3197–205. doi: 10.4049/jimmunol.1002016

43. Liu XM, Liu QG, Xu J, Pan CE. Microcirculation disturbance affects rats with acute severe pancreatitis following lung injury. *World J Gastroenterol.* (2005) 11:6208–11. doi: 10.3748/wjg.v11.i39.6208

44. Sacco P, Decleva E, Tentor F, Menegazzi R, Borgogna M, Paoletti S, et al. A suitable tool for sustained inhibition of ROS release by activated neutrophils. *Macromol Biosci.* (2017) 17:1700214. doi: 10.1002/mabi.201700214

45. Newman JH. Pulmonary hypertension. *Dtsch Arztebl Int.* (2005) 114:73–84. doi: 10.3238/arztebl.2017.0073

46. Sogami M, Era S, Murakami M, Seo Y, Watari H, Uyesaka N. Application of the transition state theory to water transport across cell membranes. *Biochim Biophys Acta.* (2001) 1511:42–8. doi: 10.1016/s0005-2736(00)00384-9

47. Towne JE, Harrod KS, Krane CM, Menon AG. Decreased expression of aquaporin AQP1 and AQP5 in mouse lung after acute viral infection. *Respir Cell Mol Biol.* (2000) 22:34–44. doi: 10.1165/ajrcmb.22.1.3818

48. Zhang X, Han D, Ding D, Yao Y. Cholecystokinin octapeptide inhibits the in vitro expression of CD14 in rat pulmonary interstitial macrophages induced by lipopolysaccharide. *Chin Med J (Engl).* (2002) 115:276–9.

49. Pana LY, Chena YF, Lia HC, Bi LM, Sun WJ, Sun GF, et al. Dachengqi decoction attenuates intestinal vascular endothelial injury in severe acute pancreatitis in vitro and in vivo. *Cell Physiol Biochem.* (2017) 44:2395–406. doi: 10.1159/000486155

50. Bhatia M. Novel therapeutic targets for acute pancreatitis and associated multiple organ dysfunction syndrome. *Curr Drug Targets Inflamm Allergy.* (2002) 1:343–51. doi: 10.2174/1568010023344517

51. Chen G, Goeddel DV. TNF-R1 signaling: a beautiful pathway. *Science.* (2002) 296:1634–5. doi: 10.1126/science.1071924

52. Rangamani P, Sirovich L. Survival and apoptotic pathways initiated by TNF-alpha: modeling and predictions. *Biotechnol Bioeng.* (2007) 97:1216–29. doi: 10.1002/bit.21307

53. Zhang X, Wu D, Jiang X. ICAM-1 and acute pancreatis complicated by acute lung injury. *J Pancreas.* (2009) 10:8–14.

54. Chen K, Kolls JK. Interluekin-17A (IL-17A). *Gene.* (2017) 614:8–14.

55. Dai SR, Li Z, Zhang JB. Serum interleukin 17 as an early prognostic biomarker ofsevere acute pancreatitis receiving continuous blood purification. *Int J Artif Organs.* (2015) 38:192–8. doi: 10.5301/ijao.5000406

56. Honda K, Wada H, Nakamura M, Nakamoto K, Inui T, Sada M, et al. IL-17A synergistically stimulates TNF-α-induced IL-8 production in human airway epi-thelial cells: a potential role in amplifying airway inflammation. *Exp Lung Res.* (2016) 42:205–16. doi: 10.1080/01902148.2016.1190796

57. Sharma AK, Mulloy DP, Le LT, Laubach VE. NADPH oxidase mediates synergistic effects of IL-17 and TNF-α on CXCL1 expression by epithelial cells after lung ischemia-reperfusion. *Am J Physiol Lung Cell Mol Physiol.* (2011) 306:L69–79. doi: 10.1152/ajplung.00205.2013

58. Shieh JM, Tseng HY, Jung F, Yang SH, Lin JC. Elevation of IL-6 and IL-33 levels in serum associated with lung fibrosis and skeletal muscle wasting in a bleomycin-induced lung injury mouse model. *Mediators Inflamm.* (2019) 2019:7947596. doi: 10.1155/2019/7947596

59. Ning F, Zheng H, Tian H, Wang T, Hao D, Han S, et al. Research on effect of adiponectin on sepsis-induced lung injury in rats through IL-6/STAT3 signaling pathway. *Panminerva Medica.* (2019) 62:184–6. doi: 10.23736/S0031-0808.19.03650-4

60. Wu XY, Tian F, Su MH, Wu M, Huang Y, Hu LH, et al. BF211, a derivative of bufalin, enhances the cytocidal effects in multiple myeloma cells by inhibiting the IL-6/JAK2/STT3 pathway. *Int Immunopharmacol.* (2019) 64:24–32. doi: 10.1016/j.intimp.2018.08.016

61. Anaka T, Narazaki T, Kishimoto M. IL-6 in inflammation, immunity, and disease. *Cold Spring Harb Perspect Biol.* (2014) 6:a016295. doi: 10.1101/cshperspect.a016295

62. Masters SL, Simon A, Aksentijevich I, Kastner DL. Horror autoinflammaticus: the molecular pathophysiology of autoinflammatory disease. *Annu Rev Immunol.* (2009) 27:621–68. doi: 10.1146/annurev.immunol.25.022106.141627

63. Yao L, Yago T, Shao B, Liu Z, Silasi-Mansat R, Setiadi H, et al. Elevated CXCL1 expression in gp130-deficient endothelial cells impairs neutrophil migration in mice. *Blood.* (2013) 122:3832–42. doi: 10.1182/blood-2012-12-473835

64. Chavez-Sanchez L, Chavez-Rueda K, Legorreta-Haquet M, Zenteno E, Ledesma-Soto Y, Montoya-Díaz E, et al. The activation of CD14, TLR4, and TLR2 by mmLDL induces IL-1β, IL-6, and IL-10 secretion in human monocytes and macrophages. *Lipids Health Dis.* (2010) 9:117. doi: 10.1186/1476-511X-9-117

65. Jin F, Liu D, Yu H, Qi J, You Y, Xu X, et al. Sialic acid-functionalized PEG-PLGA microspheres loading mitochondrial-targeting-modified curcumin for acute lung injury therapy. *Mol Pharm.* (2018) 16:71–85. doi: 10.1021/acs.molpharmaceut.8b00861

66. Cao JP, He XY, Xu HT, Zou Z, Shi XY. Autolo-gous transplantation of peripheral blood-derived circulating endothelial progenitor cells attenuates endotoxin-induced acute lung injury in rabbits by direct endothelial repair and indirect immunomodulation. *Anesthesiology.* (2010) 116:1278–87. doi: 10.1097/ALN.0b013e3182567f84

67. Ding N, Wang F, Xiao H, Xu L, She S. Mechanical ventilation enhances HMGB1 expression in an LPS-induced lung injury model. *PLoS One.* (2013) 8:e74633. doi: 10.1371/journal.pone.0074633

68. Qu L, Chen C, Chen YY, Li Y, Tang F, Huang H, et al. High-mobility group box 1 (HMGB1) and autophagy in acute lung injury (ALI): a review. *Med Sci Monitor.* (2019) 25:1828–37. doi: 10.12659/MSM.912867

69. Levy BD, Hickey L, Morris AJ, Larvie M, Keledjian R, Petasis NA, et al. Novel polyisoprenyl phosphates block phospholipase D and human neutrophil activation in vitro and murine peritoneal inflammation in vivo. *Br J Pharmacol.* (2005) 146:344–51. doi: 10.1038/sj.bjp.0706338

70. Pereda JL, Sabater L, Aparisi L, Escobar J, Sandoval J, Viña J, et al. Interaction between cytokines and oxidative stress in acute pancreatitis. *Curr Med Chem.* (2006) 13:2775–87.

71. Que RS, Cao LP, Ding GP, Hu JA, Mao KJ, Wang GF. Correlation of nitric oxide and other free radicals with the severity of acute pancreatitis and complicated systemic inflammatory response syndrome. *Pancreas.* (2010) 39:536–40. doi: 10.1097/MPA.0b013e3181c0e199

72. Copple IM, Goldring CE, Kitteringham NR. The keap1-nrf2 cellular defense pathway: mechanisms of regulation and role in protection against drug-induced toxicity. *Handb Exp Pharmacol.* (2010) 196:233–66. doi: 10.1007/978-3-642-00663-0_9

73. Al-Harbi NO, Nadeem A, Ahmad SF, AlThagfan SS, Alqinyah M, Alqahtani F, et al. Sulforaphane treatment reverses corticosteroid resistance in a mixed granulocytic mouse model of asthma by upregulation of antioxidants and attenuation of Th17 immune responses in the airways. *Eur J Pharmacol.* (2019) 855:276–84. doi: 10.1016/j.ejphar.2019.05.026

74. Wang Y, Zhang Y, Cheng J, Ni Q, Li PW, Han W, et al. Protective effects of BML-111 on cerulein-induced acute pancreatitis-associated lung injury via activation of Nrf2/ARE signaling pathway. *Inflammation.* (2014) 37:1120–33. doi: 10.1007/s10753-014-9836-y

75. Chan KH, Ng MK, Stocker R. Haem oxygenase-1 and cardiovascular disease: mechanisms and therapeutic potential. *Clin Sci (Lond).* (2011) 120:493–504. doi: 10.1042/CS20100508

76. Kuebler WM. Inflammatory pathways and microvascular responses in the lung. *Pharmacol Rep.* (2005) 57(Suppl.):196–205.

77. Zhang F, Hu L, Wu YX, Fan L, Liu WT, Wang J, et al. Doxycycline alleviates paraquat-induced acute lung injury by inhibiting neutrophil-derived matrix metalloproteinase 9. *Int Immunopharmacol.* (2019) 72:243–51. doi: 10.1016/j.intimp.2019.04.015

78. Zinter MS, Delucchi KL, Kong MY, Orwoll BE, Spicer AS, Lim MJ, et al. Early plasma matrix metalloproteinase profiles: a novel pathway in pediatric acute respiratory distress syndrome. *Am J Respir Crit Care Med.* (2019) 199:181–9. doi: 10.1164/rccm.201804-0678OC

79. Zhang X, Sun CY, Zhang YB, Guo HZ, Feng XX, Peng SZ, et al. Kegan Liyan oral liquid ameliorates lipopolysaccharide-induced acute lung injury through inhibition of TLR4-mediated NF-κB signaling pathway and MMP-9 expression. *J Ethnopharmacol.* (2016) 186:91–102. doi: 10.1016/j.jep.2016.03.057

80. Chakrabarti S, Patel KD. Matrix metalloproteinase-2 (MMP-2) and MMP-9 in pulmonary pathology. *Exp Lung Res.* (2005) 31:599–621. doi: 10.1080/019021490944232

81. Fan YX, Liu HJ, Li YX, Zhang Y, Liu W, Zhang G. Quercetin ameliorates postoperative pain by suppressing matrix metalloproteinase in microglia. *J China Pharm Univ.* (2017) 48:272–81. doi: 10.1002/ejp.1116

82. Xu XL, Ji H, Gu SY, Huang Q, Chen Y. Effects of astragaloside IV on experimental ventricular remodeling in mice and its mechanism from matrixmetalloproteinase. Aspect. *J China Pharm Univ.* (2010) 41:70–5.

83. Chen LJ, Ding YB, Ma PL. The protective effect of lidocaine on lipopolysaccharide-induced acute lung injury in rats through NF-κB and p38 MAPK signaling pathway and excessive inflammatory responses. *Eur Rev Med Pharmacol Sci.* (2018) 22:2099–108. doi: 10.26355/eurrev-201804-14743

84. Ricou B, Nicod L, Lacraz S, Welgus HG, Suter PM, Dayer JM. Matrix metalloproteinases and TIMP in acute respiratory distress syndrome. *Am J Respir Crit Care Med.* (1996) 154:346–52. doi: 10.1164/ajrccm.154.2.8756805

85. Levine B, Kroemer G. Autophagy in the pathogenesis of disease. *Cell.* (2008) 132:27–42. doi: 10.1016/j.cell.2007.12.018

86. Gukovskaya AS, Gukovsky IH, Algul A, Habtezion A. Autophagy, inflammation, and immune dysfunction in the pathogenesis of pancreatitis. *Gastroenterology.* (2017) 153:1212–26. doi: 10.1053/j.gastro.2017.08.071

87. Gukovsky I, Li N, Todoric J, Gukovskaya A, Karin M. Inflammation, autophagy, and obesity: common features in the pathogenesis of pancreatitis

and pancreatic cancer. *Gastroenterology.* (2013) 144:1199–209. doi: 10.1053/j.gastro.2013.02.007

88. Mareninova OA, Hermann K, French SW, O'Konski MS, Pandol SJ, Webster P, et al. Impaired autophagic flux mediates acinar cell vacuole formation and trypsinogen activation in rodent models of acute pancreatitis. *Clin Invest.* (2009) 119:3340–55. doi: 10.1172/JCI38674

89. Vrolyk V, Singh B. Animal models to study the role of pulmonary intravascular macrophages in spontaneous and induced acute pancreatitis. *Cell Tissue Res.* (2020) 380:207–22. doi: 10.1007/s00441-020-03211-y

90. Menger MD, Plusczyk T, Vollmar B. Microcirculatory derangements in acute pancreatitis. *J Hepatobiliary Pancreat Surg.* (2001) 8:187–94. doi: 10.1007/s005340170015

91. Frossard JL, Saluja A, Bhagat L, Lee HS, Bhatia M, Hofbauer B, et al. The role of intercellular adhesion molecule 1 and neutrophils in acute pancreatitis and pancreatitis-associated lung injury. *Gastroenterology.* (1999) 116:694–701. doi: 10.1016/s0016-5085(99)70192-7

92. Zhao X, Dib M, Wang X, Widegren B, Andersson R. Influence of mast cells on the expression of adhesion molecules on circulating and migrating leukocytes in acute pancreatitis-associated lung injury. *Lung.* (2005) 183:253–64. doi: 10.1007/s00408-004-2538-8

93. Gao ZM, Sui JD, Fan R, Qu W, Dong X, Sun D. Emodin protects against acute pancreatitis associated lung injury by Inhibiting NLPR3 inflammasome activation via Nrf2/ HO-1 signaling. *Drug Des Devel Ther.* (2020) 14:1971–82. doi: 10.2147/DDDT.S247103

94. Han X, Wang Y, Chen H, Zhang J, Xu C, Li J, et al. Enhancement of ICAM-1 via the JAK2/STAT3 signaling pathway in a rat model of severe acute pancreatitis-associated lung injury. *Exp Ther Med.* (2016) 11:788–96. doi: 10.3892/etm.2016.2988

95. Sochor M, Richter S, Schmidt A, Hempel S, Hopt UT, Keck T. Inhibition of matrix metalloproteinase-9 with doxycycline reduces pancreatitis-associated lung injury. *Digestion.* (2009) 80:65–73. doi: 10.1159/000212080

96. Yang S, Song Y, Wang Q, Liu Y, Wu Z, Duan X, et al. Daphnetin ameliorates acute lung injury in mice with severe acute pancreatitis by inhibiting the JAK2–STAT3 pathway. *Sci Rep.* (2021) 11:1–11. doi: 10.1038/s41598-021-91008-6

97. Bumbasirevic V, Radenkovic D, Jankovic Z. Severe acute pancreatitis: overall and early versus late mortality in intensive care units. *Pancreas.* (2009) 38:122–5. doi: 10.1097/MPA.0b013e31818a392f

98. Zou XP, Chen M, Wei W, Cao J, Chen L, Tian M. Effects of enteral immunonutrition on the maintenance of gut barrier function and immune function in pigs with severe acute pancreatitis. *JPEN J Parenter Enteral Nutr.* (2010) 34:554–66. doi: 10.1177/0148607110362691

99. Kylanpaa ML, Repo H, Puolakkainen PA. Inflammation and immunosuppression in severe acute pancreatitis. *World J Gastroenterol.* (2010) 16:2867–72. doi: 10.3748/wjg.v16.i23.2867

100. Huang L, Jiang Y, Sun Z, Gao Z, Wang J, Zhang D. Autophagy strengthens intestinal mucosal barrier by attenuating oxidative stress in severe acute pancreatitis. *Dig Dis Sci.* (2018) 63:910–9. doi: 10.1007/s10620-018-4962-2

101. Schietroma M, Pessia B, Carlei F, Mariani P, Amicucci G. Intestinalperme ability and systemic endotoxemia in patients with acute pancreatitis. *Ann Ital Chir.* (2016) 87:138–44.

102. Tian R, Tan JT, Wang RL, Xie H, Qian YB, Yu KL. The role of intestinal mucosa oxidative stress in gut barrier dysfunction of severe acute pancreatitis. *Eur Rev Med Pharmacol Sci.* (2013) 17:349–55.

103. Tiszlavicz Z, Szabolcs A, Takacs T, Farkas G, Kovacs-Nagy R, Szantai E, et al. Polymorphisms of beta defensins are associated with the risk of severe acute pancreatitis. *Pancreatology.* (2010) 10:483–90. doi: 10.1159/000276987

104. Arike L, Hansson GC. The densely O-Glycosylated MUC2 mucin protects the intestine and provides food for the commensal bacteria. *J Mol Biol.* (2016) 428:3221–9. doi: 10.1016/j.jmb.2016.02.010

105. Feng DX, Peng W, Chen YF, Chen T, Tian JY, Si HR, et al. Down-regulation of aquaporin 1 in rats with experimental acute necrotizing pancreatitis. *Pancreas.* (2012) 41:1092–8. doi: 10.1097/MPA.0b013e318249938e

106. Esrefoglu M. Experimental and clinical evidence of antioxidant therapy in acute pancreatitis. *World J Gastroenterol.* (2012) 18:5533–41.

107. Yang F, Xie J, Wang W, Xie Y, Sun H, Jin Y, et al. Regional arterial infusion with lipoxin A4 attenuates experimental severe acute pancreatitis. *PLoS One.* (2014) 9:e108525. doi: 10.1371/journal.pone.0108525

108. Dong Z, Shang H, Chen YQ, Xu L, She S. Sulforaphane protects pancreatic acinar cell injury by modulating Nrf2-mediated oxidative stress and NLRP3 inflammatory pathway. *Oxid Med Cell Longev.* (2016) 2016:7864150. doi: 10.1155/2016/7864150

109. Yu QH, Zhang PX, Liu Y, Liu W, Yin N. Hyperbaric oxygen preconditioning protects the lung against acute pancreatitis induced injury via attenuating inflammation and oxidative stress in a nitric oxide dependent manner. *Biochem Biophys Res Commun.* (2016) 478:93–100. doi: 10.1016/j.bbrc.2016.07.087

110. Alfieri A, Ong AC, Kammerer RA, Solanky T, Bate S, Tasab M, et al. Angiopoietin-1 regulates microvascular reactivity and protects the microcirculation during acute endothelial dysfunction: role of eNOS and VE-cadherin. *Pharmacol Res.* (2014) 80:43–51. doi: 10.1016/j.phrs.2013.12.008

111. Kim S, Kwon J. COMP-Ang1 inhibits apoptosis as well as improves the attenuated osteogenic differentiation of mesenchymal stem cells induced by advanced glycation end products. *Biochim Biophys Acta.* (2013) 1830:4928–34. doi: 10.1016/j.bbagen.2013.06.035

112. Anand SK, Singh JA, Tikoo SK. Effect of bovine adenovirus 3 on mitochondria. *Vet Res.* (2014) 45:45. doi: 10.1186/1297-9716-45-45

113. Chan DC. Dynamic organelles in disease, aging, and development. *Cell.* (2006) 125:1241–52. doi: 10.1016/j.cell.2006.06.010

114. Niklison MV, Chirou F, Dupuy L, Gallego SM, Barreiro-Arcos ML, Avila C, et al. Microcin J25 triggers cytochrome crelease through irreversible damage of mitochondrial proteins and lipids. *Int Biochem Cell Biol.* (2010) 42:273–81. doi: 10.1016/j.biocel.2009.11.002

115. Mittal A, Hickey AJ, Chai CC, Loveday BP, Thompson N, Dare A, et al. Early organ-specific mitochondrial dysfunction of jejunum and lung found in rats with experimental acute pancreatitis. *HPB (Oxford).* (2011) 13:332–41. doi: 10.1111/j.1477-2574.2010.00290.x

116. Sanna MI, Jyrki MK. Effect of acute pancreatitis on porcine intestine: a morphological study. *Uitrastruct Pathol.* (2013) 37:127–38. 2012.745638 doi: 10.3109/01913123

117. Blenkiron C, Askelund KJ, Shanbhag ST, Chakraborty M, Petrov MS, Delahunt B, et al. MicroRNAs in mesenteric lymph and plasma during acute pancreatitis. *Ann Surg.* (2014) 260:341–7. doi: 10.1097/SLA.0000000000000447

118. Zheng XL, Yang Y, Wang BJ, Tang HQ, Zhou XY. To discuss the exterior and interior relationship between lung and large intestine from the perspective of changes of the pulmonary andintestinal function under pathological state. *China J Tradit Chin Med Pharm.* (2014) 29:120–3.

119. Zhu JY, Li Y, Zhang M, Li J, Li JY, Wu FS, et al. Pharmacokinetics and pharmacodynamics of Shengjiang decoction in rats with acute pancreatitis for protecting against multiple organ injury. *World J Gastroenterol.* (2017) 23:8169–81. doi: 10.3748/wjg.v23.i46.8169

120. Liu H, Li W, Wang X, Li J, Yu W. Early gut mucosal dysfunction in patients with acute pancreatitis. *Pancreas.* (2008) 36:192–6.

121. Zhang XP, Zhang J, Song QL, Chen HQ. Mechanism of acute pancreatitis complicated with injury of intestinal mucosa barrier. *J Zhejiang Univ Sci B.* (2007) 8:888–95. doi: 10.1631/jzus.2007.B0888

122. Xu GF, Guo MZ, Tian Q, Wu GZ, Zou XP, Zhang WJ. Increased of serum high-mobility group box chromosomal protein 1 correlated with intestinal mucosal barrier injury in patients with severe acute pancreatitis. *World J Emerg Surg.* (2014) 9:61. doi: 10.1186/1749-7922-9-61

123. Chen X, Zhao HX, Bai C, Zhou XY. Blockade of high-mobility group box 1 attenuates intestinal mucosal barrier dysfunction in experimental acute pancreatitis. *Sci Rep.* (2017) 7:1–10. doi: 10.1038/s41598-017-07094-y

124. Kang R, Lotze MT, Zeh HJ, Billiar TR, Tang D. Cell death and DAMPs in acute pancreatitis. *Mol Med.* (2014) 20:466–77. doi: 10.2119/molmed.2014.00117

125. Lin Y, Lin LJ, Jin Y, Cao Y, Zhang Y, Zheng CQ, et al. Correlation between serum levels of high mobility group box-1 protein and pancreatitis: a meta-analysis. *Biomed Res Int.* (2015) 2015:430185. doi: 10.1155/2015/430185

126. Capurso G, Zerboni G, Signoretti M, Valente R, Stigliano S, Piciucchi M, et al. Role of the gut barrier in acute pancreatitis. *World J Gastroenterol.* (2012) 26:2187–93. doi: 10.3748/wjg.v26.i18.2187

127. Guo ZZ, Wang P, Yi ZH, Huang ZY, Tang CW. The crosstalk between gut inflammation and gastrointestinal disorders during acute pancreatitis. *Curr Pharm Des.* (2014) 20:1051–62. doi: 10.2174/13816128113199990414

128. Jeffery TK, Morrell NW. Molecular and cellular basis of pulmonary vascular remodeling in pulmonary hypertension. *Prog Cardiovasc Dis.* (2002) 45:173–202. doi: 10.1053/pcad.2002.130041

129. Chen GS, Huang KF, Huang CC, Wang JY. Thaliporphine derivative improves acute lung injury after traumatic brain injury. *Biomed Res Int.* (2015) 2015:729831. doi: 10.1155/2015/729831

130. Sakai H, Sagara A, Matsumoto K, Hasegawa S, Sato K, Nishizaki M, et al. 5-fluorouracil induces diarrhea with changes in the expression of inflammatory cytokines and aquaporins in mouse intestines. *PLoS One.* (2013) 8:e54788. doi: 10.1371/journal.pone.0054788

131. Kunzelmann K, Mall M. Electrolyte transport in the mammalian colon: mechanisms and implications for disease. *Physiol Rev.* (2002) 82:245–89. doi: 10.1152/physrev.00026.2001

132. Penalva JC, Martinez J, Laveda R, Esteban A, Muñoz C, Sáez J, et al. A study of intestinal permeability in relation to the inflammatory response and plasma endocab IgM levels in patients with acute pancreatitis. *J Clin Gastroenterol.* (2004) 38:512–7. doi: 10.1097/01.mcg.0000129060.46654.e0

133. Guo YY, Li HX, Zhang Y, He WH. Hypertriglyceridemia-induced acute pancreatitis: progress on disease mechanisms and treatment modalities. *Discov Med.* (2019) 27:101–9.

134. Yu J, Lan N, Zhang XY, Zhang J, Abdel-Razek O, Wang G. Surfactant prorein D dampens lung injury by suppressing NLRP3 inflammasome activation NF-κB signaling in acute pancreatitis. *Shock.* (2019) 51:557–68. doi: 10.1097/SHK.0000000000001244

135. Awla D, Abdulla A, Regn S. TLR4 but not TLR2 regulates inflammation and tissue damage in acute pancreatitis induced by retrograde infusion of taurocholate. *Inflamm Res.* (2011) 60:1093–8. doi: 10.1007/s00011-011-0370-1

136. Chen WW, Yuan CC, Lu YY. Tanshinone IIA protects against acute pancreatitis in mice by inhibiting oxidative stress via the Nrf2/ROS pathway. *Oxid Med Cell Longev.* (2020) 2020:5390482. doi: 10.1155/2020/5390482

137. Piao XH, Zou YP, Sui XD, Liu B, Meng F, Li S, et al. Hydrostatin-SN10 ameliorates pancreatitis induced lung injury by affecting IL-6 induced JAK2/STAT3 associated inflammation and oxidative stress. *Oxid Med Cell Longev.* (2019) 2019:9659757. doi: 10.1155/2019/9659757

Myxoinflammatory Fibroblastic Sarcoma of the Parotid Gland

Changhong Wei[1,2†], Xuejia Yang[2†], Pingping Guo[3†], Xiaoyu Chen[1], Chunjun Li[1], Jun Chen[1*] and Sufang Zhou[2,4*]

[1] Department of Pathology, Guangxi Medical University Cancer Hospital, Nanning, China, [2] National Center for International Research of Bio-Targeting Theranostics, Guangxi Key Laboratory of Bio-Targeting Theranostics, Collaborative Innovation Center for Targeting Tumor Diagnosis and Therapy, Guangxi Medical University, Nanning, China, [3] Department of Ultrasound Imaging, Guangxi Medical University Cancer Hospital, Nanning, China, [4] Department of Biochemistry and Molecular Biology, School of Pre-clinical Science, Guangxi Medical University, Nanning, China

*Correspondence:
Jun Chen
chenjun2826@163.com
Sufang Zhou
zsf200000@163.com

[†] These authors have contributed equally to this work

Myxoinflammatory fibroblastic sarcoma (MIFS) is a rare, low-grade malignant soft tissue tumor. Most of the previously reported cases about this tumor were diagnosed within the soft tissues. Here, we report a unique case of MIFS of the right parotid gland in a 39-year-old Chinese male. The tumor primarily consisted of an inflammatory area and a mucus-like area in a migratory distribution. A number of lymphocytes, neutrophils, viral-like cells with large nucleoli, and eosinophilic cytoplasm or Reed-Sternberg-like cells, as well as spindle cells and epithelial-like aberrant cells, were observed within the tumor. They were found to express Vimentin and CD10 protein and no other specific immunohistochemical markers. The various cytomorphology and immunohistochemical features of this tumor were highly consistent with MIFS found in other sites. Therefore, several leading pathologists ultimately confirmed the final diagnosis of MIFS in the right parotid gland after repeated deliberation. To our knowledge, this is the first case of MIFS occurring in the parotid gland. Thus, our study provides a novel basis for identifying the biological behavior of the tumor in MIFS and also allows us to better understand the pathology of this rare tumor.

Keywords: myxoinflammatory fibroblastic sarcoma, MIFS, soft tissue tumor, Vimentin, parotid gland

INTRODUCTION

Myxoinflammatory fibroblastic sarcoma (MIFS) is a rare, slow-growing, low-grade malignant soft tissue tumor (1). It was first described by Montgomery et al. (2), and several cases have since been reported around the world (3, 4). Clinically, MIFS is considered to be a superficial tumor found within the soft tissues, and generally manifests itself as a painless subcutaneous mass in the distal limb in adults. However, in recent years, a proportion of cases have been reported in several other non-extremity sites, such as the breast, buttocks, chest wall, and thighs (3, 5, 6). However, MIFS of the parotid gland has not been reported and described previously. In this study, we present a unique case of MIFS of the parotid gland in a Chinese patient with a characteristic histomorphology, consisting of inflammatory and mucin-like areas. It was characterized by the prominent morphological presentation of aberrant large cells, containing huge nucleoli with a typical immunophenotype (Vimentin protein positive), and other features that were consistent with the previously reported MIFS in other sites. The study was approved by the Institutional Review Board of the Cancer Hospital of Guangxi Medical University and was performed according to the principles of the "Declaration of Helsinki." Written informed consent for this study was obtained from the patient prior to the study.

CASE PRESENTATION

Clinical Findings

A 39-year-old male patient was diagnosed with a right submandibular mass in the outpatient clinic of our hospital 2 months ago. The physical examination showed that the neck curvature and mobility were normal, no lateral curvature was noticed, and the right lower jaw could reach the size of a 2 × 1-cm mass. Additionally, the mass was hard, had unclear boundary and blunt edge with poor activity, but no other abnormality was observed in other parts. After the patient was admitted to the hospital, the clinician used a fine needle for aspiration of cells from the tumor. The pathological examination further revealed that the nuclear atypical cells were visible, and the malignant possibility was not excluded. The ultrasound of the neck showed a substantial lesion of the right parotid gland, and the CT examination displayed a small

nodule below the parotid gland (**Figures 1A,B**), which was initially considered as a benign tumor or tumor-like lesion of the parotid gland. His laboratory tests for the blood routine analysis, liver function, renal function, blood sugar, and thyroid function were found to be within the normal range. His HIV, HBsAg, and HCV serology were also negative. Under the general anesthesia, the right parotid mass resection and right facial nerve anatomy were performed and, thereafter, submitted for the histopathological examination.

Pathologic Findings

Moreover, on the gross specimen, there was a gray-red, gray-yellow nodular mass within the parotid gland tissue, the size was 1.8 × 1.5 × 1 cm, and there was a complete capsule. The cut surface was grayish-yellow, gray, and white, soft, mucoid, and exhibited no hemorrhagic necrosis.

Histopathological microscopy showed that the tumor consisted of the different inflammatory regions as well as mucin-like regions, and the inflammatory cells were mostly lymphocytes or neutrophils. The inflammatory regions showed large nucleoli, and the cytoplasm was eosinophilic with viral-like cells or Reed-Sternberg-like cells, and it exhibited different degrees of fibrosis. The mucus region was primarily composed of spindle cells and tissue-like or epithelial-like malformed cells. The interstitial was hyaline degeneration, and small amounts of scattered multinucleated giant cells were visible in the lesion. Transitional distribution of inflammatory and mucous areas, visible large cells of nucleoli, and mitotic figures were not commonly observed, but mildly shaped spindle cells were seen in the inflammatory area. A part of the area was characterized by mucus and fibrotic regional composition, accompanied by

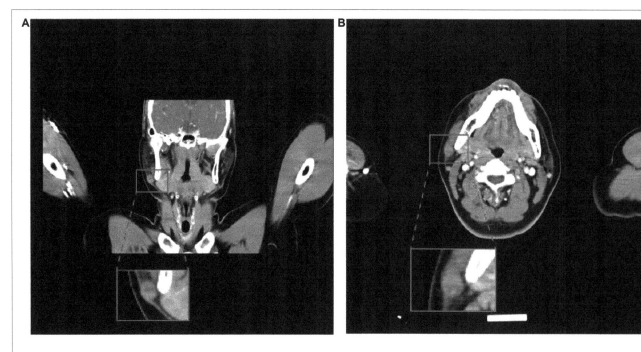

FIGURE 1 | Images of the tumor. Computed tomography showed a nodule on the lower right side of the parotid gland. **(A)** Coronal plane; **(B)** transverse plane.

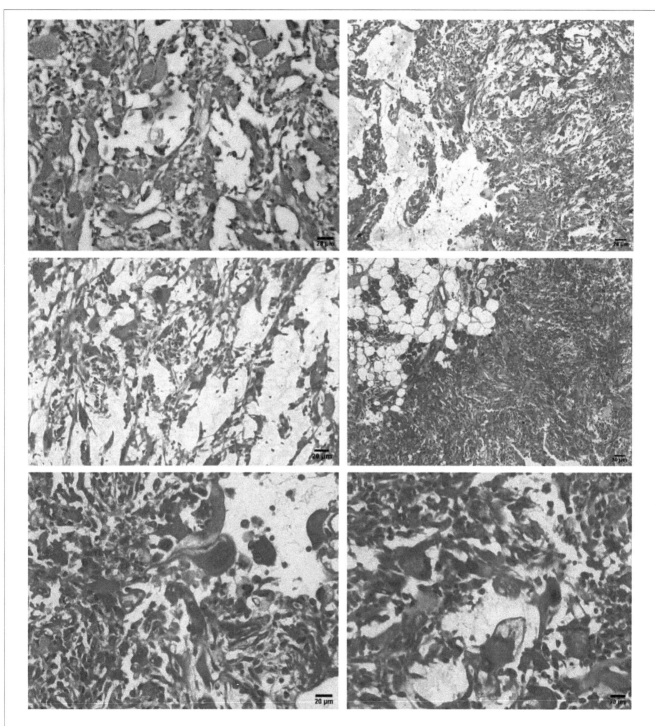

FIGURE 2 | Histology and immunohistochemistry of the tumor. **(A)** Immunohistochemical results showed Vimentin diffuse positive (+) (IHC staining, ×100). **(B)** The tumor consisted of the mucous area and the fibrous area with inflammatory cell infiltration in the mucus-like area, and the various fusiform cells can be connected to each other to form a network structure (H&E staining, ×100). **(C)** At the junction of the mucous area and the fiber area, inflammatory cell infiltration could be observed (H&E staining, ×100). **(D)** The tumor can be infiltrated into the parotid tissue (H&E staining, ×100). **(E)** Large malformed cells with large nucleoli can be noted (H&E staining, ×200). **(F)** The "inclusion body" nucleolus resembling Reed-Sternberg cells has been recognized as one of the characteristics of mucinous inflammatory fibroblastic sarcoma (H&E staining, ×200).

lymphocyte or neutrophil infiltration. The most characteristic morphological manifestations were the presence of the large cells with huge nucleoli, with interstitial inflammatory cell reactions. Moreover, visible in the mucus area were the pseudo-fat cells, spindle cells involving adipose tissue, whereas the phagocytic cells can also be seen in some areas (**Figures 2B–F, 3**).

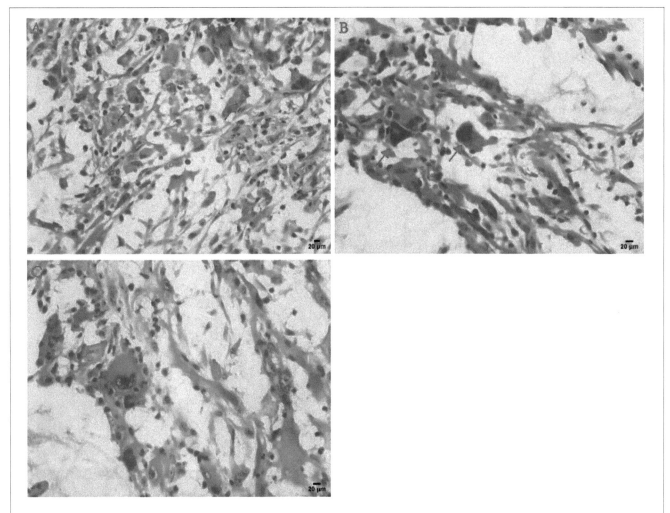

FIGURE 3 | Atypical microscopic features in MIFS. **(A)** Virus-like cells with abundant cytoplasm and nucleoli (arrows). **(B)** Large malformed cells with two enlarged nuclei shown by arrows; **(C)** R-S cell-like tumor cells with markedly large nucleoli (arrows).

Immunohistochemical Findings

Immunohistochemistry revealed that the tumor cells expressed Vimentin and CD10 (diffuse positive) (**Figures 2A, 4A**), lymphocytes expressed LCA, macrophages expressed CD163 and CD68, Ki-67 index was 10%, CK, SMA, P63, CD34, CD1a, D2-40, and S-100 were negative (**Table 1** and **Figure 4**).

According to tumor imaging, microscopic histomorphology, and comprehensive immunohistochemical analysis, the authors finally diagnosed the tumor as parotid myxoinflammatory fibroblastic sarcoma. The patient is currently in good condition and is undergoing regular follow-up in our hospital, and no recurrence or metastasis has been found.

DISCUSSION

Based on the previously published review of domestic and foreign literature, this is the first report describing the occurrence of MIFS in the parotid gland. It has been reported that MIFS usually presents as a slow-growing painless mass, mostly in adults, and the peak age of the onset is 30–50 years old, the average age is about 40 years old. A small number of cases also occur in children or adolescents, and tumors primarily arise in the soft tissue location of the distal part of the limb (1, 7). In this study, we have summarized the clinicopathological features of MIFS reported in the literature in the rare sites (non-bone and soft tissue, since 1998) (**Table 2**) (6, 8, 9). Clinically, MIFS may be similar to benign lesions and can be often misdiagnosed as the slippery membrane inflammation, ganglion cysts, or giant cell tumor of the tendon sheath. CT or MRI usually presents as diffuse enhancement, lobulated, subcutaneous mass with non-specific magnetic resonance imaging features, thereby suggesting the presence of benign or malignant lesions (1).

The rich and diverse histological performance of MIFS is a major challenge in the diagnosis of this tumor (10). For example, the ratio of mucin-like areas, fibroinflammatory areas, and the cell area can effectively vary from case to case, and the number of cells with inclusion body-like nuclei is generally considered to be the major marker of MIFS. Another major challenge in diagnosis is the presence of severe inflammatory

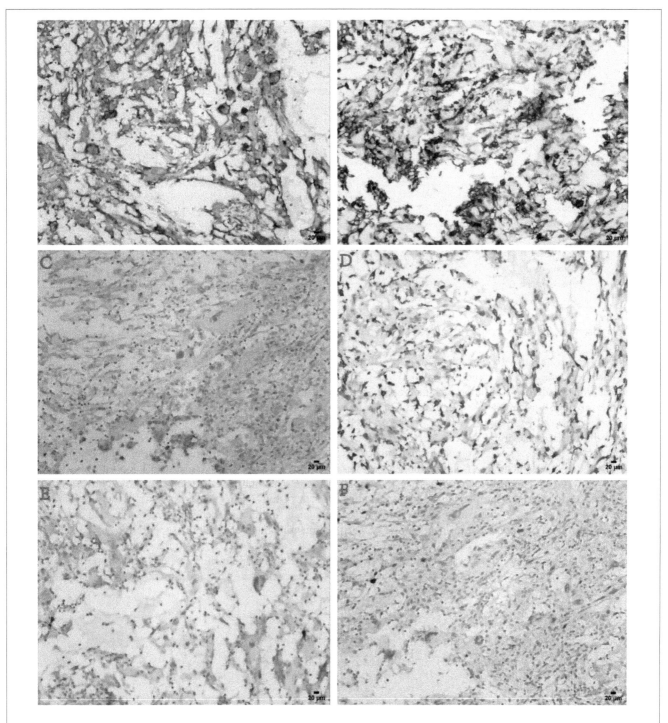

FIGURE 4 | Immunohistochemical findings in MIFS. **(A)** The tumor spindle cells and malformed cells were strongly positive for CD10. **(B)** Infiltrated inflammatory cells were strongly positive for LCA. **(C)** The reactive histiocytes were positive for CD68. **(D)** Reactive histiocytes were positive for CD163. **(E)** The tumor cells were negative for D2-40. **(F)** The tumor cells expressed low-proliferative Ki-67 (about 10%).

reactions, which are mediated primarily by the lymphocytes and lymphoid aggregates-infiltrated tumor cells. These may be mistaken for inflammatory processes or other malignant tumors, such as lymphoma mucinous fibrosarcoma (11). In the mucus background, the tumor spindle cells and epithelioid cells are usually connected to each other to form a complex network structure, and a large number of the neutrophils, macrophages, and plasma cells can be seen, but the mitotic figures and necrosis are not commonly observed in this tumor. Immunohistochemistry has been found to play a very limited

TABLE 1 | A summary of the primary antibodies used and the results of immunohistochemistry.

Antibody	Source	Dilution	Result
CKpan	Maixin, Fuzhou, China	1:100	−
Vimentin	Maixin, Fuzhou, China	1:150	+++
LCA	Maixin, Fuzhou, China	1:100	+
CD68	Maixin, Fuzhou, China	1:100	+
Ki-67	Maixin, Fuzhou, China	1:200	+ (10%)
SMA	Maixin, Fuzhou, China	1:100	−
P63	Maixin, Fuzhou, China	1:100	−
CD34	Maixin, Fuzhou, China	1:100	−
Calponin	Maixin, Fuzhou, China	1:100	−
SMMHC	Maixin, Fuzhou, China	1:100	−
CD1a	Maixin, Fuzhou, China	1:100	−
S-100	Maixin, Fuzhou, China	1:100	−
CD163	Maixin, Fuzhou, China	1:100	+
CD10	Maixin, Fuzhou, China	1:100	+
D2-40	Maixin, Fuzhou, China	1:100	−

role in the diagnosis of MIFS because it has no specific tumor markers (12).

In the present study, the main features for the diagnosis of MIFS included areas of solid spindle cells, alternating with myxoid foci with the diffuse infiltration of inflammatory cells. Unlike other previously reported cases, a random distribution of the larger atypical cells was seen in our case, including Reed-Sternberg cells, variants of virus-like cells with inclusion-like nucleoli, and large malformed cells. Immunohistochemistry has been widely used in MIFS, but no specific immunophenotype has been found. However, differential responsiveness to the various markers has been observed in the previous studies, including Vimentin, D2-40, CD68, bcl-1, CD10, and CD163 (3, 12). In the present study, we found consistent and strong immunoreactivity for Vimentin and CD10 in the tumor cells in this case. Moreover, another novel finding of our study was the low expression of the proliferative marker Ki-67, and the most characteristic

phenomenon was that, in the large malformed cells and R-S like-cells, Ki-67 was almost absent. These pieces of evidence suggested that these atypical cells were the degenerative tumor cells that were biologically inactive.

The cytogenetic analysis of MIFS further revealed complex genetic abnormalities (13), including a circular chromosome formed on the Chromosome 3, a translocation of chromosome t (1:10) (p22: q24), rearrangement of *TGFBR3* and *MGEA5* genes (14). Some other cases showed *TGFBR3* and *MGEA5* gene rearrangement, which led to an upregulation of NPM3 and FGF8, accompanied by amplification of the *VGLL3* locus (10, 15).

Most cases of MIFS have demonstrated low malignant potential. However, 22–67% of cases can potentially recur, and only a few cases can metastasize (3), but high-grade MIFS may lead to more adverse progression (16). The best treatment for MIFS is complete surgical resection to ensure that the incisal margin is negative; however, the beneficial impact of radiotherapy and chemotherapy remains unclear (17). Our patient remained in good condition after 7 months of follow-up, and no recurrence or metastasis was observed.

CONCLUSION

In summary, we report that the first case of MIFS was detected in the parotid gland. However, due to its complex histological morphology and inflammatory background, we need to distinguish it from other similar lesions, such as inflammatory myofibroblastic sarcoma and myxofibrosarcomas, to facilitate accurate diagnosis. Although no specific immunohistochemical or molecular markers are available for the diagnosis of this tumor. In addition to describing the classical histological features in this study. Our results supported the use of a distinct panel of immunohistochemical markers, including CD10 and Vimentin, might be helpful support for MIFS diagnostics in many equivocal cases. At present, the diagnosis of MIFS is still mainly based on clinicopathological diagnosis, which needs to be combined with the appropriate clinical environment

TABLE 2 | A summary of clinicopathological features of MIFS reported in the literature from the rare sites (non-bone and soft tissue, reviewed since 1998).

Author/year	Age/gender	Location	Pathological features	Treatment	Follow-up (mo)	Outcome
Current study	39/M	Parotid gland	The tumor consisted of inflammatory regions and mucin-like regions, the inflammatory cells were mostly lymphocytes or neutrophils. The most characteristic morphological manifestations are large cells with large nucleoli, with interstitial inflammatory cell reaction.	Surgery	28	No recurrence or metastasis
Jain et al. (8)	7-month-old infant	Eyeball	A mixed cellular infiltrate composed of numerous neutrophils, larger cells appeared to be binucleate (Reed-Sternberg-like or virocyte-like)	Resection	NA	NA
Auw-Haedrich et al. (6)	27/F	Iris	Tumor contained mucinous and cellular areas with high grade of polymorphy and a large variety of cell sizes and forms	Resection	15	No recurrence
Numminen et al. (9)	51/M	Nose	The tumor was heterogeneous in composition, with myxoid, relatively acellular areas alternating with cellular areas	Surgery	48	No recurrence or metastasis

NA, not available; mo, month; F, female; M, male.

and characteristic histomorphological findings to significantly improve the treatment outcome.

AUTHOR CONTRIBUTIONS

JC and SZ read and approved the final manuscript. CW performed the writing of the manuscript. XY and PG organized the material and helped with the analysis. XC carried out experiments. CL and JC performed the pathological analysis and diagnosed the patient. All authors wrote and revised the manuscript.

REFERENCES

1. Baheti AD, Tirumani SH, Rosenthal MH, Howard SA, Shinagare AB, Ramaiya NH, et al. Myxoid soft-tissue neoplasms: comprehensive update of the taxonomy and MRI features. *AJR Am J Roentgenol.* (2015) 2:374–85. doi: 10.2214/ajr.14.12888

2. Montgomery EA, Devaney KO, Giordano TJ, Weiss SW. Inflammatory myxohyaline tumor of distal extremities with virocyte or reed-sternberg-like cells: a distinctive lesion with features simulating inflammatory conditions, Hodgkin's disease, and various sarcomas. *Mod Pathol.* (1998) 4:384–91.

3. Laskin WB, Fetsch JF, Miettinen M. Myxoinflammatory fibroblastic sarcoma: a clinicopathologic analysis of 104 cases, with emphasis on predictors of outcome. *Am J Surg Pathol.* (2014) 1:1–12. doi: 10.1097/PAS.0b013e31829f3d85

4. Patne SC, Katiyar R, Gupta SK. Intramuscular myxoinflammatory fibroblastic sarcoma of the thigh. *Pathology.* (2016) 5:527–9. doi: 10.1016/j.pathol.2016.05.003

5. Gaetke-Udager K, Yablon CM, Lucas DR, Morag Y. Myxoinflammatory fibroblastic sarcoma: spectrum of disease and imaging presentation. *Skeletal Radiol.* (2016) 3:347–56. doi: 10.1007/s00256-015-2286-2

6. Auw-Haedrich C, Mentzel T, Reinhard T. Myxoinflammatory fibroblastic sarcoma of the iris. *Pathology.* (2017) 7:794–5. doi: 10.1016/j.pathol.2017.08.016

7. Kao YC, Ranucci V, Zhang L, Sung YS, Athanasian EA, Swanson D, et al. Recurrent BRAF gene rearrangements in myxoinflammatory fibroblastic sarcomas, but not hemosiderotic fibrolipomatous tumors. *Am J Surg Pathol.* (2017) 11:1456–65. doi: 10.1097/pas.0000000000000899

8. Jain E, Kini L, Alaggio R, Ranganathan S. Myxoinflammatory fibroblastic sarcoma of eyeball in an infant: a rare presentation. *Int J Surg Pathol.* (2020) 3:306–9. doi: 10.1177/1066896919879497

9. Numminen J, Bizaki A, Kujansivu J, Huovinen S, Rautiainen M. Myxoinflammatory fibroblastic sarcoma of the nose: first reported case at an unusual location (nasal dorsum), with a review of the literature. *Ear Nose Throat J.* (2016) 3:E32–5. doi: 10.1177/014556131609500304

10. Lucas DR. Myxoinflammatory fibroblastic sarcoma: review and update. *Arch Pathol Lab Med.* (2017) 11:1503–7. doi: 10.5858/arpa.2017-0219-RA

11. Chiu HY, Chen JS, Hsiao CH, Tsai TF. Transformation of myxofibrosarcoma into myxoinflammatory fibroblastic sarcoma. *J Dermatol.* (2012) 4:422–4. doi: 10.1111/j.1346-8138.2011.01297.x

12. Suster D, Michal M, Huang H, Ronen S, Springborn S, Debiec-Rychter M, et al. Myxoinflammatory fibroblastic sarcoma: an immunohistochemical and molecular genetic study of 73 cases. *Mod Pathol.* (2020) 12:2520–33. doi: 10.1038/s41379-020-0580-6

13. Arbajian E, Hofvander J, Magnusson L, Mertens F. Deep sequencing of myxoinflammatory fibroblastic sarcoma. *Genes Chromosomes Cancer.* (2020) 5:309–17. doi: 10.1002/gcc.22832

14. Liu H, Sukov WR, Ro JY. The t(1;10)(p22;q24) TGFBR3/MGEA5 translocation in pleomorphic hyalinizing angiectatic tumor, myxoinflammatory fibroblastic sarcoma, and hemosiderotic fibrolipomatous tumor. *Arch Pathol Lab Med.* (2019) 2:212–21. doi: 10.5858/arpa.2017-0412-RA

15. Ieremia E, Thway K. Myxoinflammatory fibroblastic sarcoma: morphologic and genetic updates. *Arch Pathol Lab Med.* (2014) 10:1406–11. doi: 10.5858/arpa.2013-0549-RS

16. Michal M, Kazakov DV, Hadravsky L, Kinkor Z, Kuroda N, Michal M. High-grade myxoinflammatory fibroblastic sarcoma: a report of 23 cases. *Ann Diagn Pathol.* (2015) 3:157–63. doi: 10.1016/j.anndiagpath.2015.03.012

17. Tejwani A, Kobayashi W, Chen YL, Rosenberg AE, Yoon S, Raskin KA, et al. Management of acral myxoinflammatory fibroblastic sarcoma. *Cancer.* (2010) 24:5733–9. doi: 10.1002/cncr.25567

24

Delta-Like Protein 3 Expression in Paired Chemonaive and Chemorelapsed Small Cell Lung Cancer Samples

Christiane Kuempers [1]*, Tobias Jagomast [1], Rosemarie Krupar [2], Finn-Ole Paulsen [1,3],
Carsten Heidel [1], Julika Ribbat-Idel [1], Christian Idel [4], Bruno Märkl [5], Martin Anlauf [6],
Sabina Berezowska [7,8], Markus Tiemann [9], Hans Bösmüller [10], Falko Fend [10],
Barbara Kalsdorf [11], Sabine Bohnet [12], Eva Dreyer [1], Verena Sailer [1], Jutta Kirfel [1] and
Sven Perner [1,2,13]

[1] Institute of Pathology, Luebeck, University Hospital Schleswig-Holstein, Luebeck, Germany, [2] Pathology, Research Center Borstel-Leibniz Lung Center, Borstel, Germany, [3] Department of Oncology, Hematology and Bone Marrow Transplantation With Division of Pneumology, University Medical Center Hamburg-Eppendorf, Hamburg, Germany, [4] Department of Otorhinolaryngology, Luebeck, University of Luebeck and University Hospital Schleswig-Holstein, Luebeck, Germany, [5] Medical Faculty, General Pathology and Molecular Diagnostics, University Augsburg, Augsburg, Germany, [6] Institute of Pathology, Cytology and Molecular Pathology Limburg, Limburg, Germany, [7] Department of Laboratory Medicine and Pathology, Institute of Pathology, Lausanne University Hospital and University of Lausanne, Lausanne, Switzerland, [8] Institute of Pathology, University of Bern, Bern, Switzerland, [9] Institute for Hematopathology, Hamburg, Germany, [10] Institute of Pathology and Neuropathology University Hospital Tuebingen, Tuebingen, Germany, [11] Medical Clinic, Research Center Borstel-Leibniz Lung Center, Borstel, Germany, [12] Department of Pulmonology, Luebeck, University Hospital Schleswig-Holstein, Luebeck, Germany, [13] Airway Research Center North (ARCN), Member of the German Center for Lung Research (DZL), Borstel, Germany

*Correspondence:
Christiane Kuempers
christiane.kuempers@uksh.de

Rovalpituzumab tesirine (Rova-T), an antibody-drug conjugate directed against Delta-like protein 3 (DLL3), is under development for patients with small cell lung cancer (SCLC). DLL3 is expressed on the majority of SCLC samples. Because SCLC is rarely biopsied in the course of disease, data regarding DLL3 expression in relapses is not available. The aim of this study was to investigate the expression of DLL3 in chemorelapsed (but untreated with Rova-T) SCLC samples and compare the results with chemonaive counterparts. Two evaluation methods to assess DLL3 expression were explored. Additionally, we assessed if DLL3 expression of chemorelapsed and/or chemonaive samples has prognostic impact and if it correlates with other clinicopathological data. The study included 30 paired SCLC samples, which were stained with an anti DLL3 antibody. DLL3 expression was assessed using tumor proportion score (TPS) and H-score and was categorized as DLL3 low (TPS < 50%, H-score ≤ 150) and DLL3 high (TPS ≥ 50%, H-score > 150). Expression data were correlated with clinicopathological characteristics. Kaplan–Meier curves were used to illustrate overall survival (OS) depending on DLL3 expression in chemonaive and chemorelapsed samples, respectively, and depending on dynamics of expression during course of therapy. DLL3 was expressed in 86.6% chemonaive and 80% chemorelapsed SCLC samples without significant differences between the two groups. However, the extent of expression varied in a substantial proportion of pairs (36.6% with TPS, 43.3% with H-score), defined as a shift from low to high or high to low expression. TPS and H-score provided comparable results. There were no profound correlations with clinicopathological data. Survival analysis revealed a trend toward a more favorable OS in DLL low-expressing chemonaive SCLC ($p = 0.57$) and, in turn, in DLL3 high-expressing chemorelapsed SCLC ($p = 0.42$) as well as in SCLC demonstrating a shift from low to high expression ($p = 0.56$) without being statistically significant. This is the first study to investigate DLL3 expression in a large cohort of rare paired chemonaive-chemorelapsed SCLC specimens. Comparative analysis revealed that DLL3 expression was not stable during the course of therapy, suggesting therapy-based alterations. Unlike in chemonaive samples, a high DLL3 expression in chemorelapsed samples indicated a trend for a more favorable prognosis. Our results highlight the importance to investigate DLL3 in latest chemorelapsed SCLC tumor tissue.

Keywords: delta-like protein 3, small cell lung cancer, paired, chemonaive, chemorelapsed

INTRODUCTION

Small cell lung cancer (SCLC) is known as a highly aggressive type of cancer with a miserable prognosis. It is the second most common lung cancer type and accounts for ~15% of lung cancer cases. Therapy remained essentially unchanged in recent years and is usually based on chemotherapy with etoposide and a platinating agent (1), whereas, lately, clinical activity of immunotherapies has been observed in patients with refractory or metastatic SCLC. In a phase 3 trial conducted by Horn et al. it was shown that the addition of the anti PD-L1 antibody atezolizumab to chemotherapy in the first-line treatment of extensive SCLC resulted in significantly longer overall survival (OS) and progression-free survival than chemotherapy alone (2). Almost all patients experience disease relapse within 3 months (3). Although SCLC-targeted therapy research has progressed, in contrast to non-small cell lung cancer (NSCLC) no personalized targeted therapy options have been derived so far. Thus, further research into the mechanism of SCLC and the exploration of new therapeutic targets for SCLC are indispensable (4).

A new promising target is Delta-like protein 3 (DLL3), a transmembrane protein found in most high-grade neuroendocrine carcinomas of the lung, including SCLC. Growing evidence supports a tumor-suppressor role for Notch-1 signaling in neuroendocrine tumors (5).

It is shown that the NOTCH receptor is mainly downregulated by DLL3, thereby inhibiting the NOTCH signaling pathway within the cell. Inactivation of Notch directs the lung stem cell to a neuroendocrine precursor cell and contributes via biallelic p53/RB loss to the onset of primary SCLC (6). In this context, the achaete-scute homolog 1 (Ascl1) gene transcription factor plays a major role. It controls crucial cellular mechanisms in SCLC such as cell growth and survival. DLL3 expression is understood as a direct downstream target of Ascl1, which interacts with the DLL3 gene promoter (7). This suggests that, during evolution of SCLC, Notch1 is inactivated, and Ascl1 and DLL3 are both activated and are, thus, counterparts to Notch1.

Therefore, one can assume that DLL3 could also be used in cancer chemotherapy to target and suppress tumor cells (8). Rovalpituzumab tesirine (Rova-T) is an antibody–drug conjugate composed of SC16, a humanized IgG1 antibody against DLL3. Rova-T selectively binds to DLL3 on target-expressing cells, is internalized, and upon proteolytic cleavage, releases the toxin pyrrolobenzodiazepine (PBD) leading to cell death (9).

In a phase I clinical trial, Rova-T was more effective in SCLC with DLL3 overexpression (defined as expression in at least 50% of cancer cells by immunohistochemistry) compared with SCLC with a low level of DLL3 expression (5). Hence, DLL3 might be a promising predictive marker for treatment of SCLC with Rova-T (8). Rova-T is currently under development for patients with SCLC positive for DLL3 (3).

Methods to evaluate DLL3 expression assessed via immunohistochemistry are not standardized so far. In the current study, the two applied methods (tumor proportion score and H-score) were previously described in literature, including in the above mentioned trial (5, 10) and compared with each other.

Although most SCLC recur after initial response to chemotherapy, relapsed tumors are usually not biopsied. The aim of our study was, therefore, to investigate the expression of DLL3 on chemorelapsed SCLC samples and to compare its expression to chemonaive counterparts. Differences in DLL3 expression between matched samples would suggest therapy-associated changes in the tumor cells. In case of a loss of DLL3 expression in chemorelapsed SCLC samples one could assume that a therapy with Rova-T is not promising. The results of the study could be used to derive which material should be tested in case of planned therapy with Rova-T in the recurrence situation.

MATERIALS AND METHODS
Cohort

In this multi-institutional retrospective study, tissue samples from chemonaive SCLC and paired recurrent SCLC after chemotherapy as well as from metastatic SCLC were collected. The final cohort included 42 patients and consisted of 30 paired chemonaive-chemorelapsed, 5 paired chemonaive primary-metastatic, and 7 unpaired chemorelapsed SCLC without a chemonaive counterpart. In the latter, from 3 patients, we had

---

Abbreviations: Ascl1, Achaete-scute homolog 1; DLL3, Delta-like protein 3; IHC, Immunohistochemistry; NSCLC, Non-small cell lung cancer; OS, overall survival; Rova-T, Rovalpituzumab tesirine; SCLC, Small cell lung cancer; SI, staining intensity; TPS, Tumor proportion score.

one sample each (only deriving from the primary site) and from 4 patients, we had several (up to 4) samples deriving from the primary site as well as from distant metastases (brain, lymph node, adrenal, liver, bone, contralateral lung). In the paired chemonaive-chemorelapsed subcohort, chemorelapsed tissue derived from local recurrences in 10 cases, from distant metastases in 19 cases (skin, brain, lymph node, bone, pleura, pericardium, breast, pancreas), and in one case, the location of the biopsied recurrent tumor was unknown. Chemonaive metastatic samples derived from adrenals, bone, liver, pleura, skin, and contralateral lung.

Patient Characteristics

The median age in the whole cohort was 63 years (range, 47–83 y), 27 (64.3%) patients were male, 15 (35.7%), were female. All patients received a platin-based chemotherapy, whereas none of the patients had received therapy with Rova-T or other therapeutic agents for example in the context of an immunotherapy. Follow-up data for 33 out of the 42 patients were available. From these, at time of last follow-up, 19 patients were deceased, and 14 were alive. Samples from 4 patients derived from autopsies. The basic clinicopathological data of our study cohort are summarized in **Table 1**.

This study was approved by the internal review board of the University of Luebeck (file number 16-277) and the respective local ethical committees.

Statistical Analyses

For the statistical analyses and data visualization, R software (version 4.0.2, R Foundation, Vienna, Austria; http://www.R-project.org) was used. To investigate differences of DLL3 expression between the group of chemonaive and chemorelapsed samples a Wilcoxon signed-rank test was used. To test if the two evaluation methods (TPS vs. H-score) give equivalent results, Pearson correlation was applied. The Wilcoxon rank-sum test was applied to correlate the site of the recurrent tumor and DLL3 expression. To analyze for correlation of DLL3 expression with clinicopathological characteristics, Fisher's exact test was used. Kaplan–Meier curves were used to illustrate OS in dependency of DLL3 expression and statistically proved by log-rank tests. A p-value of <0.05 was considered significant.

Immunohistochemistry (IHC)

IHC staining was performed according to the manufacturer's instructions, using the Ventana Discovery (Ventana Medical System) automated staining system. In brief, slides were incubated with the primary antibody DLL3 (clone SP347, Ventana, SN 678, RTU). Representative tumor blocks from FFPE tissue were cut in 4-μm thick sections.

DLL3 staining was considered positive if staining was membranous in at least 1% of tumor cells. Protein expression of DLL3 was assessed in two different ways: on the one hand by estimating the percentage of positive tumor cells from all tumor cells (tumor proportion score, TPS, range 0–100%) as previously described (5) and, on the other hand, semi-quantitatively using the H-score method according to Yan et al. by converting the staining intensity (SI) (range 0–3) and the TPS (range 0–100)

TABLE 1 | Patients' baseline characteristics.

	Total	Subcohort paired chemonaive-chemorelapsed
Patients		
Male	27	20
Female	15	10
Survival status		
Alive	14	8
Deceased	19	15
Unknown	9	7
Age at first diagnosis (years)		
Mean	63.6	63.8
Median	63	63
Range	47–83	47–79
Time span between diagnosis and last follow-up (days)		
Min.	13	121
Max.	2.728	1.436
Chemotherapy regime (partially known)		
Cisplatin + etopside	14/23 (60.9%)	8/16 (50%)
Carboplatin + etopside	9/23 (39.1%)	8/16 (50%)
Mean duration (days)	87.2	90.9
Min. duration (days)	30	30
Max. duration (days)	284	284
Palliative intention	21/23	15/16 (94%)
Adjuvant intention	1/23	0
Neoadjuvant intention	1/23	1/16 (6%)
Time span between chemonaive and chemorelapsed sample (days)		
Min.		48
Max.		1.294
Mean		404.1
Median		249
Time span between therapy initiation and relapse (days)		
Min.	15	92
Max.	1.297	1.297
Mean	430.9	421.7
Median	333.5	248
Tumor site		
Primary tumor + recurrent tumor same site	14	10
Primary tumor + recurrent tumor different site	27	19
Unknown	1	1
DLL3 expression (chemonaive vs. chemorelapsed sample)		
TPS 0%		4 vs. 6
TPS <1–49%		10 vs. 5
TPS ≥50%		16 vs. 19
H-Score 0		4 vs. 6
H-Score <150		16 vs. 8
H-Score ≥150		10 vs. 16
DLL3 expression dynamics		
Stable expression		19 (63.3%) with TPS vs. 17 (56.6%) with H-Score
Higher expression in chemonaive sample		4 (13.3%) with TPS vs. 4 (13.3%) with H-Score
Higher expression in chemorelapsed sample		7 (23.3%) with TPS vs. 9 (30%) with H-Score

to a H-score (range, 0–300) (10). SI was indicated as strongly positive (SI 3), moderately positive (SI 2), weakly positive (SI 1) and negative (SI 0). To dichotomize samples into positive and negative staining, TPS < 50% and H-score ≤ 150 were defined as DLL3 low expression (DLL3-low), and TPS ≥ 50% and H-score > 150 were defined as DLL3 high expression (DLL3-high) (5, 10).

RESULTS

Expression Pattern of DLL3 Protein in Unpaired Chemorelapsed SCLC Samples

In seven cases of the whole cohort, we had solely chemorelapsed samples without a chemonaive counterpart. Of these, from three patients, we had one sample each (only deriving from the primary site), and from four patients, we had several (up to four) samples deriving from the primary site as well as from distant metastases.

From the three cases with one sample, two were DLL3-high and one was DLL3-low, assessed by TPS. From the four cases with several samples, three (75%) showed a concordant DLL3 expression between the samples (two DLL3-low, one DLL3-high), and the other one showed high-DLL3 expression in the primary tumor and low-DLL3 expression in the metastatic site. Considering only the staining result of the first sample of each patient, four were DLL3-high and three DLL3-low. One of the two cases with concordant DLL3-low expression derived from an autopsy so that loss of expression may originate from autolysis.

Expression Pattern of DLL3 Protein in Paired Chemonaive Primary and Metastatic SCLC Samples

Three of the five cases with paired chemonaive primary and metastatic SCLC samples showed a concordant DLL3-high

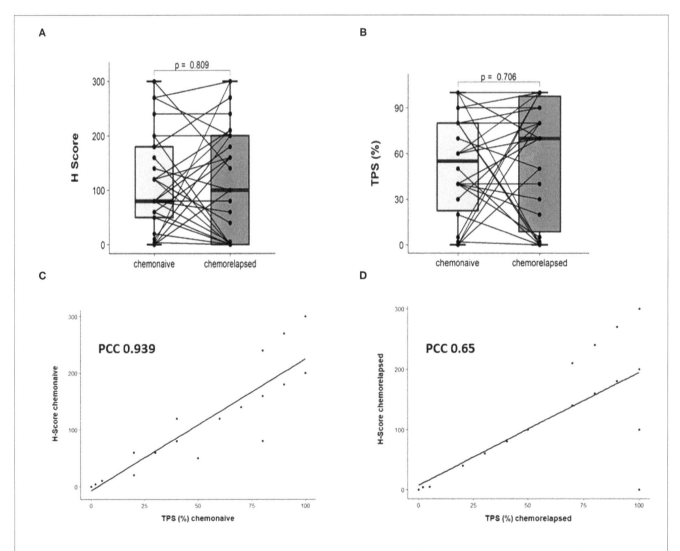

FIGURE 1 | Comparison of DLL3 expression in paired chemonaive-chemorelapsed SCLC samples. **(A)** DLL3 expression assessed by H-score. **(B)** DLL3 expression assessed by TPS. **(C)** Pearson correlation showing application of TPS and H-score on chemonaive SCLC samples. **(D)** Pearson correlation showing application of TPS and H-score on chemorelapsed SCLC samples.

staining pattern, and in two cases, we observed a high-DLL3 expression in the primary tumor and a low expression in the metastatic site, assessed by TPS. One case derived from an autopsy, and here, we investigated four samples deriving from different sites (adrenal, bone, liver, contralateral lung), all showing concordant low DLL3 expression. Here, concordant low expression might also be due to autolytic changes of the tissue.

Expression Pattern of DLL3 Protein in Paired Chemonaive-Chemorelapsed SCLC Samples

Considering only the chemonaive group, using the H-score method, 20 (66.6 %) out of 30 samples were DLL3-low, and 10 (33.3%) were DLL3-high. Out of the DLL3-low samples,

four were negative (H-score 0). In the chemorelapsed group, 14 (46.6 %) were DLL3-low and 16 (53.3%) were DLL3-high. Here, out of the DLL3-low samples, 6 were negative (H-score 0). DLL3 expression between the chemonaive and chemorelapsed groups was not significantly different (Wilcoxon signed-rank test $p = 0.809$; **Figure 1A**). Concordant staining, either DLL3-low or DLL3-high in paired chemonaive-chemorelapsed specimens, was observed in 17 out of 30 (56.6%) SCLCs. From those, in 11 cases (64.7%), both samples were DLL3-low, and 6 (35.9%) were DLL3-high. In 13 cases (43.4%) staining was not concordant, meaning that, in 9 cases, the chemonaive sample was DLL3-low and the chemorelapsed sample was DLL3-high ("DLL3 up") and that in 4 cases, the chemonaive sample was DLL3-high, and the chemorelapsed sample was DLL3-low ("DLL3 down").

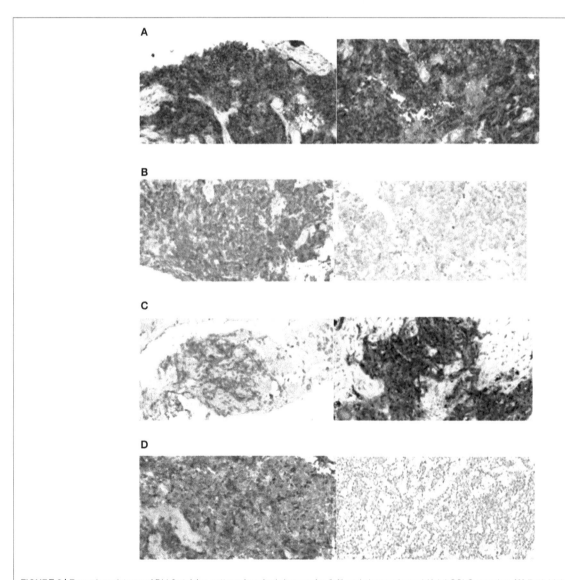

FIGURE 2 | Exemplary pictures of DLL3 staining patterns in paired chemonaive (left) and chemorelapsed (right) SCLC samples. **(A)** Both high DLL3 expression (TPS > 50%, H-score > 150), **(B)** Both low DLL3 expression (TPS < 50%, H-score < 150), **(C)** "DLL3 up" [low expression in chemonaive sample (TPS < 50%, H-score < 150) and high expression in chemorelapsed sample (TPS > 50%, H-score > 150)], **(D)** "DLL3 down" [low expression in chemorelapsed sample (TPS < 50%, H-score < 150) and high expression in chemonaive sample (TPS > 50%, H-score > 150); original magnification ×40].

With regard to TPS, 14 (46.6%) chemonaive samples were DLL3-low, and 16 (53.4%) were DLL3-high. In the chemorelapsed group, 11 (36.6%) samples were DLL3-low and 19 (63.3%) were DLL3-high. Negative samples (TPS <1%) within DLL3-low samples were identical to evaluation with H-score (4 in the chemonaive and 6 in the chemorelapsed groups, respectively). Again, DLL3 expression between the chemonaive and chemorelapsed group was not significantly different (Wilcoxon signed-rank test $p = 0.706$; **Figure 1B**). In the chemonaive group, mean TPS was 52.2%, ranging from 0 to 100%. In the chemorelapsed group, mean TPS was 57.6%, ranging from 0 to 100%. With regard to expression dynamics, 7 out of 30 samples (23.3%) showed equally low DLL3 expression, and 12 (40%) showed equally high expression, meaning that, in 63.3%, TPS was stable between chemonaive and chemorelapsed samples. In 36.7% ($n = 11$), DLL3 expression between the matched samples was different. In 7 cases (23.3%), the chemorelapsed sample had a high TPS, and the chemonaive counterpart a low TPS (DLL3 up), and in 4 cases (13.3%) the dynamic was the other way around (DLL3 down). DLL3 expression data are summarized in **Table 1**, and representative images of DLL3 protein expression assessed by IHC are provided in **Figure 2**.

Two of the cases originated from autopsies. Of these, one case showed a DLL3-down expression pattern assessed with the H-score method as well as with TPS. Again, this could be due to autolytic changes of the tissue. However, the other case showed an equally low expression without the chemorelapsed sample being completely negative (TPS 20%, SI2). Therefore, it cannot be stated in general that DLL3 expression is lost in autopsy material.

To assess both evaluation methods, we correlated TPS and H-score. Pearson correlation provided a linear dependency (PCC 0.939 for chemonaive samples, PCC 0.65 for chemorelapsed samples, **Figures 1C,D**), which proved that both methods were equally applicable. Because the TPS is easier to use in everyday diagnostic practice and probably shows less interobserver variability, only TPS was used for further statistical analysis.

We next evaluated if there was a correlation between tumor site and DLL3 expression. We found no significant differences between local pulmonal and distant recurrences (Wilcoxon rank-sum test $p = 0.32$; **Figure 3**).

Correlation of DLL3 With Clinicopathological Characteristics in the Paired Chemonaive-Chemorelapsed SCLC Cohort

There was no significant correlation of DLL3 expression level estimated in chemonaive samples with regard to gender, T-status, N-status, M-status, UICC-status, or time to recurrence. The only significant result was shown with regard to age: DLL3-high SCLCs were more frequent in younger patients (median age 57 years) and SCLC with low DLL3 expression more frequent in older patients (median age 67) ($p = 0.024$) (**Table 2**). We performed the same analysis for the DLL3 expression level estimated in chemorelapsed samples and, however, found no

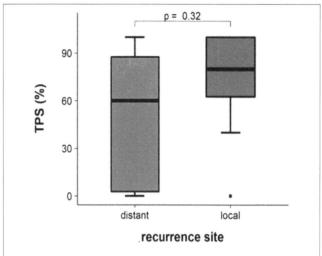

FIGURE 3 | DLL3 expression in chemorelapsed samples in dependency of site of recurrent tumor.

significant result for any of the above mentioned parameters (not shown).

Correlation of DLL3 With OS in the Paired Chemonaive-Chemorelapsed SCLC Cohort

The median age of this subcohort was 63 years (range, 47–79), 20 (66.6%) were male, 10 (33.3%), were female. From 23 out of the 30 patients, data concerning survival status was available. The median follow-up time for the patients with SCLCs was 354 days (range, 121–1,436). At the time of last follow-up, 15 patients were deceased and eight were alive.

We analyzed whether DLL3 expression (TPS low vs. high) in chemorelapsed or chemonaive samples could predict OS. Although results are not significant, Kaplan–Meier curves show a trend for better OS if DLL is highly expressed in chemorelapsed samples (log-rank $p = 0.57$) and less expressed in chemonaive samples (log-rank $p = 0.42$) (**Figures 4A,B**), whereas a low DLL3 status in chemorelapsed samples and a high DLL3 expression status in chemonaive samples seem to be more unfavorable. Next, we aimed to analyze if the dynamics of DLL3 expression during therapy has an impact on OS. As the above mentioned results already suggest, upregulation of DLL3 expression in matched samples after therapy reveals a trend for a better OS, whereas the worst survival rates were seen in cases with a downregulated DLL3 expression (log-rank test $p = 0.56$; **Figure 4C**). Survival curves indicating cases in which DLL3 expression stayed stable, either both low or high, lay in between the two curves indicating an upregulated or downregulated DLL3-status and show also a trend for a more favorable survival in high DLL3 expressing tumors.

DISCUSSION

SCLC is one of the most aggressive tumors with so far very limited therapeutic options (5, 9). Essentially all patients with

TABLE 2 | Association analysis between DLL3 expression assessed in chemonaive samples and clinicopathological characteristics of paired chemonaive-chemorelapsed SCLC cohort.

DLL3 expression assessed in chemonaive sample	Total (*n* = 30)	TPS ≥ 50% (*n* = 16)	TPS < 50% (*n* = 14)	*p*-value
Gender				0.26
Male	20 (66.7%)	9 (56.2%)	11 (78.6%)	
Female	10 (33.3%)	7 (43.8%)	3 (21.4%)	
Age				0.024
Missing	1	1	0	
Median (IQR)	65 (57, 70)	57 (55, 68)	67 (61, 75)	
T-Stage				0.58
Missing	16	8	8	
T(1, 2)	4 (28.6%)	3 (37.5%)	1 (16.7%)	
T(3,4)	10 (71.4%)	5 (62.5%)	5 (83.3%)	
N-Status				1
Missing	16	8	8	
N–	2 (14.3%)	1 (12.5%)	1 (16.7%)	
N+	12 (85.7%)	7 (87.5%)	5 (83.3%)	
M-Status				1
Missing	16	8	8	
M–	4 (28.6%)	2 (25.0%)	2 (33.3%)	
M+	10 (71.4%)	6 (75.0%)	4 (66.7%)	
UICC-Stage				1
Missing	16	8	8	
<IV	4 (28.6%)	2 (25.0%)	2 (33.3%)	
IV	10 (71.4%)	6 (75.0%)	4 (66.7%)	
Time to recurrence (months)				0.693
Missing		1	0	
Mean (SD)	12.8 (11.6)	10.4 (7.6)	15.4 (14.5)	
Median (IQR)	8 (5, 16)	8 (6, 14)	8.5 (4, 23.5)	

extensive-stage SCLC and the majority of patients with limited-stage SCLC suffer relapse within months of completing initial standard therapy (11). As SCLC is rarely biopsied following the initial diagnosis, dynamics of expression of therapeutically relevant biomarkers in relapsed disease are poorly understood. Because DLL3 is largely expressed in SCLC and regarded as a potential biomarker for response to Rova-T treatment (8), we aimed to investigate DLL3 expression in chemorelapsed SCLC samples and to compare its expression with matched chemonaive SCLC samples, correlate its expression with clinicopathological data, and perform survival analysis stratified according to DLL3-high or DLL3-low status and dynamics of DLL3 expression during the course of therapy. Possible differences in expression may further indicate if chemonaive or chemorelapsed SCLC specimens should be investigated in cases of a planned therapy with Rova-T. To our knowledge, there are hardly any published studies that investigated DLL3 expression in chemorelapsed SCLC samples and paired chemonaive-chemorelapsed SCLC samples, respectively.

In line with data from the literature, we as well found DLL3 expression in the majority of our SCLC samples. The evaluation method to assess DLL3 expression is not standardized, and there are so far no international standards for cut-off values to determine expression of DLL3 (4).

When comparing the DLL3 expression data of our study with those from the literature, it is important to consider not only the evaluation method, but also the diversity of the DLL3 antibodies used. Brcic et al. (12) investigated four different DLL3 antibodies (VenA (clone SP347; Ventana, Roche, Tucson, AZ, USA), NovA (NBP2–24669; Novus Biological, Littleton, CA, USA), TherA (PA5–26336; Thermo Fisher Scientific, Waltham, MA, USA), and AbcA (ab103102; Abcam, Cambridge, MA, USA)) for their reliability to detect DLL3 expression in high-grade neuroendocrine tumors of the lung. Comparison of VenA [the antibody used in the current study and in the clinical trial (5)] with the other three antibodies demonstrated poor results for overall agreement, positive and negative agreement, and Kappa values. The authors concluded that using VenA as a reference antibody, none of the other three antibodies can reliably be used for the DLL3 test. This, of course, makes comparison of DLL3 expression data between studies difficult. **Table 3** gives an overview of some recent studies dealing with DLL3 expression in SCLC, including their cohort sizes, evaluation methods, used

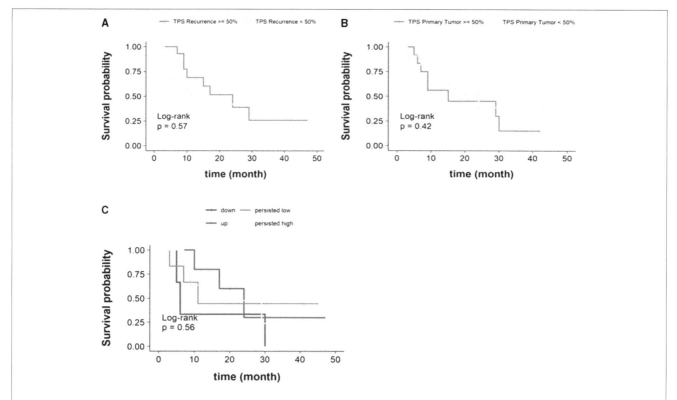

FIGURE 4 | Overall survival according to DLL3 expression status. **(A)** Kaplan–Meier curves stratified according to DLL3-high or DLL3-low status assessed with TPS in chemorelapsed specimens (log-rank $p = 0.57$). **(B)** Kaplan–Meier curves stratified according to DLL3-high or DLL3-low status assessed with TPS in chemonaive specimens (log-rank $p = 0.42$). **(C)** Kaplan–Meier curves stratified according to dynamics of DLL3 expression in the course of therapy. Persisted DLL3-low was defined as TPS < 50% in chemonaive and chemorelapsed samples, persisted DLL3-high was defined as TPS ≥50% in chemonaive and chemorelapsed samples, "up" was defined as a switch from TPS < 50% to ≥ 50%, and "down" was defined as a switch from TPS ≥50% to <50% in the course of therapy (log-rank test $p = 0.56$).

DLL3 antibodies, used cutoffs, and assessed expression data of DLL3 in SCLC.

We assessed DLL3 expression in two different ways, using the H-score and TPS, both known from prior studies (5, 10). We adopted 50% as the cutoff for TPS from a phase I trial conducted by Rudin et al. (5) and, with that, found expression of DLL3 in majority of chemonaive samples (86.6%) out of which 46.6% were DLL3-low and 53.4% DLL3-high. In the study from Rudin et al. (5), the range was higher with 74.4% being highly positive (29/39) and 25.6% (10/39) being weakly positive. The same cutoff was used by Tanaka et al., who investigated 63 presumably chemonaive SCLC samples and found 83% (52/63) positive for DLL3 with 20 samples (32%) being highly positive (3). The data in the literature vary; nevertheless, overall, a quite high rate of highly DLL3 expressing SCLC can be observed. In the group of chemorelapsed SCLC, we found similar DLL3 expression to that in the chemonaive group with 80% being positive, but with a slightly higher proportion of DLL3-high cases (63.3%, 19/30). DLL3 expression between chemonaive and chemorelapsed was stable in more than half of the cases (63.3%) and shifted from low to high or vice versa in 36.7%. However, DLL3 expression between chemonaive and chemorelapsed SCLC samples was not significantly different (Wilcoxon signed-rank test $p = 0.706$; **Figure 1B**) indicating no essential therapy-induced differences.

For evaluation with H-score, we adopted the cutoff of 150 from Yan et al. (10), who investigated 335 presumably chemonaive (*de novo*) SCLC samples and found a low expression (H-score ≤ 150) in 37.6% and a high expression (H-score > 150) in 62.4%. We found contrasting results with this method with a low expression in 66.6% (20/30) in the chemonaive group and a high expression in 33.3% (10/30) in the chemorelapsed group. In the chemorelapsed group instead, expression data were then again similar to those from above mentioned study with a shift to more highly positive SCLC cases [(53.3%, 16/30) vs. 46.6% (14/30) DLL3 low expressing samples]. However, the data are hardly comparable due to the significant differences in the size of the cohorts (335 vs. 30).

Concordant staining in paired chemonaive-chemorelapsed specimens, either both DLL3-low or DLL3-high, was found in only approximately half of the cases (56.6%), meaning that a significant portion (43.4%) showed a shift of DLL3 expression during course of therapy. However, also with this method, we found no significantly different DLL3 expressions between the two groups (Wilcoxon signed-rank test $p = 0.809$; **Figure 1A**).

With both evaluation methods, the proportion of matched samples showing deviating DLL3 expression, meaning a shift from low to high expression or vice versa, during course of therapy was considerable (43.4% with H-score, 36.7% with

TABLE 3 | Overview of recent studies on DLL3 expression in SCLC.

Study	Tissue related to therapy	Cohort size (n)	DLL3 antibody	Evaluation method	Cutoff	DLL 3 expression
Yan et al. (10)	Chemonaive ("de novo")	335	ab103102; Abcam, Cambridge, UK	H-Score	≤150 low vs. > 150 high	37.6% low (126/335)
						62.4% high (209/335)
Tanaka et al. (3)	not applicable	63	Stemcentrx, South San Francisco, CA, USA	TPS	<1%, 1–49%, ≥50%	<1%: 17% negative (11/63)
	Presumably Chemonaive					1–49%: 51% (32/63)
						≥50%: 32% (20/63)
Xie et al. (13)	not applicable	44	Clone SP346, Ventana-Roche Diagnostics, Indianapolis, IN, USA	TPS plus four-level SI, but cut-off based on TPS	<50% low, ≥50% high	20.5% low (9/44)
						79.5% high (35/44)
Regzedmaa et al. (8)	Chemonaive	38	No SAB1302862, Sigma-Aldrich, Shanghai, China	TPS scored as 1 (≤25%), 2 (26–50%), 3 (51–75%), 4 (>75%) multiplied with four-level SI	Median	47.4% low (18/38)
						52.6% high (20/38)
Huang et al. (14)	Chemonaive ("firstly diagnosed")	72	ab103102, Abcam, Cambridge, MA, USA	TPS scored as 1 (1–9%), 2 (10–49%), 3 (50–79%), 4 (≥80%) multiplied with four-level SI	<6 low, ≥6 high	68% low (49/72)
						32% high (23/72)
Furata et al. (15)	Chemonaive ("primary")	93	SP347; Spring Bioscience, Pleasanton, CA	TPS	<75% low, ≥75% high	53% low (49/93)
						47% high (44/93)
Rudin et al. (5)	not applicable	39	Stemcentrx, South San Francisco, CA, USA	TPS	<50% low, ≥50% high	25.6% low (10/39)
						74.4% high (29/39)
Rojo et al. (16)	Diverse (independent and paired)	1,050	Clone SP347, Ventana, Tucson	TPS Negative (0–24%), positive (≥25%), non-high positive (25–74%), high positive (≥75%)	Positive (≥25 %)	15% negative (155/1050)
						85% positive (895/1050)

TPS). This indicates that DLL3 expression might be influenced by therapy and cannot be considered as stable. Unlike other predictive biomarkers, such as, e.g., PD-L1 with a required TPS of 50% for therapy of NSCLC with Pembrolizumab, so far, a high (≥50%) DLL3 expression of SCLC is not implemented as a prerequisite for therapy with Rova-T. However, if this were the case, our data demonstrate that it does matter which samples are chosen to assess DLL3 expression. There is only a little literature concerning DLL3 expression in paired chemonaive-chemorelapsed SCLC samples. Rojo et al. (16) investigated, in addition to a huge number of independent SCLC samples, also 36 paired SCLC samples, defining "paired" as two specimens from the same patient and same primary disease site or as a first specimen obtained at diagnosis and the second obtained at relapse/recurrence. Of these, only two samples corresponded to paired chemonaive-chemorelapsed samples as we had examined. Moreover, they used a different cutoff than we did with

≥25% positive tumor cells defined as positive DLL3 expression (**Table 3**). With that, they found 88% concordance between paired specimens without specifically addressing the paired chemonaive-chemorelapsed samples. Due to the significant deviation in size of the cohorts, results of this study are hardly comparable with our results.

To our knowledge, the above mentioned study by Yan et al. (10) is the only one using the H-score method with a cutoff of 150. Furthermore, combining a four-level SI and TPS to a H-score should show higher interobserver variability than just using TPS. We, therefore, assessed the two evaluation methods, and after Pearson correlation provided a linear dependency that indicated equality, we have then focused on TPS for further analyses.

We next investigated if the site of the biopsied recurrent tumor has an impact on DLL3 expression. In 33.3% (10/30) chemorelapsed tissue derived from local pulmonal recurrences and in 63.3% (19/30) from distant metastases. Concordant with the literature (3, 10), we found no significant differences of DLL3 expression between local pulmonal and distant recurrences (Wilcoxon rank-sum test $p = 0.32$; **Figure 3**). Yan et al., for instance, compared intertumoral expression of DLL3 on the basis of 37 paired biopsies of primary and metastatic sites and found concordant staining in all cases (10).

Apart from age when considering the chemonaive samples, we found no association of DLL3 expression with clinicopathological data in our cohort (**Table 2**). Our observation that DLL3 expression actually does not associate with clinicopathological data broadly fit with those from the literature. For instance, Tanaka et al. (3) also found no significant association between DLL3 expression and age, sex, smoking history, or disease stage, and Yan et al. (10) found no significant association with age, distant metastasis status, or TNM stage. In the latter study, DLL3 expression was higher in TTF-1 expressing SCLC samples ($p = 0.006$), smokers ($p = 0.023$), and males ($p = 0.041$), whereas high DLL3 expression was associated with female sex ($p = 0.03$) in a study conducted by Xie et al. (13). Furata et al. found that DLL3-high expression (defined as TPS $\geq 75\%$) was significantly more prevalent in patients with lymph node metastases and advanced c-stage (15). These few significant correlations found in our study and in the literature are, due to their diversity, primarily a coincidence and might not have a causal relationship.

We next investigated if DLL3 expression has an impact on OS. Kaplan–Meier curves do not show significant results, but a trend for a better OS if DLL is highly expressed in chemorelapsed samples (log-rank $p = 0.57$) and low expressed in chemonaive samples (log-rank $p = 0.42$) (**Figures 4A,B**), whereas a low DLL3 status in chemorelapsed samples and a high DLL3 expression status in chemonaive samples seem to be more unfavorable. Several other studies also analyzed the relationship of DLL3 expression and OS, and the corresponding results are partly contradictory. Some studies found no statistically significant difference of OS between DLL3 low and high expressing tumors (3, 15), whereas Regzedmaa et al. found that high expression of DLL3 assessed on chemonaive SCLC correlated significantly with poorer patient outcomes ($p = <0.001$) (8). Yan et al. also found that patients with chemonaive SCLC having a high DLL3 expression level exhibited a lower OS compared with patients with DLL3-low expressing SCLC ($p = 0.007$). In this study, expression of DLL3 and TTF-1 was investigated in combination, and additionally, it was found that the group of SCLC with low expression of DLL3 in combination with missing TTF-1 expression showed improved OS (10). Huang et al. also found a high level of DLL3 to be correlated with low OS rate ($p < 0.01$) (14). Despite lacking significance, our survival curves also indicate that there is a trend for better survival if chemonaive samples show low DLL3 expression (**Figure 4B**). Xie et al. found that high DLL3 expression was associated with better OS in SCLC ($p = 0.049$). At first glance, the results seem contradictory. However, in this study, only a few cases showed low DLL3 expression, and after adjusting for age, tumor size, and stage, DLL3 expression was no longer associated with OS (13).

Due to our samples being matched, we then analyzed if the dynamics of DLL3 expression in the course of therapy associates with survival. As the above mentioned results

already suggest, upregulation of DLL3 expression in matched samples after therapy reveals a trend for better overall survival, whereas the worst survival rates were seen in cases with a downregulated DLL3 expression (log-rank test $p = 0.56$; **Figure 4C**). Survival curves indicating cases in which DLL3 expression was concordant in chemonaive and chemorelapsed samples, either both low or high, lay in between the two curves, indicating survival in dependency of an upregulated or downregulated DLL3-status. Here, a trend that stable high expression is associated with a more favorable survival than stable low expression can be derived. This might suggest that DLL3 expression assessed in chemorelapsed samples is more meaningful regarding OS due to beforehand we could show that a low expression in chemonaive samples and a high expression of DLL3 only in chemorelapsed samples indicated a better OS (**Figures 4A,B**).

In a study from Tendler et al. (7), it was found that subjects with Notch1 low expressing chemorelapsed SCLC samples showed a better prognosis and higher sensitivity to chemotherapy. Assuming that Notch1 and DLL3 are opponents during the evolution of SCLC, one could expect a high DLL3 expression if Notch 1 shows a low expression. Thus, our result for a trend for better prognosis in DLL3 high expressing chemorelapsed SCLC is in line with that of Tendler et al.

To our knowledge, our study is the first investigating DLL3 expression in a large cohort of paired chemonaive-chemorelapsed SCLC samples, which is why our results concerning OS in relation to the dynamics of DLL3 expression cannot be compared with data in the literature. Our survival data is not significant. This might be due to the relatively small cohort size, which, at the same time, represents a limitation of our study. However, against the background that, in most cases, recurrent SCLC is not biopsied at all, our cohort is exceptional. Another limitation of our study is that recent literature (17, 18) on DLL3 seems to diminish its value as a potential therapeutic agent, which also weakens the value of the present work.

To sum up, the current study delivers, for the first time, data concerning DLL3 expression in a large cohort of rare paired chemonaive and chemorelapsed SCLC samples, which is exceptional due to relapsed SCLC are usually not being biopsied. However, investigation of chemorelapsed tumor tissue is essential because it might provide hints why early recurrences, characteristic for SCLC, occur. As the first, we show that, in a large proportion of paired chemonaive-chemorelapsed SCLC samples, DLL3 expression is not stable during the course of therapy, indicating therapy-associated alterations. This demonstrates that it is worth assessing protein expression of biomarkers in general and here, especially of DLL3 in chemorelapsed samples, meaning in the latest tumor tissue. This should, at the same time, be an incentive to gain tumor tissue by biopsy in relapses. Due to the manner of assessing expression of DLL3 not being standardized, we tested two evaluation methods and applied TPS and H-score. Both approaches delivered comparable results, but because TPS should be more practical in routine diagnostics than the H-score method, we have continued working with TPS. As in other studies, we found that the majority of SCLC samples expressed DLL3 and also did not find any profound correlations with clinicopathological data or tumor site. Concordant with data from the literature, our survival analysis revealed a trend for a better OS if DLL is low expressed (<50%) in chemonaive samples. Interestingly, this does not seem to apply to chemorelapsed SCLC because, for those, we could observe a trend for a more favorable survival in the event of a high expression (≥50%). In line with that, cases showing a shift from a low to a high expression of DLL3 during the course of therapy indicated the most favorable survival data. These results should not be overstated due to the size of our cohort not being powered to detect association with survival data. However, the study definitely shows the importance of research of chemorelapsed tumor tissue.

REFERENCES

1. Saunders LR, Bankovich AJ, Anderson WC, Aujay MA, Bheddah S, Black K, et al. A DLL3-targeted antibody-drug conjugate eradicates high-grade pulmonary neuroendocrine tumor-initiating cells *in vivo*. *Sci Transl Med.* (2015) 7:302ra136. doi: 10.1126/scitranslmed. aac9459

2. Horn L, Mansfield AS, Szczesna A, Havel L, Krzakowski M, Hochmair MJ, et al. First-Line Atezolizumab plus chemotherapy in extensive-stage small-cell lung cancer. *N Engl J Med.* (2018) 379:2220–9. doi: 10.1056/NEJMoa18 09064

3. Tanaka K, Isse K, Fujihira T, Takenoyama M, Saunders L, Bheddah S, et al. Prevalence of Delta-like protein 3 expression in patients with small cell lung cancer. *Lung Cancer Amst Neth.* (2018) 115:116–20. doi: 10.1016/j.lungcan.2017.11.018

4. Chen B, Li H, Liu C, Wang S, Zhang F, Zhang L, et al. Potential prognostic value of delta-like protein 3 in small cell lung cancer: a meta-analysis. *World J Surg Oncol.* (2020) 18:226. doi: 10.1186/s12957-020-02004-5

5. Rudin CM, Pietanza MC, Bauer TM, Ready N, Morgensztern D, Glisson BS, et al. Rovalpituzumab tesirine, a DLL3-targeted antibody-drug conjugate, in recurrent small-cell lung cancer: a first-in-human, first-in-class, open-label, phase 1 study. *Lancet Oncol.* (2017) 18:42–51. doi: 10.1016/S1470-2045(16)30565-4

6. Leonetti A, Facchinetti F, Minari R, Cortellini A, Rolfo CD, Giovannetti E, et al. Notch pathway in small-cell lung cancer: from preclinical evidence to therapeutic challenges. *Cell Oncol Dordr.* (2019) 42:261–73. doi: 10.1007/s13402-019-00441-3

7. Tendler S, Kanter L, Lewensohn R, Ortiz-Villalón C, Viktorsson K, De Petris L. The prognostic implications of Notch1, Hes1, Ascl1, and DLL3 protein expression in SCLC patients receiving platinum-based chemotherapy. *PLoS ONE.* (2020) 15:e0240973. doi: 10.1371/journal.pone.02 40973

8. Regzedmaa O, Li Y, Li Y, Zhang H, Wang J, Gong H, et al. Prevalence of DLL3, CTLA-4 and MSTN expression in patients with small cell lung cancer. *OncoTargets Ther.* (2019) 12:10043–55. doi: 10.2147/OTT.S2 16362

9. Morgensztern D, Besse B, Greillier L, Santana-Davila R, Ready N, Hann CL, et al. Efficacy and safety of rovalpituzumab tesirine in third-line and beyond patients with DLL3-expressing, relapsed/refractory small-cell lung cancer: results from the phase II TRINITY study. *Clin Cancer Res.* (2019) 25:6958–66. doi: 10.1158/1078-0432.CCR-19-1133

10. Yan L-X, Liu Y-H, Li Z, Luo D-L, Li Y-F, Yan J-H, et al. Prognostic value of delta-like protein 3 combined with thyroid transcription factor-1 in small-cell lung cancer. *Oncol Lett.* (2019) 18:2254–61. doi: 10.3892/ol.2019. 10538

11. Pietanza MC, Byers LA, Minna JD, Rudin CM. Small cell lung cancer: will recent progress lead to improved outcomes? *Clin Cancer Res.* (2015) 21:2244–55. doi: 10.1158/1078-0432.CCR-14-2958

12. Brcic L, Kuchler C, Eidenhammer S, Pabst D, Quehenberger F, Gazdar AF, et al. Comparison of four DLL3 antibodies performance in high grade neuroendocrine lung tumor samples and cell cultures. *Diagn Pathol.* (2019) 14:549–61. doi: 10.1186/s13000-019-0827-z

13. Xie H, Boland JM, Maleszewski JJ, Aubry MC, Yi ES, Jenkins SM, et al. Expression of delta-like protein 3 is reproducibly present in a subset of small cell lung carcinomas and pulmonary carcinoid tumors. *Lung Cancer Amst Neth.* (2019) 135:73–9. doi: 10.1016/j.lungcan.2019. 07.016

14. Huang J, Cao D, Sha J, Zhu X, Han S. DLL3 is regulated by LIN28B and miR-518d-5p and regulates cell proliferation, migration and chemotherapy response in advanced small cell lung cancer. *Biochem Biophys Res Commun.* (2019) 514:853–60. doi: 10.1016/j.bbrc.2019. 04.130

15. Furuta M, Sakakibara-Konishi J, Kikuchi H, Yokouchi H, Nishihara H, Minemura H, et al. Analysis of DLL3 and ASCL1 in surgically resected small cell lung cancer (HOT1702). *Oncologist.* (2019) 24:e1172–9. doi: 10.1634/theoncologist.2018-0676

16. Rojo F, Corassa M, Mavroudis D, Öz AB, Biesma B, Brcic L, et al. International real-world study of DLL3 expression in patients with small cell lung cancer. *Lung Cancer Amst Neth.* (2020) 147:237–43. doi: 10.1016/j.lungcan.2020. 07.026

17. Blackhall F, Jao K, Greillier L, Cho BC, Penkov K, Reguart N, et al. Efficacy and safety of rovalpituzumab tesirine compared with topotecan as second-line therapy in DLL3-high SCLC: results from the phase 3 TAHOE study. *J Thorac Oncol.* (2021) 16:1547–58. doi: 10.1016/j.jtho.2021. 02.009

18. Johnson ML, Zvirbule Z, Laktionov K, Helland A, Cho BC, Gutierrez V, et al. Rovalpituzumab tesirine as a maintenance therapy after first-line platinum-based chemotherapy in patients with extensive-stage-SCLC: results from the phase 3 MERU study. *J Thorac Oncol.* (2021) 16:1570–81. doi: 10.1016/j.jtho.2021. 03.012

AUTHOR CONTRIBUTIONS

SP and CK planned the research project and evaluated the samples. ED performed the immunohistochemical stainings. TJ performed the statistical analysis. F-OP, CH, BK, SBo, BM, MA, SBe, MT, HB, and FF provided patients' follow-up data. CK, TJ, RK, F-OP, CH, BM, JR-I, CI, MA, SBe, MT, HB, FF, BK, SBo, VS, JK, and SP wrote and/or revised the manuscript. All authors have read and agreed to the published version of the manuscript.

ACKNOWLEDGMENTS

The authors thank ED for the excellent technical assistance.

Permissions

The contributors of this book come from diverse backgrounds, making this book a truly international effort. This book will bring forth new frontiers with its revolutionizing research information and detailed analysis of the nascent developments around the world.

We would like to thank all the contributing authors for lending their expertise to make the book truly unique. They have played a crucial role in the development of this book. Without their invaluable contributions this book wouldn't have been possible. They have made vital efforts to compile up to date information on the varied aspects of this subject to make this book a valuable addition to the collection of many professionals and students.

This book was conceptualized with the vision of imparting up-to-date information and advanced data in this field. To ensure the same, a matchless editorial board was set up. Every individual on the board went through rigorous rounds of assessment to prove their worth. After which they invested a large part of their time researching and compiling the most relevant data for our readers.

The editorial board has been involved in producing this book since its inception. They have spent rigorous hours researching and exploring the diverse topics which have resulted in the successful publishing of this book. They have passed on their knowledge of decades through this book. To expedite this challenging task, the publisher supported the team at every step. A small team of assistant editors was also appointed to further simplify the editing procedure and attain best results for the readers.

Apart from the editorial board, the designing team has also invested a significant amount of their time in understanding the subject and creating the most relevant covers. They scrutinized every image to scout for the most suitable representation of the subject and create an appropriate cover for the book.

The publishing team has been an ardent support to the editorial, designing and production team. Their endless efforts to recruit the best for this project, has resulted in the accomplishment of this book. They are a veteran in the field of academics and their pool of knowledge is as vast as their experience in printing. Their expertise and guidance has proved useful at every step. Their uncompromising quality standards have made this book an exceptional effort. Their encouragement from time to time has been an inspiration for everyone.

The publisher and the editorial board hope that this book will prove to be a valuable piece of knowledge for researchers, students, practitioners and scholars across the globe.

List of Contributors

Li-Hua Gong, Wen Zhang, Rong-Fang Dong, Xiao-Qi Sun, Ming Zhang and Yi Ding
Department of Pathology, Beijing Jishuitan Hospital, The Fourth Medical College of Peking University, Beijing, China

Yong-Bin Su
Department of Radiology, Beijing Jishuitan Hospital, The Fourth Medical College of Peking University, Beijing, China

Wei-Feng Liu
Department of Orthopedic Oncology Surgery, Beijing Jishuitan Hospital, Fourth Medical College of Peking University, Beijing, China

Sarah E. Coupland
Department of Molecular and Clinical Cancer Medicine, University of Liverpool, Liverpool, United Kingdom
Liverpool Clinical Laboratories, Liverpool University Hospitals NHS Foundation Trust, Liverpool, United Kingdom

Lance N. Sandle
The Royal College of Pathologists, London, United Kingdom

Michael Osborn
Department of Cellular Pathology, Charing Cross Hospital, North West London Pathology Hosted at Imperial College NHS Trust, London, United Kingdom

Hiba A. Al Dallal, Brock A. Martin and Alaleh E. Shandiz
Department of Pathology and Laboratory Medicine, University of Louisville, Louisville, KY, United States

Siddharth Narayanan
Department of Pediatrics, Nationwide Children's Hospital, Columbus, OH, United States

Hanah F. Alley
Department of Neurology, University of Louisville, Louisville, KY, United States

Michael J. Eiswerth
Department of Internal Medicine, University of Louisville, Louisville, KY, United States

Forest W. Arnold
Division of Infectious Diseases, University of Louisville, Louisville, KY, United States

Costanza Chiapponi, Hakan Alakus and Christiane J. Bruns
Department of General, Visceral, Cancer and Transplant Surgery, University Clinic of Cologne, Cologne, Germany

Matthias Schmidt
Department for Nuclear Medicine, University Clinic of Cologne, Cologne, Germany

Michael Faust
Policlinic for Endocrinology, Diabetes and Prevention Medicine, University Clinic of Cologne, Cologne, Germany

Reinhard Büttner, Marie-Lisa Eich and Anne M. Schultheis
Institute for Pathology, University Clinic of Cologne, Cologne, Germany

Tania Rossi, Ivan Vannini, Giulia Gallerani and Francesco Fabbri
Biosciences Laboratory, IRCCS Istituto Romagnolo per lo Studio dei Tumori (IRST) "Dino Amadori", Meldola, Italy

Michela Palleschi
Department of Medical Oncology, IRCCS Istituto Romagnolo per lo Studio dei Tumori (IRST) "Dino Amadori", Meldola, Italy

Davide Angeli and Michela Tebaldi
Unit of Biostatistics and Clinical Trials, IRCCS Istituto Romagnolo per lo Studio dei Tumori (IRST) "Dino Amadori", Meldola, Italy

Giovanni Martinelli
Scientific Directorate, IRCCS Istituto Scientifico Romagnolo per lo Studio dei Tumori (IRST) "Dino Amadori", Meldola, Italy

Maurizio Puccetti
Azienda Unità Sanitaria Locale Imola, Imola, Italy

Francesco Limarzi
Pathology Unit, Morgagni-Pierantoni Hospital, Forlì, Italy

Roberta Maltoni
Healthcare Administration, IRCCS Istituto Romagnolo per lo Studio dei Tumori (IRST) "Dino Amadori", Meldola, Italy

Umberto Maccio, Holger Moch and Zsuzsanna Varga
Department of Pathology and Molecular Pathology, University Hospital of Zürich, University of Zurich, Zurich, Switzerland

Annelies S. Zinkernagel and Silvio D. Brugger
Department of Infectious Diseases and Hospital Epidemiology, University Hospital of Zürich, University of Zurich, Zurich, Switzerland

Reto Schuepbach and Daniel Andrea Hofmaenner
Institute of Intensive Care, University Hospital Zurich, University Hospital of Zürich, Zurich, Switzerland

Elsbeth Probst-Mueller
Department of Immunology, University Hospital of Zürich, Zurich, Switzerland

Karl Frontzek
Institute of Neuropathology, University Hospital Zurich, Zurich, Switzerland

Samantha Sarcognato, Diana Sacchi, Monia Niero and Giovanna Gallina
Department of Pathology, Azienda ULSS2 Marca Trevigiana, Treviso, Italy

Luca Fabris
Department of Molecular Medicine – DMM, University of Padova, Padova, Italy

Giacomo Zanus
4th Surgery Unit, Azienda ULSS2 Marca Trevigiana, Treviso, Italy
Department of Surgery, Oncology and Gastroenterology – DISCOG, University of Padova, Padova, Italy

Enrico Gringeri
Department of Surgery, Oncology and Gastroenterology – DISCOG, University of Padova, Padova, Italy

Maria Guido
Department of Pathology, Azienda ULSS2 Marca Trevigiana, Treviso, Italy
Department of Medicine – DIMED, University of Padova, Padova, Italy

Fang Liu
Department of Respiratory Medicine, Wei fang People's Hospital, The First Affiliated Hospital of Wei fang Medical University, Wei fang, China

Hengxiao Lu and Tongzhen Xu
Department of Thoracic Surgery, Wei fang People's Hospital, The First Affiliated Hospital of Wei fang Medical University, Wei fang, China

Liqian Chen
Department of Pathology, Wei fang People's Hospital, The First Affiliated Hospital of Wei fang Medical University, Wei fang, China

Junfeng Geng
Department of Thoracic Surgery, Shanghai Chest Hospital, Shanghai Jiao Tong University, Shanghai, China

Hongtao Kang, Die Luo, Weihua Feng, Shaoqun Zeng, Tingwei Quan and Xiuli Liu
Britton Chance Center for Biomedical Photonics, Wuhan National Laboratory for Optoelectronics, Huazhong University of Science and Technology, Wuhan, China
Ministry of Education (MOE) Key Laboratory for Biomedical Photonics, School of Engineering Sciences, Huazhong University of Science and Technology, Wuhan, China

Junbo Hu
Department of Pathology, Hubei Maternal and Child Health Hospital, Wuhan, China

Henrik Sahlin Pettersen and Elin Synnøve Røyset
Department of Pathology, St. Olavs Hospital, Trondheim University Hospital, Trondheim, Norway
Department of Clinical and Molecular Medicine, Faculty of Medicine and Health Sciences, NTNU - Norwegian University of Science and Technology, Trondheim, Norway
Clinic of Laboratory Medicine, St. Olavs Hospital, Trondheim University Hospital, Trondheim, Norway

Ingunn Bakke
Department of Clinical and Molecular Medicine, Faculty of Medicine and Health Sciences, NTNU - Norwegian University of Science and Technology, Trondheim, Norway
Clinic of Laboratory Medicine, St. Olavs Hospital, Trondheim University Hospital, Trondheim, Norway

Ilya Belevich and Eija Jokitalo
Electron Microscopy Unit, Institute of Biotechnology, Helsinki Institute of Life Science, University of Helsinki, Helsinki, Finland

Erik Smistad and Ingerid Reinertsen
Department of Health Research, SINTEF Digital, Trondheim, Norway
Department of Circulation and Medical Imaging, Faculty of Medicine and Health Sciences, NTNU - Norwegian University of Science and Technology, Trondheim, Norway

Melanie Rae Simpson
Department of Public Health and Nursing, Faculty of Medicine and Health Sciences, NTNU - Norwegian University of Science and Technology, Trondheim, Norway
The Clinical Research Unit for Central Norway, Trondheim, Norway

André Pedersen
Department of Clinical and Molecular Medicine, Faculty of Medicine and Health Sciences, NTNU - Norwegian University of Science and Technology, Trondheim, Norway
Department of Health Research, SINTEF Digital, Trondheim, Norway
The Cancer Foundation, St. Olavs Hospital, Trondheim University Hospital, Trondheim, Norway

Dörthe Schaffrin-Nabe and Rudolf Voigtmann
Praxis für Hämatologie und Onkologie, Bochum, Germany

Stefan Schuster
Datar Cancer Genetics Europe GmbH, Eckersdorf, Germany

Andrea Tannapfel
Institute of Pathology, Ruhr-University Bochum, Bochum, Germany

Marcelo Luiz Balancin, Camila Machado Baldavira, Tabatha Gutierrez Prieto, Cecília Farhat, Aline Kawassaki Assato, Alexandre Muxfeldt Ab'Saber and Vera Luiza Capelozzi
Laboratory of Genomics and Histomorphometry, Department of Pathology, University of São Paulo Medical School (USP), São Paulo, Brazil

Juliana Machado-Rugolo
Laboratory of Genomics and Histomorphometry, Department of Pathology, University of São Paulo Medical School (USP), São Paulo, Brazil
Health Technology Assessment Center (NATS), Clinical Hospital (HCFMB), Medical School of São Paulo State University (UNESP), Botucatu, Brazil

Ana Paula Pereira Velosa and Walcy Rosolia Teodoro
Rheumatology Division of the Hospital das Clinicas da Faculdade de Medicina da Universidade de São Paulo, FMUSP, São Paulo, Brazil

Teresa Yae Takagaki
Division of Pneumology, Instituto do Coração (Incor), University of São Paulo Medical School (USP), São Paulo, Brazil

Sergio Decherchi
Computational and Chemical Biology, Fondazione Istituto Italiano di Tecnologia, Genoa, Italy

Elena Pedrini, Marina Mordenti and Luca Sangiorgi
Department of Rare Skeletal Disorders, IRCCS Istituto Ortopedico Rizzoli, Bologna, Italy

Andrea Cavalli
Computational and Chemical Biology, Fondazione Istituto Italiano di Tecnologia, Genoa, Italy
Department of Pharmacy and Biotechnology (FaBiT), Alma Mater Studiorum – University of Bologna, Bologna, Italy

Severine Banek, Luis Kluth, Clarissa Wittler and Felix K.H. Chun
Department of Urology, University Hospital Frankfurt, Goethe University, Frankfurt, Germany

Florestan J. Koll
Department of Urology, University Hospital Frankfurt, Goethe University, Frankfurt, Germany
Frankfurt Cancer Institute (FCI), University Hospital, Goethe University, Frankfurt, Germany
University Cancer Center (UCT) Frankfurt, University Hospital, Goethe University, Frankfurt, Germany

Nina Becker
University Cancer Center (UCT) Frankfurt, University Hospital, Goethe University, Frankfurt, Germany
Dr. Senckenberg Institute of Pathology, University Hospital Frankfurt, Frankfurt, Germany

Alina Schwarz, Jens Köllermann, Katrin Bankov, Claudia Döring and Henning Reis
Dr. Senckenberg Institute of Pathology, University Hospital Frankfurt, Frankfurt, Germany

Peter J. Wild
Frankfurt Cancer Institute (FCI), University Hospital, Goethe University, Frankfurt, Germany
Dr. Senckenberg Institute of Pathology, University Hospital Frankfurt, Frankfurt, Germany
Frankfurt Institute for Advanced Studies, Frankfurt, Germany

Taek Chung
Department of Biomedical Systems Informatics, Yonsei University College of Medicine, Seoul, South Korea

Young Nyun Park
Department of Pathology, Graduate School of Medical Science, Brain Korea 21 Project, Yonsei University College of Medicine, Seoul, South Korea

Daniel Wai-Hung Ho, Wai-Ling Macrina Lam, Lo-Kong Chan and Irene Oi-Lin Ng
Department of Pathology and State Key Laboratory of Liver Research, University of Hong Kong, Hong Kong, Hong Kong SAR, China

Kumutnart Chanprapaph, Suthinee Rutnin and Poonkiat Suchonwanit
Division of Dermatology, Department of Medicine, Faculty of Medicine, Ramathibodi Hospital, Mahidol University, Bangkok, Thailand

Saranya Khunkhet
Division of Dermatology, Department of Medicine, Faculty of Medicine, Ramathibodi Hospital, Mahidol University, Bangkok, Thailand
Skin Center, Srinakharinwirot University, Bangkok, Thailand

Stijn E. Verleden
Antwerp Surgical Training, Anatomy and Research Centre (ASTARC), Antwerp University, Antwerp, Belgium
Division of Pneumology, University Hospital Antwerp, Edegem, Belgium
Department of Thoracic and Vascular Surgery, University Hospital Antwerp, Edegem, Belgium

Veronique Verplancke
Division of Pneumology, University Hospital Antwerp, Edegem, Belgium

Paul E. Van Schil and Jeroen M. H. Hendriks
Antwerp Surgical Training, Anatomy and Research Centre (ASTARC), Antwerp University, Antwerp, Belgium
Department of Thoracic and Vascular Surgery, University Hospital Antwerp, Edegem, Belgium

Peter Braubach, Edith Plucinski, Mark P. Kuhnel, Florian P. Laenger and Danny Jonigk
Member of the German Center for Lung Research (DZL), Biomedical Research in Endstage and Obstructive Lung Disease Hannover (BREATH), Hannover, Germany
Institute for Pathology, Hannover Medical School, Hannover, Germany

Christopher Werlein
Institute for Pathology, Hannover Medical School, Hannover, Germany

Annemiek Snoeckx and Haroun El Addouli
Division of Radiology, University Hospital Antwerp and University of Antwerp, Edegem, Belgium

Tobias Welte
Member of the German Center for Lung Research (DZL), Biomedical Research in Endstage and Obstructive Lung Disease Hannover (BREATH), Hannover, Germany
Division of Pneumology, Hannover Medical School, Hannover, Germany

Axel Haverich
Member of the German Center for Lung Research (DZL), Biomedical Research in Endstage and Obstructive Lung Disease Hannover (BREATH), Hannover, Germany
Division of Thoracic Surgery, Hannover Medical School, Hannover, Germany

Sabine Dettmer
Member of the German Center for Lung Research (DZL), Biomedical Research in Endstage and Obstructive Lung Disease Hannover (BREATH), Hannover, Germany
Department of Radiology, Hannover Medical School, Hannover, Germany

Patrick Pauwels
Division of Pathology, University Hospital Antwerp, Edegem, Belgium

Therese Lapperre and Johanna M. Kwakkel-Van-Erp
Division of Pneumology, University Hospital Antwerp, Edegem, Belgium
Laboratory of Experimental Medicine and Pediatrics (LEMP), Antwerp University, Antwerp, Belgium

Maximilian Ackermann
Institute of Pathology and Department of Molecular Pathology, Helios University Clinic Wuppertal, University of Witten-Herdecke, Witten, Germany
Institute of Functional and Clinical Anatomy, University Medical Center of the Johannes Gutenberg University Mainz, Mainz, Germany

Helen C. Causton
Department of Pathology and Cell Biology, Columbia University Irving Medical Center, New York, NY, United States

Franziska Kellers, Aurélie Fernandez, Mario Schindeldecker, Katrin E. Tagscherer, Wilfried Roth and Sebastian Foersch
Institute of Pathology, University Medical Center Mainz, Mainz, Germany

Björn Konukiewitz
Institute of Pathology, Christian-Albrecht University of Kiel, Kiel, Germany

Achim Heintz
Department of General, Visceral and Vascular Surgery, Catholic Hospital Mainz, Mainz, Germany

Moritz Jesinghaus
Department of Pathology, University Hospital Marburg, Marburg, Germany

Alison E. Burkett, Sophia B. Sher, Chirag R. Patel, Isam Ildin-Eltoum, Deepti Dhall, Goo Lee, Prachi Bajpai and Paul V. Benson
Department of Pathology, University of Alabama at Birmingham, Birmingham, AL, United States

Camilla Margaroli
Division of Pulmonary, Allergy and Critical Care Medicine, Department of Medicine, University of Alabama at Birmingham, Birmingham, AL, United States

Shajan Peter
Division of Gastroenterology, Department of Medicine, University of Alabama at Birmingham, Birmingham, AL, United States

Upender Manne and Sameer Al Diffalha
Department of Pathology, University of Alabama at Birmingham, Birmingham, AL, United States
O'Neal Compressive Cancer Center, Birmingham, AL, United States

Dongling Liu
School of Pharmacy, Gansu University of Chinese Medicine, Lanzhou, China

Zhandong Wang and Dan Yang
School of Traditional Chinese and Western Medicine, Gansu University of Chinese Medicine, Lanzhou, China

Linlin Wen
School of Traditional Chinese and Western Medicine, Gansu University of Chinese Medicine, Lanzhou, China
County People's Hospital, Pingliang, China

Yang Hai
Gansu University of Chinese Medicine/Scientific Research and Experimental Center, Lanzhou, China

Yanying Zhang and Bing Song
Gansu University of Chinese Medicine/Scientific Research and Experimental Center, Lanzhou, China
Gansu Provincial Engineering Laboratory for Research and Promotion of Quality Standardization of Authentic Medicinal Materials in Gansu Province/Provincial Key Laboratory of Pharmaceutical Chemistry and Quality Research in Colleges and Universities in Gansu Province/Gansu Provincial Laboratory Animal Industry Technology Center, Lanzhou, China

Yongfeng Wang and Min Bai
Gansu Provincial Engineering Laboratory for Research and Promotion of Quality Standardization of Authentic Medicinal Materials in Gansu Province/Provincial Key Laboratory of Pharmaceutical Chemistry and Quality Research in Colleges and Universities in Gansu Province/Gansu Provincial Laboratory Animal Industry Technology Center, Lanzhou, China

Changhong Wei
Department of Pathology, Guangxi Medical University Cancer Hospital, Nanning, China
National Center for International Research of Bio-Targeting Theranostics, Guangxi Key Laboratory of Bio-Targeting Theranostics, Collaborative Innovation Center for Targeting Tumor Diagnosis and Therapy, Guangxi Medical University, Nanning, China

Xiaoyu Chen, Chunjun Li and Jun Chen
Department of Pathology, Guangxi Medical University Cancer Hospital, Nanning, China

Xuejia Yang
National Center for International Research of Bio-Targeting Theranostics, Guangxi Key Laboratory of Bio-Targeting Theranostics, Collaborative Innovation Center for Targeting Tumor Diagnosis and Therapy, Guangxi Medical University, Nanning, China

Pingping Guo
Department of Ultrasound Imaging, Guangxi Medical University Cancer Hospital, Nanning, China

Sufang Zhou
National Center for International Research of Bio-Targeting Theranostics, Guangxi Key Laboratory of Bio-Targeting Theranostics, Collaborative Innovation Center for Targeting Tumor Diagnosis and Therapy, Guangxi Medical University, Nanning, China
Department of Biochemistry and Molecular Biology, School of Pre-clinical Science, Guangxi Medical University, Nanning, China

Christiane Kuempers, Tobias Jagomast, Carsten Heidel, Julika Ribbat-Idel, Eva Dreyer, Verena Sailer and Jutta Kirfel
Institute of Pathology, Luebeck, University Hospital Schleswig-Holstein, Luebeck, Germany

Rosemarie Krupar
Pathology, Research Center Borstel-Leibniz Lung Center, Borstel, Germany